Marie Emywiele OTR/L

HAND SPLINTING
PRINCIPLES AND METHODS

HAND SPLINTING

PRINCIPLES AND METHODS

Elaine Ewing Fess, M.S., O.T.R., F.A.O.T.A.
Hand Therapist, Founding active member of American Society of Hand Therapists;
Consultant in Private Practice, Zionsville, Indiana

Cynthia A. Philips, M.A., O.T.R.
Hand Therapist, Founding active member of American Society
of Hand Therapists; Chief Occupational Therapist, Newton-Wellesley
Hospital, Newton, Mass.; Adjunct Assistant Professor,
Department of Occupational Therapy, Sargent College of Allied
Health Professions, Boston University, Boston, Massachusetts

with contributions by **James W. Strickland, M.D.**
and **Judith Bell-Krotoski, O.T.R., F.A.O.T.A.**
Founding active member of American Society of Hand Therapists

SECOND EDITION

with 902 *illustrations*
Craig Gosling, Art Director

THE C. V. MOSBY COMPANY

St. Louis • Washington, D.C. • Toronto   1987

A TRADITION OF PUBLISHING EXCELLENCE

Editor: Eugenia A. Klein
Developmental Editor: Kathryn H. Falk
Editing Supervisor: Bob Kelly
Editing, Production, and Book Design: Top Graphics
Cover Design: Liz Fett

SECOND EDITION

The C.V. Mosby Company
11830 Westline Industrial Drive, St. Louis, Missouri 63146

Library of Congress Cataloging-in-Publication Data

Fess, Elaine Ewing
    Hand splinting.

    Bibliography: p.
    Includes index.
    1. Hand—Wounds and injuries. 2. Splints (Surgery)
I. Philips, Cynthia A. II. Title. [DNLM: 1. Hand
Injuries—therapy. 2. Splints. WE 830 F413h]
RD559.F47 1987   617'.575059   86-23601
ISBN 0-8016-1578-X

C/MV/MV 9 8 7 6 5 4   02/A/274

DEDICATION TO SECOND EDITION

In every field of endeavor there are those whose foresight, dedication, and leadership leave a lasting imprint on both present and future practitioners. Dr. James Hunter, Mrs. Evelyn Mackin, and Dr. Lawrence Schneider are such individuals.

In 1976, based on their own successful experiences using a team approach to assist their patients in achieving full rehabilitative potential, Dr. Hunter, Mrs. Mackin, and Dr. Schneider launched the first of a series of educational meetings on hand rehabilitation where surgeons and therapists participated on an equal basis, sharing their expertise and voicing mutual concerns to learn from each other for the benefit of their patients. For the time, this was a truly unique, almost radical, concept.

Now, ten years later, their generous and dedicated leadership has produced ten hand rehabilitation meetings, leading to an international network of therapists and surgeons and setting a strong precedent for the future. A spin off of the meetings, their book, *Rehabilitation of the Hand*, ed. 2, in which chapters are authored by both surgeons and therapists, is considered a classic in the field.

Their steadfast belief in the value and abilities of therapists has significantly altered the profession, laying a strong foundation for the treatment of hands that have been debilitated by disease or injury. In recognition of their contributions to the field of hand rehabilitation, we dedicate the second edition of *Hand Splinting Principles and Methods* to James M. Hunter, M.D., Evelyn J. Mackin, L.P.T., and Lawrence H. Schneider, M.D.

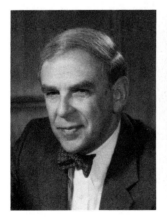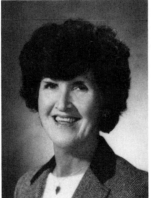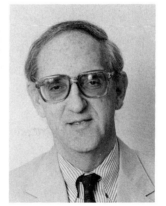

DEDICATION TO FIRST EDITION

The authors dedicate this book to Kay Bradley Carl, O.T.R., whose ingenious and creative efforts resulted in the original splint manual used in the Occupational Therapy Program, Division of Allied Health Sciences, Indiana University School of Medicine. It is from this manual that this book takes its philosophic and structural orientation.

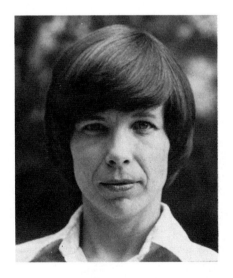

Foreword to first edition

The emergence of hand surgery as a specialty and the advances in the science and art of hand surgery since World War II have been truly phenomenal. Societies for surgery of the hand have attracted some of the most skillful and dedicated surgeons and have served as a forum for discussion and criticism, new concepts, and the testing and trial of competing ideas.

At first, this exciting advance in hand surgery was not accompanied by a parallel advance in techniques of conservative and nonoperative management of the hand. Not only has this led to a tendency to operate on patients who might have been better treated conservatively, but many patients who have rightly and properly been operated on have failed to obtain the best results of their surgery because of inadequate or poorly planned preoperative and postoperative management.

It is encouraging to note that just in the last decade interest has surged in what is being called "hand rehabilitation." This term is used to cover the whole range of con-servative management of the hand. It represents an area in which the surgeon and ther-apist work closely together, with each bringing their special experience and expertise to the common problem. Hand rehabilitation centers are multiplying, and a new group, the Society of Hand Therapists, has been formed in association with the American Society for Surgery of the Hand to bring together those physical therapists and occupational therapists who specialize in the hand.

Pioneers in the new movement are Elaine Fess, Karan Gettle, and James Strickland, and their work has concentrated on the neglected field of hand splinting. Little research has been done on the actual effect of externally applied forces on joints and tissues of the hand. Experienced surgeons and therapists have developed an intuitive "feel" for what can be accomplished, but there is little in the literature to assist the young surgeon in what to prescribe or to help a young therapist know the hazards that can turn a good prescription into a harmful application. In this situation, Elaine Fess, Karan Gettle, and James Strickland have put their own experience down on paper and made it available to all of us. It is obvious that they have a great deal of experience. It is also clear that they have gone far beyond the "cookbook" stage of previous splinting manuals. They have researched and studied their subject thoroughly, and we are fortunate indeed to have the result of that study presented so clearly and illustrated so well.

What pleases me most about this book is that it deals first with principles and only then with specific design. It begins with an emphasis on anatomy and topography and then with mechanical principles; after chapters on principles of design and fit and construction, the authors discuss specific splints. In addition, there is a good chapter on specific problems and how to handle them.

It is a measure of how far we still have to go in the science of splinting that the authors do not feel able to recommend actual specific forces by numbers to use in dynamic splints. My own feeling is that the boundary between art and science is numbers. Even in hand surgery we are not yet able to say that a specific tendon should be attached with a tension of 200 grams, so why should we expect a therapist to fix a rubber band at a specific level of tension? One day we will take these extra steps toward precision. When data are available, Elaine Fess, Karan Gettle, and James Strickland will be the first to put it into their next book. They have jumped into a clear position of leadership with this book. I am sure they will stay ahead of each new advance as it comes along.

Paul W. Brand, F.R.C.S.
Clinical Professor of Surgery and Orthopaedics,
Louisiana State University; Chief, Rehabilitation Branch,
United States Public Health Service Hospital,
Carville, Louisiana

Preface to second edition

Designing and fitting a hand splint is a serious undertaking that requires careful consideration and integration of many factors. One must beware of attempts to oversimplify splinting concepts to the point of rotely designating a given splint for a specific type of hand problem. Pathologic, physiologic, psychologic, sociologic, and technical factors must be taken into account to produce splints that are truly efficacious. It is important to remember that although their diagnoses may be similar, no two patients have identical splinting requirements.

Like the artist who, rather than limiting himself to primary colors, blends and shades in subtle interpretation, the astute hand specialist integrates a multitude of factors in creating a hand splint. Reflecting patient capacity and life-style, a splint must be created from the hand out. Splint components should be carefully chosen to combat specific pathology, allowing the splint to take shape bit by bit according to the problems and needs identified. The final configuration is secondary to efficient functioning of each component. This approach results in a wide variety of finished splints that are uniquely designed to meet individual patient requirements. Grossly, many hand splints seem to perform similar functions (Fig. 1), but upon close examination it is apparent that unique differences exist, and these differences have serious implications for use. Those who persist in dispensing splints without regard to patient idiosyncracies function as technicians rather than integral members of a professional team and, unfortunately, may seriously jeopardize their patient's chances to obtain full rehabilitative potential. "Cookbook" approaches to splinting are never appropriate when dealing with patients whose hands have been compromised by disease or injury.

As with the first edition, *Hand Splinting: Principles and Methods,* ed. 2 identifies basic concepts that, when followed, help clinicians create appropriate and well functioning hand splints. In addition to updating and expanding existing chapters, we have added new chapters to address the physiologic basis for splinting, hand assessment, use of dynamic assists for mobilization of joints, splinting the arthritic hand, serial casting, and pattern construction. Founded on anatomy, kinesiology, physics, and clinical experience, these chapters emphasize a scientific approach to hand splinting. Through the

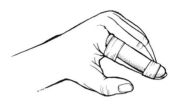

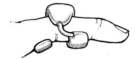

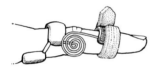

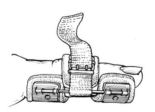

Although each of these splints is designed to extend the proximal interphalangeal joint(s), they differ considerably in configuration and purpose of application.

Those responsible for splint preparation must understand the subtle differences in splints with seemingly similar functions to use them appropriately.

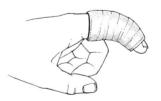

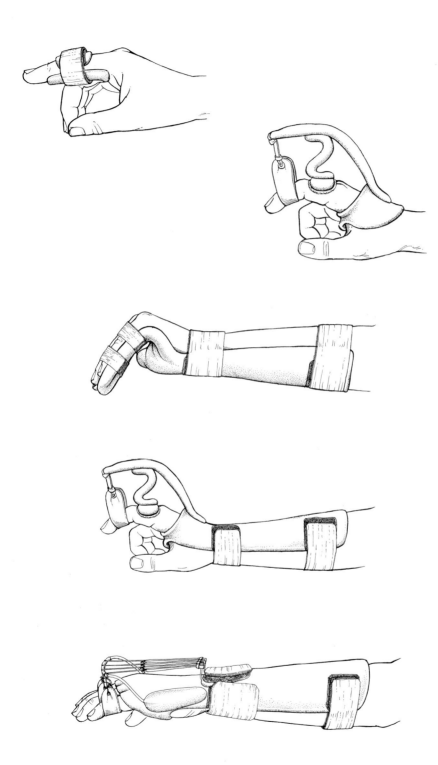

generosity of numerous hand specialists throughout the United States, Canada, Europe, Japan, and the Middle East who contributed photographs, the illustrative scope of the second edition is increased considerably. To facilitate accessibility, an index of illustrated splints arranged according to classification type is also included. In addition, currently available splinting materials have been grouped according to physical properties, and a variety of hand assessment forms may be found in the updated appendices.

We wish to acknowledge the significant contributions made by Karan Harmon (Gettle), O.T.R., and James W. Strickland, M.D., to the first edition of *Hand Splinting: Principles and Methods*. Without Karan's enthusiasm and energy the first edition would have never been written. Her tireless dedication and good humor made the long hours and frustrations of writing bearable. Jim Strickland's intellectual honesty and exceptional clinical and surgical knowledge set the high standards of excellence for the first edition. His commitment to teaching and his never condescending assistance to a fledgling and sometimes flailing writer will always be appreciated. We are most grateful for his excellent contributions to this second edition, the chapters on anatomy and biologic basis of splinting.

Craig Gosling's expertise as a gifted medical illustrator is apparent throughout both editions of *Hand Splinting: Principles and Methods*. His clever cartoons in the second edition help emphasize important concepts and provide a humorous highlight to each chapter. We wish to thank Craig and members of the Indiana University Medical Center Illustration Department, including photographers Dave Jaynes, John Murphy, and Joe Demma.

We also wish to thank Judy Bell-Krotoski, O.T.R., F.A.O.T.A., for her invaluable chapter on serial casting, and David Thompson, Ph.D., for his very much appreciated addition to the mechanics chapter on shear forces.

A splinting book cannot be written without crediting Paul Brand, M.D., for his pioneering work and leadership in documenting and measuring splinting forces. A generous and tireless teacher, Dr. Brand's contributions to understanding the positive ramifications of prolonged gentle stress on soft tissue are of unparalleled significance. His work will influence splinting theory for many decades to come.

We appreciate the timely assistance of John Kirk and Alice Shafer, M.S., O.T.R./ L., F.A.O.T.A., for helping organize the information on splinting materials; and we wish to thank WFR/Aquaplast Corporation, Johnson and Johnson, AliMed Inc., Roylan Medical Products, and Jobst for their generous donations of splinting materials and information.

Finally, we wish to recognize the special contributions of Mr. and Mrs. Arthur C. Kaufmann. Through their enthusiastic support of the educational programs produced by the Philadelphia Hand Rehabilitation Center, therapists and surgeons throughout the world have been given a unique opportunity for sharing and learning. We thank them for their generous hospitality over the years and for their dedicated commitment to the field of hand rehabilitation.

E.E.F.
C.A.P.

We would like to acknowledge the following therapists who generously shared their splinting expertise by contributing photographs and ideas:

Barbara Allen, O.T.R./L.*
Norma Arras, M.A., O.T.R./L.*
Shandra Artzberger, M.S., O.T.R.*
Janet Bailey, O.T.R./L.*
Karen Priest Barrett, O.T.R.*
Jane Bear-Lehnan, M.S., O.T.R.*
Rivka Ben Porath, O.T.*
Theresa Bielawski, O.T.(C)*
Kay Colello-Abraham, O.T.R.*
Ruth Coopee, O.T.R.
Carolina deLeeuw, M.A., O.T.R.*
Lisa Dennys, B.Sc., O.T.*
Jolene Eastburn, O.T.R./L.*
Susan Emerson, M.Ed., O.T.R.*
Roslyn Brown Evans, O.T.R.*
Joan Farrell, O.T.R., P.A.*
Bonnie Fehring, L.P.T.*
Sharon Flinn-Wagner, M.Ed., O.T.R./L.*
Kenneth Flowers, L.P.T.*
Lynnlee Fullenwider, O.T.R.*
Susan Glaser-Morales, O.T.R.*
Christine Heaney, B.Sc., O.T.
Renske Houck-Romkes, O.T.

Joanne Kassimir, O.T.R.*
Janet Kinnunen, O.T.R.
Elaine Lacroix, M.H.S.M., O.T.R.*
K. Patricia MacBain, O.T.
Gretchen Maurer, O.T.R.*
Bobbie-Ann Neel, O.T.R.
Barbara Raff, O.T.R.*
Donna Reist, O.T.R./L.*
Joyce Ellison Roalef, O.T.R./L.*
Patricia Samuels, O.T.R.
Karen Schultz, M.S., O.T.R., C.V.E.*
Kathryn Hutcherson Schultz, O.T.R., C.V.E.*
Kimiko Shiina, O.T.R.*
Linda Shuttleton, O.T.R.*
Barbara Sopp, O.T.R./L.
Elizabeth Spencer, O.T.R.*
Erica Stern, M.S., O.T.R.
Linda Tresley, O.T.R.*
Robin Miller Wagman, O.T.R./L.*
Jill White, M.A., O.T.R.*
Diana Williams, O.T.R.*
Joanne Zitter, O.T.R./L.*

*Member, American Society of Hand Therapists.

Elaine Ewing Fess
Cynthia A. Philips

Preface to first edition

Webster's Unabridged Dictionary describes splints as "rigid or flexible appliances used for the prevention of movement of a joint or for the fixation of displaced or movable parts." However, in current medical practice the boundaries of this definition have been expanded to include a greater variety of devices that not only prevent joint motion but also maintain or enhance it. It is now recognized that such appliances can serve many important roles in the management of disease and injury of the hand. Splints may be employed to prevent deformity of, immobilize, mobilize, position, or protect the wrist and digital joints with the intent of restoring maximum function. Design and construction of splints have ranged from abject simplicity to complex appliances reminiscent of Rube Goldberg contraptions.

Medical science treatises devoted to the management of injuries and disease of the upper extremity have contained illustrations of clever devices designed to prevent or correct deformities. Interestingly, modern literature has done little more than elaborate on these devices with techniques developed for the simplified preparation of more comfortable splints made possible by the development of new materials. Unfortunately, there has been an appalling lack of a scientific approach to the design and preparation of hand splints. Devices constructed without an adequate understanding of the underlying pathologic conditions of the hand, the realistic goals expected of a given splint, and the mechanics that must be correctly used to achieve these goals will often prove to be failures.

Although many hand splints have been proposed with great concern for individual anatomic and pathologic differences, others are mass produced commercially for application to a wide spectrum of clinical conditions. An appreciation of the enormous variation in hand size and configuration and for the almost endless number of possible conditions that may exist in the upper extremity should lead one to worry about the potential pitfalls of the rote application of such standardized devices.

Although the proper use of hand splints is now considered an essential part of the management of patients with acute or chronic disease or injury of the hand and upper extremity, an approach to the preparation of these splints must be made with a thorough understanding of the underlying anatomic alterations and the realistic therapeutic consid-erations—be they medical, surgical, or rehabilitative—that comprise the total treatment program. The patient's management cannot be fragmented into these various compo-nents, but requires a close working relationship among patient, surgeon, and therapist to provide an integrated approach that achieves maximum functional benefit. It is not enough for the person engaged in the preparation of a hand splint to create that splint from a prescription supplied at long range by a surgeon who has undertaken the initial management or reconstructive effort of a given hand problem. The insufficient infor-mation created by this "communication gap" will almost inevitably lead not only to an incorrectly prepared splint, but also to confusion on the part of the patient and therapist as to the exact goals and realistic expectations of such a device. We cannot overempha-size, therefore, the need for an excellent line of communication between surgeon and therapist, with extensive instruction to the patient not only with regard to splint use, but also to the desired objectives of splinting. Only through this close working relationship can the correct preparation and use of splints be expected.

In *Hand Splinting: Principles and Methods,* we have reviewed the anatomy and kinesiology of the hand to provide a sound, basic understanding of the important under-lying structures and their function. We have discussed the mechanical principles that must be employed in the preparation of hand splints. A classification and description of the nomenclature of various splints and splint components is also provided, together with an extensive examination of the principles of splint fit, construction, and design. A breakdown of splint considerations by anatomic area is provided, as well as a review of the use of splints for special problems and the importance of exercise. A survey of the materials and equipment, splint checkout and referral forms, work area examples, and American Society for Surgery of the Hand Clinical Assessment Recommendations are included in the appendices.

Hand Splinting: Principles and Methods is presented in a learning theory hierarchy in which basic principles are discussed and examples given. Once readers progress through the fundamental early chapters, they are provided with the opportunity to use this acquired information by analyzing splints that are incorrectly designed, constructed, or fitted. Immediate feedback is given for each splint so that readers may compare their analysis with ours.

We concede at the onset that a particular splint may not be best for any one clinical situation and that in many cases one may choose from a wide variety of splints to try to accomplish a given therapeutic goal. Nonetheless, it is important for the person pre-paring the splint to thoroughly understand the exact purpose for the splint being prepared, the necessary mechanics to achieve it, and the available design options. We have at-tempted to leave these specific splint selection decisions to readers and to simply review the various possibilities, with discussion of the various advantages and disadvantages of each. The philosophy of the book is predicated on the design of individual splints for specific problems from basic splint components. We emphasize that there are no rote splinting solutions to combating pathologic conditions of the hand and that each splint is created on an individual basis using the principles of mechanics, fit, construction, and design. Although we acknowledge a redundancy in the discussion of many of the principles and specific splint considerations, we believe that this approach will provide the best ultimate understanding of the important role of splinting in the management of hand disease and injury.

We gratefully acknowledge the continued help and support our families have given us during the writing of *Hand Splinting: Principles and Methods*. Sherran Schmalfeldt, Geanora Westlake, and Jan Casner deserve recognition for the many hours spent in typing the manuscript. Craig Gosling, Carol Stahl, Joe Demma, and Tom Rohyans must be commended for their excellent illustrations and photographs. Special appreciation goes to Kenneth Dunipace, Ph.D., for proofreading the mechanics chapter. We also thank Roylan Manufacturing Company, Johnson and Johnson, and Abbey Rents, who generously donated materials for many of the splints illustrated. Finally, we express our admiration and gratitude to the patients of the Hand Rehabilitation Center of Indiana in Indianapolis, without whose assistance this book could not have been written.

Elaine Ewing Fess
Karan S. Gettle
James W. Strickland

Contents

xix

PART ONE

Fundamental concepts

CHAPTER 1

Anatomy and kinesiology of the hand

James W. Strickland*

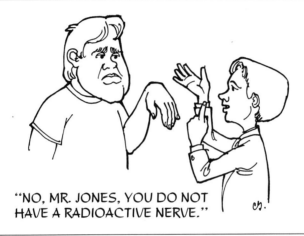

"NO, MR. JONES, YOU DO NOT HAVE A RADIOACTIVE NERVE."

One cannot expect to adequately participate in the treatment of disorders of the hand and arm without a solid working knowledge of the intricate anatomic and kinesiologic relationships of the upper extremity. The preparation of externally applied splinting devices to the forearm, wrist, and hand necessitates a thorough understanding of and respect for the underlying anatomic structures. Only through comprehension of the normal anatomy of the human hand can one adequately develop an appreciation for the anatomic alterations that accompany injury and disease. It is appropriate, therefore, that the first chapter in a book devoted to hand splinting be concerned with the anatomy and kinesiology of the hand. Since it is impossible in this chapter to review in great detail

I am extremely grateful to Gary W. Schnitz for many of the excellent illustrations used in this chapter.
*Clinical Professor of Orthopaedic Surgery and Director, Hand Surgery Rotation, Indiana University School of Medicine; Chief of Hand Surgery Service, St. Vincent Hospital and Hand Care Center, Indianapolis, Indiana.

the enormous amount of literature that has been written about the anatomic, kinesiologic, and biomechanical aspects of the hand, readers are directed to the bibliography for more extensive reading on these subjects.

The anatomy of the hand must be approached in a systematic fashion with individual consideration of the osseous structures, joints, musculotendinous units, blood supply, nerve supply, and surface anatomy. However, it is obvious that the systems do not function independently, but that the integrated presence of all these structures is required for normal hand function. In presenting this material, I stray into the important mechanical and kinesiologic considerations that result from the unique anatomic arrangement of the hand and briefly try to indicate the problems resulting from various forms of pathologic conditions in certain areas. Surface anatomy and a description of the basic patterns of hand function are also included at the end of this chapter.

OSSEOUS STRUCTURES

The unique arrangement and mobility of the bones of the hand (Fig. 1-1) provide a structural basis for its enormous functional adaptability. The osseous skeleton consists of eight carpal bones divided into two rows: the proximal row articulates with the distal radius and ulna (with the exception of the pisiform, which lies palmar to and articulates with the triquetrum); the distal four carpal bones in turn articulate with the five meta-

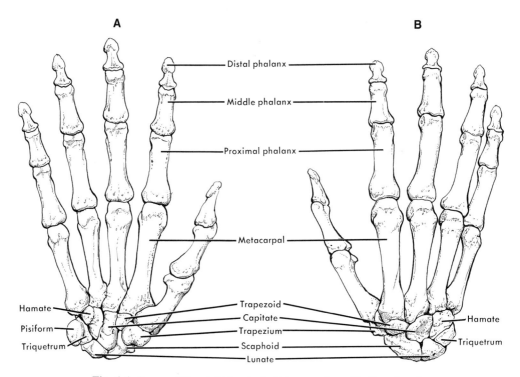

Fig. 1-1. Bones of the right hand. **A,** Palmar surface. **B,** Dorsal surface.

carpals. Two phalanges complete the first ray, or thumb unit, and three phalanges each comprise the index, long, ring, and small fingers. These 27 bones, together with the intricate arrangement of supportive ligaments and contractile musculotendinous units, are arranged to provide both mobility and stability to the various joints of the hand. Although the exact anatomic configuration of the bone of the hand need not be memorized in detail, it is important to develop a knowledge of the position and names of the carpal bones, metacarpals, and phalanges and an understanding of their kinesiologic patterns to proceed with the management of many hand problems.

The bones of the hand are arranged in three arches (Fig. 1-2), two transversely oriented and one which is longitudinal. The proximal transverse arch, the keystone of which is the capitate, lies at the level of the distal part of the carpus and is reasonably fixed, whereas the distal transverse arch passing through the metacarpal heads is more mobile. The two transverse arches are connected by the rigid portion of the longitudinal arch consisting of the second and third metacarpals, the index and long fingers distally, and the central carpus proximally. The longitudinal arch is completed by the individual digital rays, and the mobility of the first, fourth, and fifth rays around the second and third allows the palm to flatten or cup itself to accommodate objects of various sizes and shapes.

To a large extent the intrinsic muscles of the hand are responsible for changes in the

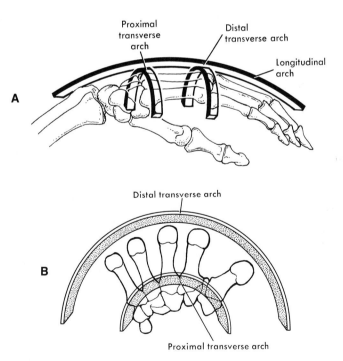

Fig. 1-2. A, Skeletal arches of the hand. The proximal transverse arch passes through the distal carpus; the distal transverse arch, through the metacarpal heads. The longitudinal arch is made up of the four digital rays and the carpus proximally. **B,** Proximal and distal transverse arches.

configuration of the osseous arches, and collapse in the arch system resulting from injury to the osseous skeleton or paralysis of the intrinsic muscles can contribute to severe disability and deformity. Flatt (1972) has pointed out that grasp is dependent on the integrity of the mobile longitudinal arches and that, when destruction at the carpometacarpal joint, metacarpophalangeal joint, or proximal interphalangeal joint interrupts the integrity of these arches, crippling deformity may result.

JOINTS

The multiple complex articulations between the distal radius and ulna, the eight carpal bones, and the metacarpal bases comprise the wrist joint, whose proximal position makes it the functional key to the motion at the more distal digital joints of the

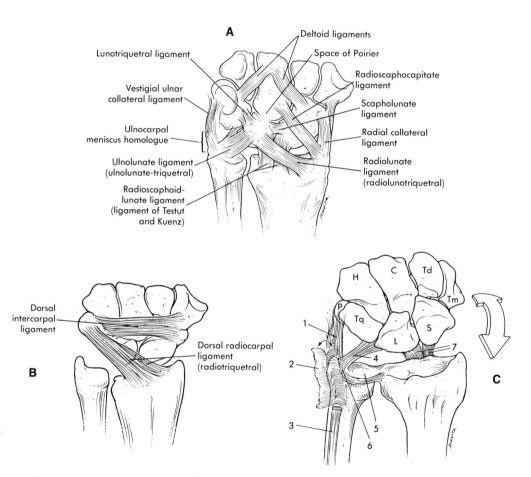

Fig. 1-3. Ligamentous anatomy of the wrist. **A,** Palmar wrist ligaments. **B,** Dorsal wrist ligaments. **C,** Dorsal view of the flexed wrist, including the triangular fibrocartilage. *1,* Ulnar collateral ligament; *2,* retinacular sheath; *3,* tendon of extensor carpi ulnaris; *4,* ulnolunate ligament; *5,* triangular fibrocartilage; *6,* ulnocarpal meniscus homologue; *7,* palmar radioscaphoid lunate ligament. *P,* Pisiform; *H,* hamate; *C,* capitate; *Td,* trapezoid; *Tm,* trapezium; *Tq,* triquetrum; *L,* lunate; *S,* scaphoid.

hand. Functionally the carpus transmits forces through the hand to the forearm. The proximal carpal row consisting of the scaphoid (navicular), lunate, and triquetrum articulates distally with the trapezium, trapezoid, capitate, and hamate; there is a complex motion pattern which relies both on ligamentous and contact surface constraints. The major ligaments of the wrist (Fig. 1-3) are the palmar and intracapsular ligaments. There are three strong radial palmar ligaments: the radioscaphocapitate or "sling" ligament, which supports the waist of the scaphoid; the radiolunate ligament, which supports the lunate; and the radioscapholunate ligament, which connects the scapholunate articulation with the palmar portion of the distal radius. This ligament functions as a checkrein for the scaphoid flexion and extension. The ulnolunate ligament arises intraarticularly from the triangular articular meniscus of the wrist joint and inserts on the lunate and, to a lesser extent, the triquetrum. The radial and ulnar collateral ligaments are capsular ligaments, and V-shaped ligaments from the capitate to the triquetrum and scaphoid have been termed the deltoid ligaments. Dorsally, the radiocarpal ligament connects the radius to the triquetrum and acts as a dorsal sling for the lunate, maintaining the lunate in apposition to the distal radius. Further dorsal carpal support is provided by the dorsal intracarpal ligament. These strong ligaments combine to provide carpal stability while permitting the normal range of wrist motion.

The distal ulna is covered with an articular cartilage (Fig. 1-3, *C*) over its most dorsal, palmar, and radial aspects, where it articulates with the sigmoid or ulnar notch of the radius. The triangular fibrocartilage complex describes the ligamentous and cartilaginous structure that suspends the distal radius and ulnar carpus from the distal ulna. Blumfield and Champoux (1984) have indicated that the optimal functional wrist motion to accomplish most activities of daily living is from 10 degrees of flexion to 35 degrees of extension.

Taleisnik (1976) has emphasized the importance of considering the wrist in terms of longitudinal columns (Fig. 1-4). The central, or flexion extension column consists of the lunate and the entire distal carpal row; the lateral, or mobile, column comprises the

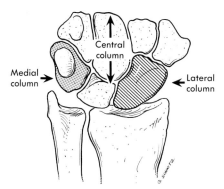

Fig. 1-4. Columnar carpus. The scaphoid is the mobile or lateral column. The central or flexion extension, column comprises the lunate and the entire distal carpal row. The medial, or rotational, column comprises the triquetrum alone.

scaphoid alone; and the medial, or rotation, column is made up of the triquetrum. Wrist motion is produced by the muscles that attach to the metacarpals, and the ligamentous control system provides stability only at the extremes of motion. The distal carpal row of the carpal bones is firmly attached to the hand and moves with it. Therefore during dorsiflexion the distal carpal row dorsiflexes, during palmar flexion it palmar flexes, and during radial and ulnar deviation it deviates radially or ulnarly. As the wrist ranges from radial to ulnar deviation, the proximal carpal row rotates in a dorsal direction, and a simultaneous translocation of the proximal carpus occurs in a radial direction at the radiocarpal and midcarpal articulations. This combined motion of the carpal rows has been referred to as the rotational shift of the carpus. It was once taught that palmar flexion takes place to a greater extent at the radiocarpal joint and secondarily in the midcarpal joint; but since dorsiflexion occurs primarily at the midcarpal joint and only secondarily at the radiocarpal articulation, this now appears to be a significant oversimplification. The complex carpal kinematics are beyond the scope of this chapter, and the reader is referred to the works of Weber (1982) and Taleisnik (1976) to gain a thorough understanding of this difficult subject.

The articulation between the base of the first metacarpal and the trapezium (Fig. 1-5) is a highly mobile joint with a configuration thought to be similar to that of a saddle. The base of the first metacarpal is concave in the anteroposterior plane and convex in the lateral plane, with a reciprocal concavity in the lateral plane and an anteroposterior convexity on the opposing surface of the trapezium. This arrangement allows for the positioning of the thumb in a wide arc of motion (Fig. 1-6), including flexion, extension, abduction, adduction, and opposition. The ligamentous arrangement about this joint, while permitting the wide circumduction, continues to provide stability at the extremes of motion, allowing the thumb to be brought into a variety of positions for pinch and grasp, but maintaining its stability during these functions. The articulations formed by the ulnar half of the hamate and the fourth and fifth metacarpal bases allow a modest amount of motion (15 degrees at the fourth carpometacarpal joint and 25 to 30 degrees of flexion and extension at the fifth carpometacarpal joint). A resulting ''palmar descent'' of these metacarpals occurs during strong grasp.

The metacarpophalangeal joints of the fingers are diarthrodial joints with motion permitted in three planes and combinations thereof (Fig. 1-7). The cartilaginous surfaces

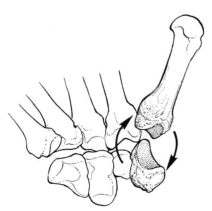

Fig. 1-5. Saddle-shaped carpometacarpal joint of the thumb. A wide range of motion *(arrows)* is permitted by the configuration of this joint.

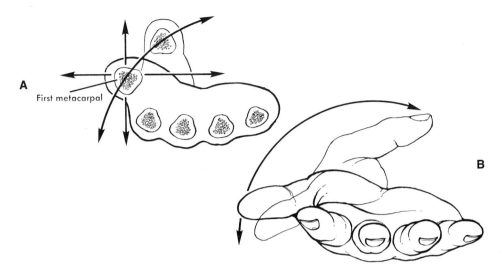

First metacarpal

Fig. 1-6. A, Multiple planes of motion *(arrows)* that occur at the carpometacarpal joint of the thumb. **B,** The thumb moves *(arrow)* from a position of adduction against the second metacarpal to a position of extension abduction away from the hand and fingers and can then be rotated into positions of opposition and flexion.

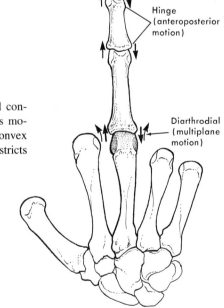

Hinge (anteroposterior motion)

Diarthrodial (multiplane motion)

Fig. 1-7. Joints of the phalanges. The diarthrodial configuration of the metacarpophalangeal joint permits motion in multiple planes, whereas the biconcave-convex hinge configuration of the interphalangeal joints restricts motion to the anteroposterior plane.

of the metacarpal head and the bases of the proximal phalanges are enclosed in a complex apparatus consisting of the joint capsule, collateral ligaments, and the anterior fibrocartilage or palmar plate (Fig. 1-8). The capsule extends from the borders of the base of the proximal phalanx proximally to the head of the metacarpals beyond the cartilaginous joint surface. The collateral ligaments, which reinforce the capsule on each side of the metacarpophalangeal joints, run from the dorsolateral side of the metacarpal head to the palmar lateral side of the proximal phalanges. These ligaments form two bundles, the more central of which is referred to as the *cord portion of the collateral ligament* and inserts into the side of the proximal phalanx; the more palmar portion joins the palmar plate and is termed the *accessory collateral ligament.* These collateral ligaments are somewhat loose with the metacarpophalangeal joint in extension, allowing for considerable ''play'' in the side-to-side motion of the digits (Fig. 1-9). With the metacarpophalangeal joints in full flexion, however, the cam configuration of the metacarpal head tightens the collateral ligaments and limits lateral mobility of the digits. This alteration in tension becomes an important factor in immobilization of the metacarpophalangeal joints for any length of time, since the secondary shortening of the lax collateral ligaments that may occur when these joints are immobilized in extension will result in severe limitation of metacarpophalangeal joint flexion by these structures.

The palmar fibrocartilaginous plate on the palmar side of the metacarpophalangeal joint is firmly attached to the base of the proximal phalanx and loosely attached to the anterior surface of the neck of the metacarpal by means of the joint capsule at the neck of the metacarpal. This arrangement allows the palmar plate to slide proximally during metacarpophalangeal joint flexion. The flexor tendons pass along a groove anterior to the plate. The palmar plates are connected by the transverse intermetacarpal ligaments, which connect each plate to its neighbor.

The metacarpophalangeal joint of the thumb differs from the others in that the head of the first metacarpal is flatter, and its cartilaginous surface does not extend as far

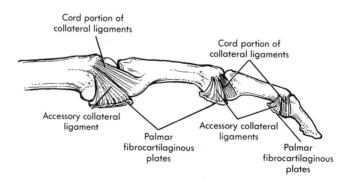

Fig. 1-8. Ligamentous structures of the digital joints. The collateral ligaments of the metacarpophalangeal and interdigital joints are composed of a strong cord portion with bony origin and insertion. The more palmarly placed accessory collateral ligaments originate from the proximal bone and insert into the palmar fibrocartilaginous plate. The palmar plates have strong distal attachments to resist extension forces.

laterally or posteriorly. Two small sesamoid bones are also adjacent to this joint, and the ligamentous structure differs somewhat. A few degrees of abduction and rotation are permitted by the ligament arrangement of the metacarpophalangeal joint at the thumb, which is of considerable functional importance in delicate precision functions. There is considerable variation in the range of motion present at the thumb metacarpophalangeal joints. The amount of motion varies from as little as 30 degrees to as much as 90 degrees.

The digital interphalangeal joints are hinge joints (Fig. 1-7) and, like the metacarpophalangeal joints, have capsular and ligamentous enclosure. The articular surface of the proximal phalangeal head is convex in the anteroposterior plane with a depression in the middle between the two condyles, which articulates with the phalanx distal to it. The bases of the middle and distal phalanges appear as a concave surface with an elevated ridge dividing two concave depressions. A cord portion of the collateral liga-

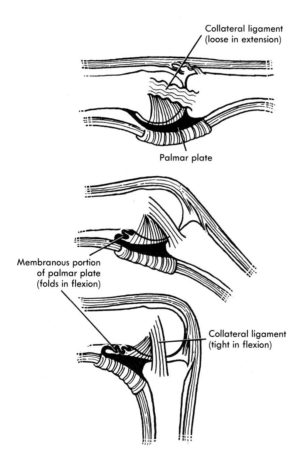

Collateral ligament
(loose in extension)

Palmar plate

Membranous portion
of palmar plate
(folds in flexion)

Collateral ligament
(tight in flexion)

Fig. 1-9. At the metacarpophalangeal joint level the collateral ligaments are loose in extension but become tightened in flexion. The proximal membranous portion of the palmar plate moves proximally to accommodate for flexion. (Modified from Wynn Parry, C.B., et al.: Rehabilitation of the hand, ed. 3, London, 1973, Butterworth & Co. [Publishers], Ltd.)

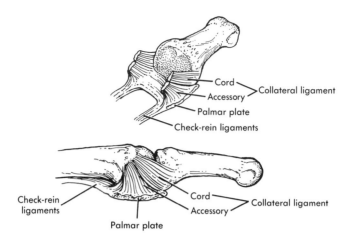

Fig. 1-10. Strong, three-sided ligamentous support system of the proximal interphalangeal joint with cord and accessory collateral ligaments and the fibrocartilaginous plate, which is anchored proximally by the check-rein ligamentous attachment. (Modified from Eaton, R.G.: Joint injuries of the hand, Springfield, Ill., 1971, Charles C Thomas, Publisher.)

ment and an accessory collateral ligament are present, and the collateral ligaments run on each side of the joint from the dorsolateral aspect of the proximal phalanx in a palmar and lateral direction to insert into the distally placed phalanx and its fibrocartilage plate (Fig. 1-10). A strong fibrocartilaginous (palmar) plate is also present, and the collateral ligaments of the proximal and distal interphalangeal joints are tightest with the joints in near full extension.

The stability of the proximal interphalangeal joint is ensured by a three-sided supporting cradle produced by the junction of the palmar plate with the base of the middle phalanx and the accessory collateral ligament structures (Fig. 1-10). The confluence of ligaments is strongly anchored by proximal and lateral extensions referred to as the *check-rein ligaments*. This system has been described as a three-dimensional hinge that results in remarkable palmar and lateral restraint.

A wide range of pathologic conditions may result from the interruption of the supportive ligament system of the intercarpal or digital joints. At the wrist level, interruption of key radiocarpal or intercarpal ligaments may result in occult patterns of wrist instability that are often difficult to diagnose and treat. In the digits, disruption of the collateral ligaments or the fibrocartilaginous palmar plates will produce joint laxity or deformity, which is more obvious. Rupture or attenuation of these supporting structures may result not only from trauma, but may also occur more insidiously with chronic disease processes such as arthritis.

MUSCLES AND TENDONS

The muscles acting on the hand can be grouped as extrinsic, when their muscle bellies are in the forearm, or intrinsic, when the muscles originate distal to the wrist joint. It is important to thoroughly understand both systems. Although their contributions to hand function are distinctly different, the integrated function of both systems is important to the satisfactory performance of the hand in a wide variety of tasks. A schematic representation of the origin and insertion of the extrinsic flexor and extensor muscle tendon units of the hand is provided in Fig. 1-11. The important nerve supply to each muscle group is reviewed in this figure and again when discussing the nerve supply to the upper extremity.

Extrinsic muscles

The extrinsic flexor muscles (Fig. 1-11) of the forearm form a prominent mass on the medial side of the upper part of the forearm: the most superficial group comprises the pronator teres, the flexor carpi radialis, the flexor carpi ulnaris, and the palmaris longus; the intermediate group the flexor digitorum superficialis; and the deep extrinsics the flexor digitorum profundus and the flexor pollicis longus. The pronator, palmaris, wrist flexors, and superficialis tendons arise from the area about the medial epicondyle, the ulnar collateral ligament of the elbow, and the medial aspect of the coronoid process. The flexor pollicis longus originates from the entire middle third of the palmar surface of the radius and the adjacent interosseous membrane, and the flexor digitorum profundus originates deep to the other muscles of the forearm from the proximal two thirds of the ulna on the palmar and medial side. The deepest layer of the palmar forearm is completed distally by the pronator quadratus muscle.

The flexor carpi radialis tendon inserts on the base of the second metacarpal, whereas the flexor carpi ulnaris inserts into both the pisiform and fifth metacarpal base. The superficialis tendons lie superficial to the profundus tendons as far as the digital bases, where they bifurcate and wrap around the profundi and rejoin over the distal half of the proximal phalanx as Camper's chiasma (Fig. 1-11). The superficialis tendon again splits for a dual insertion on the proximal half of the middle phalanges (Fig. 1-12). The profundi continue through the superficialis decussation to insert on the base of the distal phalanx. The flexor pollicis longus inserts on the base of the distal phalanx of the thumb.

At the wrist the nine long flexor tendons enter the carpal tunnel beneath the protective roof of the deep transverse carpal ligament in company with the median nerve. In this canal the common profundus tendon to the long, ring, and small fingers divides into the individual tendons that fan out distally and proceed toward the distal phalanges of these digits (Fig. 1-13). At approximately the level of the distal palmar crease the paired profundus and superficialis tendons to the index, long, ring, and small fingers and the flexor pollicis longus to the thumb enter the individual flexor sheaths that house them throughout the remainder of their digital course. These sheaths with their predictable annular pulley arrangement (Fig. 1-14) serve not only as a protective housing for the flexor tendons, but also provide a smooth gliding surface by virtue of their synovial lining and an efficient mechanism to hold the tendons close to the digital bone and joints. There is an increasing recognition that disruption of this valuable pulley system can produce substantial mechanical alterations in digital function, resulting in imbalance and deformity.

Extension of the wrist and fingers is produced by the extrinsic extensor muscle

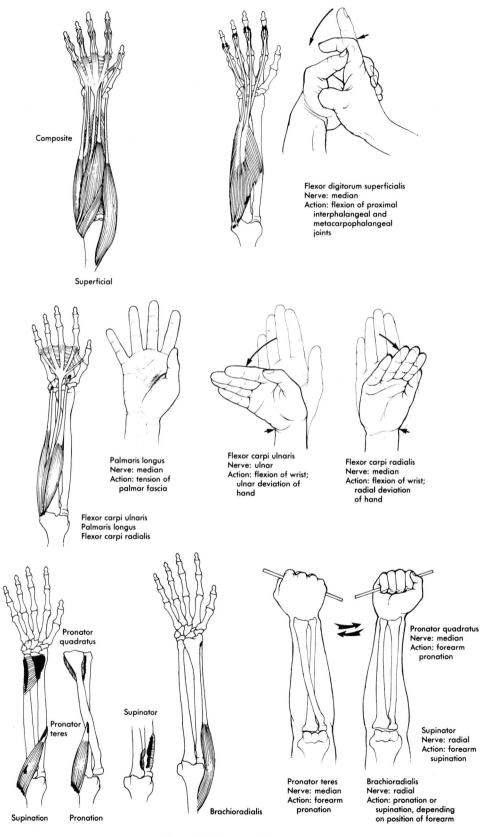

Composite

Superficial

Flexor digitorum superficialis
Nerve: median
Action: flexion of proximal
interphalangeal and
metacarpophalangeal
joints

Palmaris longus
Nerve: median
Action: tension of
palmar fascia

Flexor carpi ulnaris
Nerve: ulnar
Action: flexion of wrist;
ulnar deviation of
hand

Flexor carpi radialis
Nerve: median
Action: flexion of wrist;
radial deviation
of hand

Flexor carpi ulnaris
Palmaris longus
Flexor carpi radialis

Pronator
quadratus

Pronator
teres

Supinator

Supination   Pronation

Brachioradialis

Pronator quadratus
Nerve: median
Action: forearm
pronation

Supinator
Nerve: radial
Action: forearm
supination

Pronator teres
Nerve: median
Action: forearm
pronation

Brachioradialis
Nerve: radial
Action: pronation or
supination, depending
on position of forearm

Fig. 1-11. For legend see p. 15.

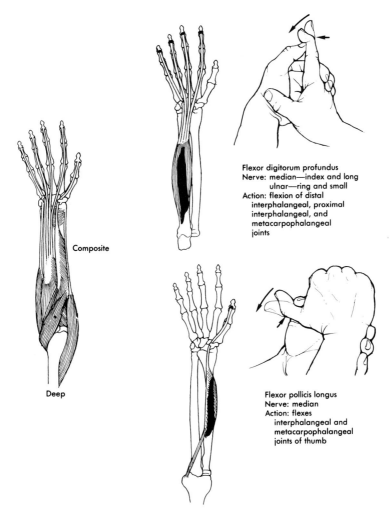

Flexor digitorum profundus
Nerve: median—index and long
        ulnar—ring and small
Action: flexion of distal
        interphalangeal, proximal
        interphalangeal, and
        metacarpophalangeal
        joints

Flexor pollicis longus
Nerve: median
Action: flexes
        interphalangeal and
        metacarpophalangeal
        joints of thumb

Fig. 1-11. Extrinsic flexor muscles of the arm and hand. (Dark areas represent origins and insertions of muscles.) (Modified from Marble, H.C.: The hand, a manual and atlas for the general surgeon, Philadelphia, 1960, W.B. Saunders Co.)

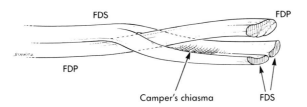

Fig. 1-12. Anatomy of the relationship between the flexor digitorum superficialis *(FDS)* flexor digitorum profundus *(FDP)* and the proximal portion of the flexor tendon sheath. The superficialis tendon divides and passes around the profundus tendon to reunite at Campers' chiasma. The tendon once again divides prior to insertion on the base of the middle phalanx.

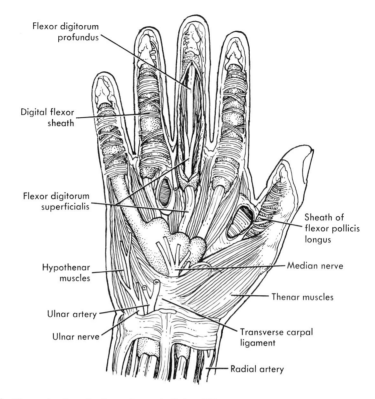

Flexor digitorum profundus

Digital flexor sheath

Flexor digitorum superficialis

Hypothenar muscles

Ulnar artery

Ulnar nerve

Sheath of flexor pollicis longus

Median nerve

Thenar muscles

Transverse carpal ligament

Radial artery

Fig. 1-13. Flexor tendons in the palm and digits. Fibroosseous digital sheaths with their pulley arrangement are shown, as is a division of the superficialis tendon about the profundus in the proximal portion of the sheath.

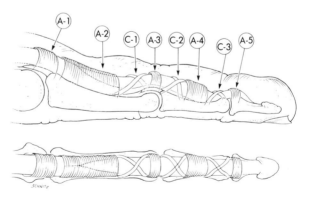

Fig. 1-14. Components of the digital flexor sheath. The sturdy annular pulleys (**A**) are important biomechanically in guaranteeing the efficient digital motion by keeping the tendons closely applied to the phalanges. The thin pliable cruciate pulleys (**C**) permit the flexor sheath to be flexible while maintaining its integrity. (Modified from Doyle, J.R., and Blythe, W.: The finger flexor tendon sheath and pulleys: anatomy and reconstruction. In American Academy of Orthopaedic Surgeons: Symposium on tendon surgery in the hand, St. Louis, 1975, The C.V. Mosby Co.)

tendon system, which consists of the two radial wrist extensors, the extensor carpi ulnaris, the extensor digitorum communis, and the extensor digiti quinti proprius (extensor digiti minimi) (Fig 1-15). These muscles originate in common from the lateral epicondyle and the lateral epicondylar ridge and from a small area posterior to the radial notch of the ulna. The brachioradialis originates from the epicondylar line proximal to the lateral epicondyle, and, because it inserts on the distal radius, it does not truly contribute to wrist or digit motion. The extensor carpi radialis longus and brevis insert proximally on the bases of the second and third metacarpals, respectively, and the extensor carpi ulnaris inserts on the base of the fifth metacarpal. The long digital extensors terminate by insertions on the bases of the middle phalanges after receiving and giving fibers to the intrinsic tendons to form the lateral bands that are destined to insert on the bases of the distal phalanx. Digital extension, therefore, results from a combination of the contribution of both the extrinsic and intrinsic extensor systems. The extensor pollicis longus and brevis tendons, together with the abductor pollicis longus, originate from the dorsal forearm and, by virtue of their respective insertions into the distal phalanx, proximal phalanx, and first metacarpal of the thumb, provide extension at all three levels. The extensor pollicis longus approaches the thumb obliquely around a small bony tubercle on the dorsal radius (Lister's tubercle) and therefore functions not only as an extensor but as a strong secondary adductor of the thumb. The extensor indicis proprius also originates more distally than the extensor communis tendons from an area near the origin of the thumb extensor and long abductor. It lies on the ulnar aspect of the communis tendon to the index finger and inserts with it in the dorsal approaches of that digit. The extensor digiti quinti proprius arises near the lateral epicondyle to occupy a superficial position on the dorsum of the forearm with its paired tendons lying on the fifth metacarpal ulnar to the communis tendon to the fifth finger. It inserts into the extensor apparatus of that digit.

At the wrist, the extensor tendons are divided into six dorsal compartments (Fig. 1-16). The first compartment consists of the tendons of the abductor pollicis longus and extensor pollicis brevis, and the second compartment houses the two radial wrist extensors, the extensor carpi radialis longus and brevis. The third compartment is composed of the tendon of the extensor pollicis longus, and the fourth compartment allows passage of the four communis extensor tendons and the extensor indicis proprius tendon. The extensor digiti quinti proprius travels through the fifth dorsal compartment, and the sixth houses the extensor carpi ulnaris.

Intrinsic muscles

The important intrinsic musculature of the hand can be divided into muscles comprising the thenar eminence, those comprising the hypothenar eminence, and the remaining muscles between the two groups (Fig. 1-17). The muscles of the thenar eminence consist of the abductor pollicis brevis, the flexor pollicis brevis, and the opponens pollicis, which originate in common from the transverse carpal ligament and the scaphoid and trapezium bones. The abductor brevis inserts into the radial side of the proximal phalanx and the radial wing tendon of the thumb, as does the flexor pollicis brevis, whereas the opponens inserts into the whole radial side of the first metacarpal.

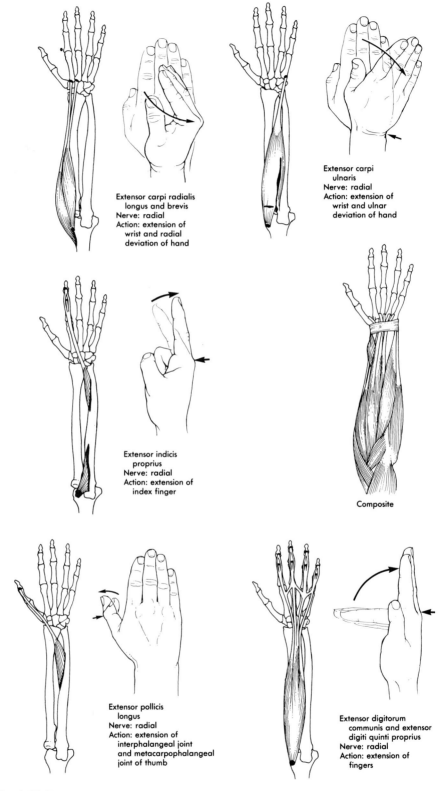

Extensor carpi radialis longus and brevis
Nerve: radial
Action: extension of wrist and radial deviation of hand

Extensor carpi ulnaris
Nerve: radial
Action: extension of wrist and ulnar deviation of hand

Extensor indicis proprius
Nerve: radial
Action: extension of index finger

Composite

Extensor pollicis longus
Nerve: radial
Action: extension of interphalangeal joint and metacarpophalangeal joint of thumb

Extensor digitorum communis and extensor digiti quinti proprius
Nerve: radial
Action: extension of fingers

Fig. 1-15. Extensor muscles of the forearm and hand. (Modified from Marble, H.C.: The hand, a manual and atlas for the general surgeon, Philadelphia, 1960, W.B. Saunders Co.)

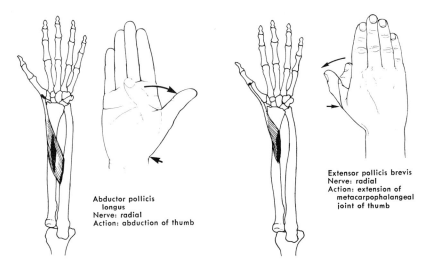

Abductor pollicis
longus
Nerve: radial
Action: abduction of thumb

Extensor pollicis brevis
Nerve: radial
Action: extension of
  metacarpophalangeal
  joint of thumb

Fig. 1-15, cont'd. Extensor muscles of the forearm and hand.

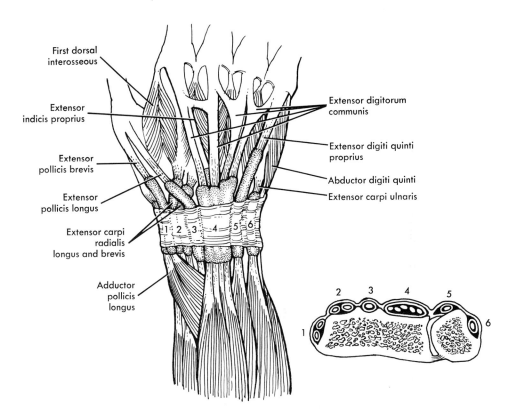

First dorsal
interosseous

Extensor
indicis proprius

Extensor
pollicis brevis

Extensor
pollicis longus

Extensor carpi
radialis
longus and brevis

Adductor
pollicis
longus

Extensor digitorum
communis

Extensor digiti quinti
proprius

Abductor digiti quinti

Extensor carpi ulnaris

Fig. 1-16. Arrangement of the extensor tendons in the compartments of the wrist. (Modified from Lampe, E.W.: Surgical anatomy of the hand. In Clinical symposia, New York, 1969, CIBA Pharmaceutical Co., Division of CIBA-GEIGY Corp.; illustrated by F.H. Netter.)

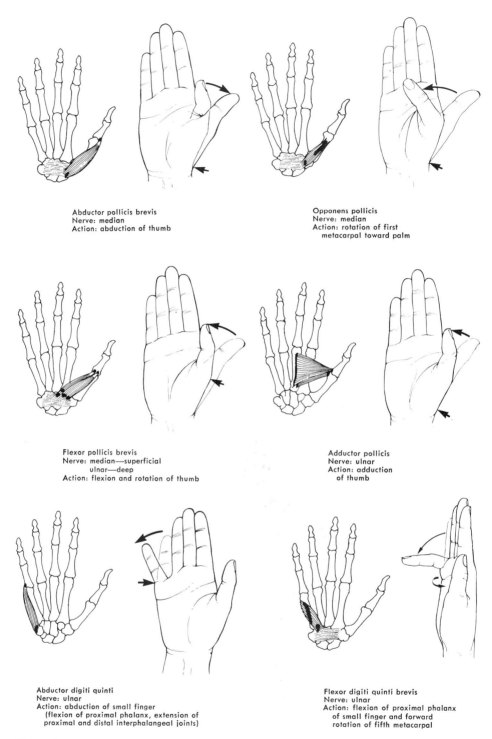

Abductor pollicis brevis
Nerve: median
Action: abduction of thumb

Opponens pollicis
Nerve: median
Action: rotation of first
        metacarpal toward palm

Flexor pollicis brevis
Nerve: median—superficial
        ulnar—deep
Action: flexion and rotation of thumb

Adductor pollicis
Nerve: ulnar
Action: adduction
        of thumb

Abductor digiti quinti
Nerve: ulnar
Action: abduction of small finger
        (flexion of proximal phalanx, extension of
        proximal and distal interphalangeal joints)

Flexor digiti quinti brevis
Nerve: ulnar
Action: flexion of proximal phalanx
        of small finger and forward
        rotation of fifth metacarpal

Fig. 1-17. Intrinsic muscles of the hand. (Modified from Marble, H.C.: The hand, a manual and atlas for the general surgeon, Philadelphia, 1960, W.B. Saunders Co.)

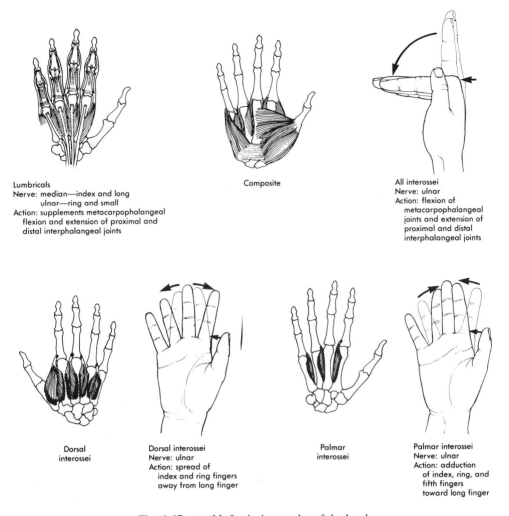

Lumbricals
Nerve: median—index and long
      ulnar—ring and small
Action: supplements metacarpophalangeal
  flexion and extension of proximal and
  distal interphalangeal joints

Composite

All interossei
Nerve: ulnar
Action: flexion of
  metacarpophalangeal
  joints and extension of
  proximal and distal
  interphalangeal joints

Dorsal
interossei

Dorsal interossei
Nerve: ulnar
Action: spread of
  index and ring fingers
  away from long finger

Palmar
interossei

Palmar interossei
Nerve: ulnar
Action: adduction
  of index, ring, and
  fifth fingers
  toward long finger

Fig. 1-17, cont'd. Intrinsic muscles of the hand.

The flexor pollicis brevis has a superficial portion that is innervated by the median nerve and a deep portion that arises from the ulnar side of the first metacarpal and is often innervated by the ulnar nerve. The hypothenar eminence in a similar manner is made up of the abductor digiti quinti, the flexor digiti quinti brevis, and the opponens digiti quinti, which originate primarily from the pisiform bone and the pisohamate ligament and insert into the joint capsule of the fifth metacarpophalangeal joint, the ulnar side of the base of the proximal phalanx of the fifth finger, and the ulnar border of the aponeurosis of this digit. The strong thenar musculature is responsible for the ability to position the thumb in opposition so that it may meet the adjacent digits for pinch and grasp functions, whereas the hypothenar group allows a similar but less pronounced rotation of the fifth metacarpal.

Of the seven interosseous muscles (Fig. 1-18, *A*), four are considered in the dorsal group (Fig. 1-18, *B*), and three as palmar interossei (Fig. 1-18, *C*). The four dorsal interossei originate from the adjacent sides of the metacarpal bones, and, because of their bipinnate nature with two individual muscle bellies, have separate insertions into the tubercle and the lateral aspect of the proximal phalanges and into the extensor expansion. The more palmarly placed three palmar interossei (Fig. 1-18, *C*) have similar insertions and origins and are responsible for adducting the digits together, as opposed to the spreading or abducting function of the dorsal interossei. In addition, four lumbrical tendons (Fig. 1-19, *A*) arising from the radial side of the palmar portion of the flexor digitorum profundus tendons pass through their individual canals on the radial side of the digits to provide an additional contribution to the complex extensor assemblage of the digits. The arrangement of the extensor mechanism, including the transverse sagittal band fibers at the metacarpophalangeal joint and the components of the extensor hood mechanism that gain fibers from both the extrinsic and intrinsic tendons, can be seen in Fig. 1-19, *B* and *C*.

An oversimplification of the function of the intrinsic musculature in the digits would be that they provide strong flexion at the metacarpophalangeal joints and extension at the proximal and distal interphalangeal joints. The lumbrical tendons, by virtue of their origin from the flexor profundi and insertion into the digital extensor mechanism, function as a governor between the two systems, resulting in a loosening of the antagonistic profundus tendon during interphalangeal joint extension. The interossei are further responsible for spreading and closing of the fingers and, together with the extrinsic flexor and extensor tendons, are invaluable to digital balance. A composite, well-integrated pattern of digital flexion and extension is reliant on the smooth performance of both systems, and a loss of intrinsic function will result in severe deformity.

Perhaps the most important intrinsic muscle, the adductor pollicis (Fig. 1-18, *A*), originates from the third metacarpal and inserts on the ulnar side of the base of the proximal phalanx of the thumb and into the ulnar wing expansion of the extensor mechanism. This muscle, by virtue of its strong adducting influence on the thumb and its stabilizing effect on the first metacarpophalangeal joint, functions together with the first dorsal interosseous to provide strong pinch. The adductor pollicis, deep head of the flexor pollicis brevis, ulnar two lumbricals, and all interossei, as well as the hypothenar muscle group, are innervated by the ulnar nerve. Loss of ulnar nerve function has a profound influence on hand function.

Muscle balance and biomechanical considerations

When there is normal resting tone in the extrinsic and intrinsic muscle groups of the forearm and hand, the wrist and digital joints will be maintained in a balanced position. With the forearm midway between pronation and supination, the wrist dorsiflexed, and the digits in moderate flexion, the hand is in the optimum position from which to function.

It may be seen that muscles are usually arranged about joints in pairs so that each musculotendinous unit has at least one antagonistic muscle to balance the involved joint. To a large extent the wrist is the key joint and has a strong influence on the long extrinsic muscle performance at the digital level. Maximal digital flexion strength is facilitated by dorsiflexion of the wrist, which lessens the effective amplitude of the antagonistic extensor tendons while maximizing the contractural force of the digital flexors. Conversely, a posture of wrist flexion will markedly weaken grasping power.

At the digital level, metacarpophalangeal joint flexion is a combination of extrinsic flexor power supplemented by the contribution of the intrinsic muscles, whereas proximal interphalangeal joint extension results from a combination of extrinsic extensor and

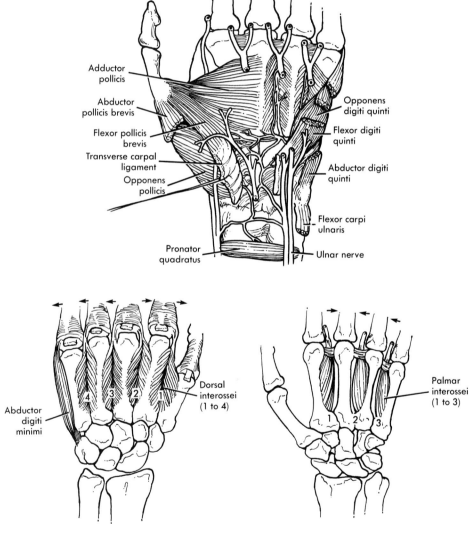

Fig. 1-18. Position and function of the intrinsic muscles of the hand. (Modified from Lampe, E.W.: Surgical anatomy of the hand. In Clinical symposia, New York, 1969, CIBA Pharmaceutical Co., Division of CIBA-GEIGY Corp.; illustrated by F.H. Netter.)

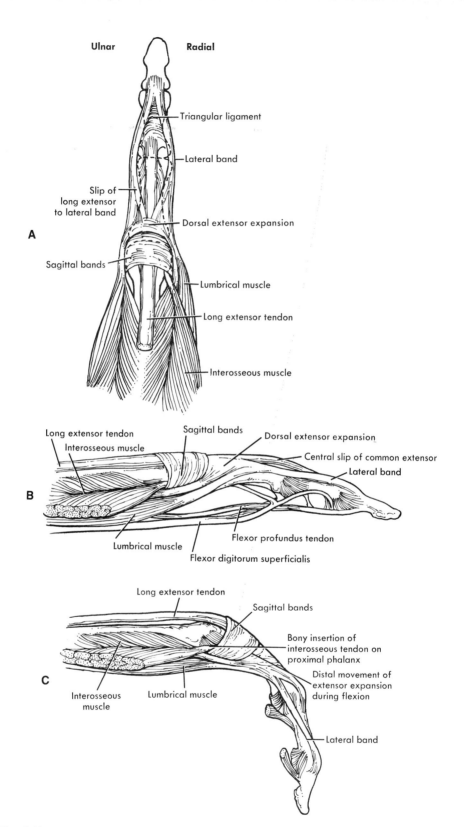

Fig. 1-19. Extensor mechanism of the digits. **B** and **C,** Distal movement of the extensor expansion with metacarpophalangeal joint flexion is shown. (Modified from Lampe, E.W.: Surgical anatomy of the hand. In Clinical symposia, New York, 1969, CIBA Pharmaceutical Co., Division of CIBA-GEIGY Corp.; illustrated by F.H. Netter.)

intrinsic muscle power. At the distal interphalangeal joint the intrinsic muscles provide a majority of the extensor power necessary to balance the antagonistic flexor digitorum profundus tendon.

The distance that a tendon moves when its muscle contracts is defined as the amplitude of the tendon and has been measured in numerous studies. In actuality the effective amplitude of any muscle will be limited by the motion permitted by the joint or joints on which its tendon acts. It has been suggested that the amplitude of wrist movers (flexor carpi ulnaris, flexor carpi radialis, extensor carpi radialis longus, extensor carpi radialis brevis, and extensor carpi ulnaris), is approximately 30 mm with the amplitude of finger extensors averaging 50 mm; the thumb flexor, 50 mm; and the finger flexors 70 mm (Fig. 1-20). Although these amplitudes have been thought to be important considerations when deciding on appropriate tendon transfers, Brand (1974) has shown that the potential excursion of a given tendon such as the extensor carpi radialis longus may be considerably greater than the excursion which was required to produce full motion of the joints on which it acted in its original position.

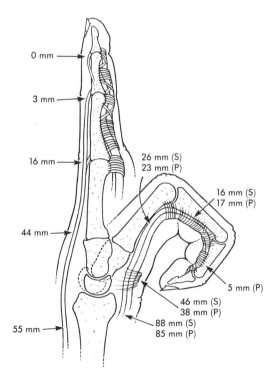

Fig. 1-20. Excursion of the flexor and extensor tendons at various levels. The numbers on the dorsum of the extended finger represent the excursion in millimeters required at each level to bring all distal joints from full flexion into full extension. The numbers shown by arrows on the palmar aspect of the flexed digit represent the excursion in millimeters for the superficialis *(S)* and the profundus *(P)* required at each level to bring the finger from full extension to full flexion. (From Verdan, C.: An introduction to tendon surgery, In Verdan, C., editor: Tendon surgery of the hand, London, 1979, Churchill Livingston.)

Table 1-1. Work capacity of muscles*

Muscle	Mkg
Flexor carpi radialis	0.8
Extensor carpi radialis longus	1.1
Extensor carpi radialis brevis	0.9
Extensor carpi ulnaris	1.1
Abductor pollicis longus	0.1
Flexor pollicis longus	1.2
Flexor digitorum profundus	4.5
Flexor digitorum superficialis	4.8
Brachioradialis	1.9
Flexor carpi ulnaris	2.0
Pronator teres	1.2
Palmaris longus	0.1
Extensor pollicis longus	0.1
Extensor digitorum communis	1.7

*From Von Lanz, T., and Wachsmuth, W.: Praktische anatomie. In Boyes, J.H., editor: Bunnell's surgery of the hand, ed. 5, Philadelphia, 1970, J.B. Lippincott Co.

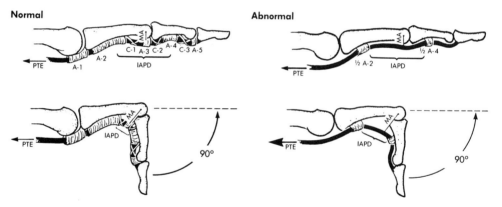

Fig. 1-21. Biomechanics of the finger flexor pulley system. **A,** The arrangement of the annular and cruciate pulleys of the flexor tendon sheath. **A** and **B,** Normal moment arm *(MA),* the intraannular pulley distance *(IPD)* between the A-2 and A-4 pulleys, and the profundus tendon excursion *(PTE),* which occurs within the intact digital fibroosseous canal as the proximal interphalangeal joint is flexed to 90 degrees. Annular pulleys: A-1, A-2, A-3, A-4, and A-5; cruciate pulleys: C-1, C-2, C-3. **C** and **D,** Biomechanical alteration resulting from excision of the distal half of the A-2 pulley together with the C-1, A-3, C-2, and proximal portion of the A-4 pulley. The moment arm is increased, and a greater profundus tendon excursion is required to produce 90 degrees of flexion because of the bow-stringing that results from the loss of pulley support. (From Strickland, J.W.: Management of acute flexor tendon injuries, Orthopaedic Clinics of North America, vol. 14, Philadelphia, 1983, W.B. Saunders Co.)

Efforts have been made to determine the power of individual forearm and hand muscles, and a formula based on the physiologic cross section is generally accepted as the best method for determining this value. The number of fibers in cross section determines the absolute muscle power of a given muscle, whereas the force of muscle action times the distance or amplitude of a given muscle determines the work capacity of the muscle. Therefore a large extrinsic muscle with relatively long fibers such as the flexor digitorum profundus is found to be capable of much more work than is a muscle with shorter fibers such as a wrist extensor. Table 1-1 is an indicator of the work capacities of the various forearm muscles. It can be seen that the flexor digitorum profundus and superficialis have a significantly greater work capacity than do the remaining extrinsic muscles. The abductor pollicis longus, palmaris longus, extensor pollicis longus, extensor carpi radialis brevis, and flexor carpi radialis have less than one fourth the capacity of these muscles.

Several mechanical considerations are important in understanding the effect of a muscle on a given joint. The moment arm of a particular muscle is the perpendicular distance between the muscle or its tendon and the axis of the joint. The greater the displacement of an unrestrained tendon from the joint on which it acts, the greater will be the angulatory effect created by the increased length of the moment arm. Therefore a tendon positioned close to a given joint either by position of the joint or by a restraining pulley will have a much shorter moment arm than will a tendon that is allowed to displace away from the joint (Fig. 1-21).

In simplifying the biomechanics of musculotendinous function, Brand (1974) has emphasized that the ''moment'' of a given muscle is the power of the muscle to turn a joint on its axis. It is determined by multiplying the strength (tension) of the muscle by the length of the moment arm. Again, it can be seen that the distance of tendon displacement away from the joint is the critical factor and that it does not matter where the tendon insertion lies. The importance of the various anatomic restraints of the extrinsic musculotendinous units at the wrist and in the digits is magnified by these mechanical factors.

NERVE SUPPLY

In considering the nerve supply to the forearm, hand, and wrist, it is important to realize that these nerves are a direct continuation of the brachial plexus and that at least a working knowledge of the multiple ramifications of the plexus is necessary if one is to fully appreciate the more distal motor and sensory contributions of the nerves of the upper extremity. Injuries at either the spinal cord or plexus level or to the major peripheral nerves in the upper extremity result in a substantial functional impairment for which splinting may be necessary.

The median, ulnar, and radial nerves, as well as the terminal course of the musculocutaneous, are responsible for the sensory and motor transmission to the forearm, wrist, and hand. The superficial sensory distribution is shared by the median, radial, and ulnar nerves in a fairly constant pattern (Fig. 1-22). This chapter is concerned with the most frequent distribution of these nerves, although it is acknowledged that variations are common.

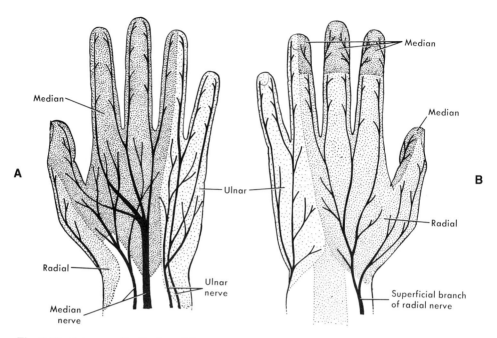

Fig. 1-22. Cutaneous distribution of the nerves of the hand. **A,** Palmar surface. **B,** Dorsal surface.

The palmar side of the hand from the thumb to a line passed longitudinally from the tip of the ring finger to the wrist receives sensory innervation from the median nerve. The remainder of the palm as well as the ulnar half of the ring finger and the entire small finger receive sensory innervation from the ulnar nerve. On the dorsal side the ulnar nerve, distribution again includes the ulnar half of the dorsal hand and the ring and small fingers, whereas the radial side is supplied by the superficial branch of the radial nerve. Some innervation to an area distal to the proximal interphalangeal joints is supplied by the palmar digital nerves originating from the median nerve. The area around the dorsum of the thumb over the metacarpophalangeal joint is frequently supplied by the end branches of the lateral antebrachial cutaneous nerve.

The extrinsic and intrinsic musculature of the forearm and hand is supplied by the median, ulnar, and radial nerves (Fig. 1-23). The long wrist and digital flexors, with the exception of the flexor carpi ulnaris and the profundi to the ring and small fingers, are all supplied by the median nerve. The pronators of the forearm and the muscles of the thenar eminence, with the exception of the deep head of the flexor pollicis brevis and the adductor pollicis, which are innervated by the ulnar nerve, are also supplied by the median nerve. All muscles of the hypothenar eminence, all interossei, the third and fourth lumbrical muscles, the deep head of the flexor pollicis brevis, the adductor pollicis brevis, as well as the flexor carpi ulnaris and the ulnar-most two profundi, are supplied by the ulnar nerve. The radial nerve supplies all long extensors of the hand and wrist as well as the long abductor and short extensor of the thumb and the brachioradialis.

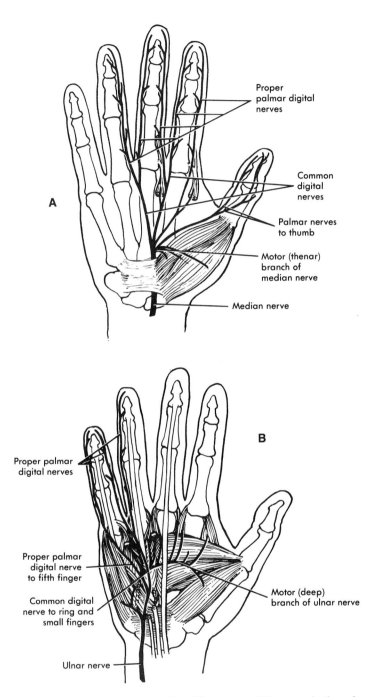

Fig. 1-23. Distribution of the median (**A**) and ulnar (**B**) nerves in the palm.

When considering sensibility, one should remember that the hand is an extremely important organ for the detection and transmission to the brain of information relating to the size, weight, texture, and temperature of objects with which it comes in contact. The types of cutaneous sensation have been defined as touch, pain, hot, and cold. Although most of the nervous tissue in the skin is found in the dermal network, smaller branches course through the subcutaneous tissue following blood vessels. Several types of sensory receptors have been described, and in most areas of the hand there is an interweaving of nerve fibers that allows each area to receive nerve input from several sources. In addition, deep sensibility from nerve endings in muscles and tendons is important in the recognition of joint position.

The high interruption of the median nerve above the elbow will result in a paralysis of the flexor carpi radialis, the flexor digitorum superficialis, the flexor pollicus longus, the profundi to the index and long fingers, and the lumbricals to the index and long fingers. In addition, pronation will be weakened as a result of the loss of innervation of both the pronator teres and quadratus muscles, and most importantly, the patient will lose the ability to oppose the thumb because of paralysis of the median nerve–innervated thenar muscle group. A more distal interruption of the median nerve at the wrist level produces loss of opposition, and both lesions result in a critical impairment of sensation in the important distribution of that nerve to the palmar aspect of the thumb, index, long, and radial half of the ring finger.

High ulnar nerve interruption produces paralysis of the flexor carpi ulnaris, the flexor profundi and lumbricals to the ring and small fingers, and, most important, the interossei, adductor pollicis brevis, and deep head of the flexor pollicis brevis. The resulting loss of the antagonistic flexion at the metacarpophalangeal joints of the ring and small fingers permits hyperextension at this level by the unopposed long extensor tendons, often resulting in a claw deformity. The loss of the strong adducting and stabilizing influence of the adductor pollicis combined with the paralysis of the first dorsal interosseous muscle results in profound weakness of pinch and produces a collapse deformity of the thumb, necessitating interphalangeal joint hyperflexion for pinch (Froment's sign). More distal lesions of the ulnar nerve usually result in a greater degree of claw deformity due to the sparing of the profundi function of the ring and small fingers. Sensory loss following ulnar nerve interruption involves the palmar ring (ulnar half) and small fingers.

Radial nerve lesions at or proximal to the elbow result in a complete wrist drop and inability to extend the fingers at the metacarpophalangeal joints. It should be remembered that paralysis of this nerve does not result in inability to extend the interphalangeal joints of either the thumb or digits because of the contribution to that function by the intrinsic muscles. The sensory deficit over the dorsoradial aspect of the wrist and hand resulting from radial nerve interruption is of much less significance than are lesions to nerves innervating the palmar side.

Various combinations of paralyses involving more than one nerve of the upper extremity are frequently encountered; those of the median and ulnar nerve are the most common. High lesions of these two nerves produce paralyses of both the extrinsic and intrinsic muscle groups with total sensory loss over the palmar aspect of the hand. More

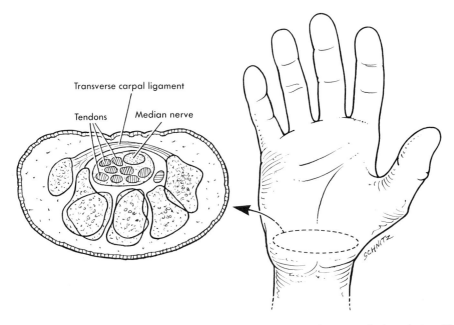

Fig. 1-24. Cross sectional anatomy of the carpal tunnel shows its anatomic boundaries. The carpus and the palmar roof formed by the transverse carpal ligament are shown, as is the position of the median nerve. An increased volume in this passageway most frequently resulting from thickening or inflammation around the nine flexor tendons can result in compression of the median nerve and the condition known as carpal tunnel syndrome.

distal combined median and ulnar lesions will have their effect primarily on the intrinsic muscles, resulting in the most disabling deformities with metacarpophalangeal hyperextension, interphalangeal flexion, and thumb collapse. An inefficient pattern of digital flexion consisting of a slow distal-to-proximal, rolling grasp will result from the loss of the integrated intrinsic participation.

A number of entrapment phenomena are now recognized that may cause complete or partial paralyses, purely sensory deficits, or a combination of these alterations in any of the three major peripheral nerves of the upper extremity. Ulnar nerve compression at the elbow and median nerve compression in the carpal tunnel (Fig. 1-24) are among the more frequent entrapment entities.

BLOOD SUPPLY

The blood supply to the hand is carried by the radial and ulnar arteries and their branches (Fig. 1-25). The ulnar artery, which can often be palpated just lateral to the pisiform, reaches the wrist in company with the ulnar nerve immediately lateral to the flexor carpi ulnaris tendon. The artery divides at the wrist into a large branch that forms the superficial arterial arch of the hand and a smaller branch that forms the lesser part of the deep palmar arch. As it passes between the pisiform and the hamate (canal of Guyon), the ulnar artery is particularly vulnerable to repetitive trauma, which may result

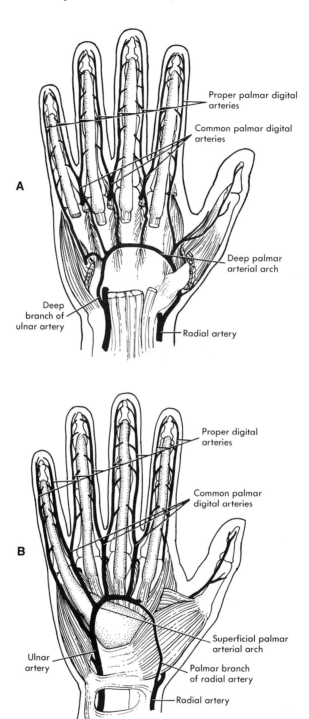

Fig. 1-25. Vascular anatomy of the hand. **A,** The deep arch is supplied by the radial artery. **B,** The superficial arch is supplied by the ulnar artery.

in thrombosis, giving rise to symptoms of vascular embarrassment and occasionally sensory abnormalities of the ulnar nerve by virtue of its close proximity to this structure.

The radial artery, which may be palpated near the proximal palmar wrist crease, divides into a small superficial branch, which continues distally over the thenar eminence to complete the superficial arterial arch. The larger deep radial branch passes from dorsal to palmar between the heads of the first dorsal interosseous and around the base of the thumb, where it reaches the palm to join the ulnar artery and form the deep palmar arch.

The superficial arterial arch gives off common palmar digital branches that bifurcate into proper digital branches immediately below the central part of the palmar fascia. The palmar metacarpal branches of the deep arch empty into the common palmar digital branches of the superficial arch just proximal to their bifurcation into the phalangeal arteries. It is believed by many that the superficial arterial arch is larger and more important than is the deep arch.

Although little emphasis is placed on the venous drainage of the hand, it is important to remember that the hand, like the remainder of the upper extremity, is drained by two sets of veins: a superficial group located on the superficial fascia and a deep group that travels with the arteries. The superficial venous system is the more important, and the majority of these draining vessels form a large network over the dorsum of the hand. The dorsal venous arch receives digital veins from the fingers and becomes continuous proximally with the cephalic and basilic veins on the radial and ulnar borders of the wrist. It is easy to see why injuries over the dorsum of the hand that interrupt or are prejudicial to the flow of venous drainage can result in marked congestion and edema.

SKIN AND SUBCUTANEOUS FASCIA

The palmar skin with its numerous small fibrous connections to the underlying palmar aponeurosis is a highly specialized, thickened structure with very little mobility. Numerous small blood vessels pass through the underlying subcutaneous tissues into the dermis. In contrast, the dorsal skin and subcutaneous tissue are much more loose with few anchoring fibers and a high degree of mobility. Most of the lymphatic drainage from the palmar aspect of the fingers, web areas, and hypothenar and thenar eminences flows in lymph channels on the dorsum of the hand. Clinical swelling, which frequently accompanies injury or infection, is usually a result of impaired lymph drainage.

The central, triangularly shaped palmar aponeurosis (Fig. 1-26) provides a semirigid barrier between the palmar skin and the important underlying neurovascular and tendon structures. It fuses medially and laterally with the deep fascia covering the hypothenar and thenar muscles, and fasciculi extending from this thick fascial barrier extend to the proximal phalanges to fuse with the tendon sheaths on the palmar, medial, and lateral aspects. In the distal palm, septa from this palmar fascia extend to the deep transverse metacarpal ligaments forming the sides of the annular fibrous canals, allowing for the passage of the ensheathed flexor tendons and the lumbrical muscles as well as the neurovascular bundles.

Dorsally the deep fascia and extensor tendons fuse to form the roof for the dorsal

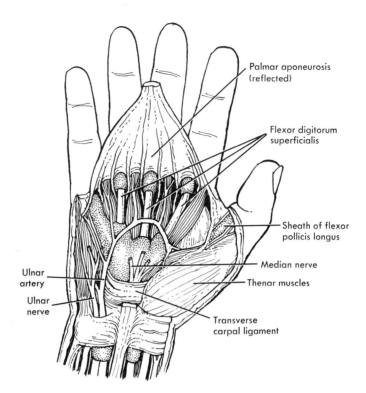

Palmar aponeurosis
(reflected)

Flexor digitorum
superficialis

Sheath of flexor
pollicis longus

Median nerve

Thenar muscles

Ulnar
artery

Ulnar
nerve

Transverse
carpal ligament

Fig. 1-26. Palmar aponeurosis reflected distally reveals septa and underlying palmar anatomy. (Modified from Lampe, E.W.: Surgical anatomy of the hand. In Clinical symposia, New York, 1969, CIBA Pharmaceutical Co., Division of CIBA-GEIGY Corp.; illustrated by F.H. Netter.)

subaponeurotic space, which, although not as thick as its palmar counterpart, may prove restrictive to underlying fluid accumulations or intrinsic muscle swelling.

SUPERFICIAL ANATOMY

It is particularly important for the person engaged in splint preparation to thoroughly understand the surface anatomy of the forearm and hand, including the various landmarks that represent underlying anatomic structures. Respect for bony prominences and a knowledge of the position of underlying joints will be particularly important if one is to prepare splint devices that are comfortable and either immobilize or allow motion at various levels. Figs. 1-27 to 1-29 indicate the various contours of the forearm, wrist, and palm and the underlying structures that are responsible for these contours. In addition, the palmar creases of the surface of the wrist and palm are depicted in relation to their underlying joint structures (Fig. 1-30) to indicate the anatomic borders that must be respected in the preparation of splints designed to allow motion at either the wrist, metacarpophalangeal, or interphalangeal joint level.

Perhaps the most vulnerable of the bony prominences of the wrist and hand are the styloid processes of the radius and ulna. By virtue of their subcutaneous position, these areas are particularly vulnerable to poorly contoured splints. Great care must be taken to avoid appliances that place unequal pressure against these osseous structures.

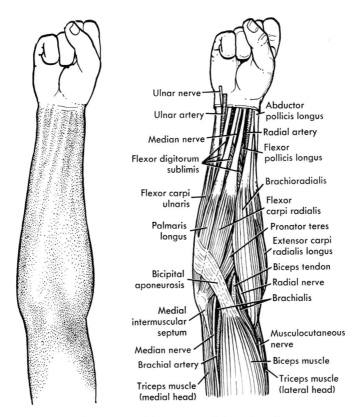

Fig. 1-27. Topographic anatomy of the palmar forearm.

Labels for Fig. 1-27:
Ulnar nerve
Ulnar artery
Median nerve
Flexor digitorum sublimis
Flexor carpi ulnaris
Palmaris longus
Bicipital aponeurosis
Medial intermuscular septum
Median nerve
Brachial artery
Triceps muscle (medial head)
Abductor pollicis longus
Radial artery
Flexor pollicis longus
Brachioradialis
Flexor carpi radialis
Pronator teres
Extensor carpi radialis longus
Biceps tendon
Radial nerve
Brachialis
Musculocutaneous nerve
Biceps muscle
Triceps muscle (lateral head)

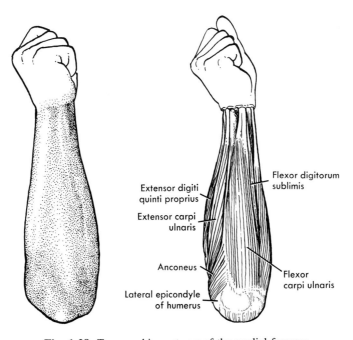

Fig. 1-28. Topographic anatomy of the medial forearm.

Labels for Fig. 1-28:
Extensor digiti quinti proprius
Extensor carpi ulnaris
Anconeus
Lateral epicondyle of humerus
Flexor digitorum sublimis
Flexor carpi ulnaris

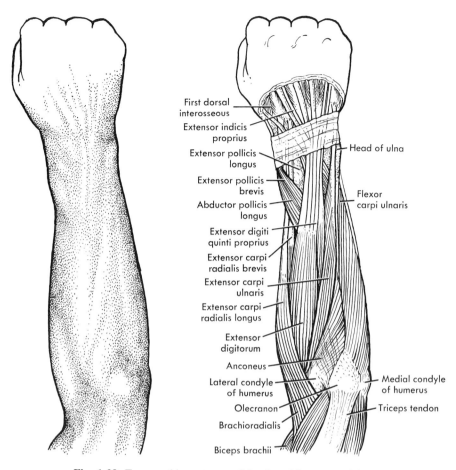

Fig. 1-29. Topographic anatomy of the dorsal forearm and hand.

Labels, clockwise from upper left:
First dorsal interosseous
Extensor indicis proprius
Extensor pollicis longus
Extensor pollicis brevis
Abductor pollicis longus
Extensor digiti quinti proprius
Extensor carpi radialis brevis
Extensor carpi ulnaris
Extensor carpi radialis longus
Extensor digitorum
Anconeus
Lateral condyle of humerus
Olecranon
Brachioradialis
Biceps brachii
Head of ulna
Flexor carpi ulnaris
Medial condyle of humerus
Triceps tendon

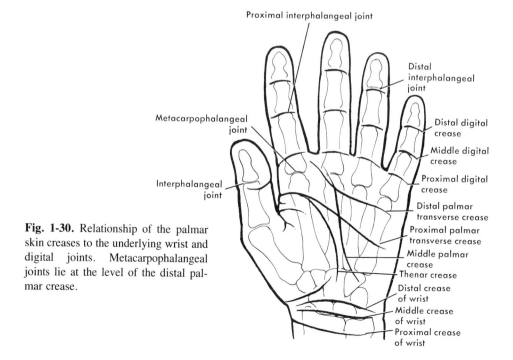

Fig. 1-30. Relationship of the palmar skin creases to the underlying wrist and digital joints. Metacarpophalangeal joints lie at the level of the distal palmar crease.

Labels:
Proximal interphalangeal joint
Metacarpophalangeal joint
Interphalangeal joint
Distal interphalangeal joint
Distal digital crease
Middle digital crease
Proximal digital crease
Distal palmar transverse crease
Proximal palmar transverse crease
Middle palmar crease
Thenar crease
Distal crease of wrist
Middle crease of wrist
Proximal crease of wrist

FUNCTIONAL PATTERNS

The prehensile function of the hand depends on the integrity of the kinetic chain of bones and joints extending from the wrist to the distal phalanges. Interruptions of the transverse and longitudinal arch systems formed by these structures will always result in instability, deformity, or functional loss at a more proximal or distal level. Similarly, the balanced synergism-antagonism relationship between the long extrinsic muscles and the intrinsic muscles is a requisite for the composite functions required for both power and precision functions of the hand. It is important to recognize that the hand cannot function well without normal sensory input from all areas.

Many attempts have been made to classify the different patterns of hand function, and various types of grasp and pinch have been described. Perhaps the more simplified analysis of power grasp and precision handling as proposed by Napier (1968) and refined by Flatt (1972) is the easiest to consider.

As generally stated, power grip is a combination of strong thumb flexion and adduction with the powerful flexion of the ring and small fingers on the ulnar side of the hand. The radial half of the hand employing the delicate tripod of pinch between the thumb, index, and long fingers is responsible for more delicate precision function.

An analysis of hand functions requires that one consider the thumb and the remainder of the hand as two separate parts. Rotation of the thumb into an opposing position is a requirement of almost any hand function, whether it be strong grasp or delicate pinch. The wide range of motion permitted at the carpometacarpal joint is extremely important in allowing the thumb to be correctly positioned. Stability at this joint is a requirement of almost all prehensile activities and is ensured by a unique ligamentous arrangement, which allows mobility in the midposition and provides stability at the extremes. As can be seen in Fig. 1-31, the thumb moves through a wide arc from the side of the index finger tip to the tip of the small finger, and the adaptation that occurs between the thumb and digits as progressively smaller objects are held occurs primarily at the metacarpophalangeal joints of the digits and the carpometacarpal joint of the thumb.

For power grip the wrist is in an extended position that allows the extrinsic digital flexors to press the object firmly against the palm while the thumb is closed tightly around the object. The thumb, ring, and small fingers are the most important participants in this strong grasp function, and the importance of the ulnar border digits cannot be minimized (Fig. 1-32).

In precision grasp, wrist position is less important, and the thumb is opposed to the semiflexed fingers with the intrinsic tendons providing most of the finger movement. When the intrinsic muscles are paralyzed, the balance of each finger is markedly disturbed. The metacarpophalangeal joint loses its primary flexors, and the interphalangeal joints lose the intrinsic contribution to extension. A dyskinetic finger flexion results in which the metacarpophalangeal joints lag behind the interphalangeal joints in flexion. When the hand is closed on an object, only the fingertips make contact rather than the uniform contact of the fingers, palm, and thumb that occurs with normal grip (Fig. 1-33).

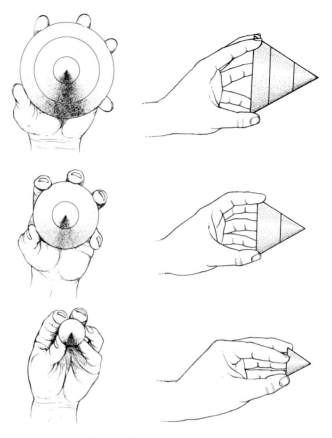

Fig. 1-31. Progressive alterations in precision grasp with changes in object size. Adaptation takes place primarily at the carpometacarpal joint of the thumb and the metacarpophalangeal joints of the digits.

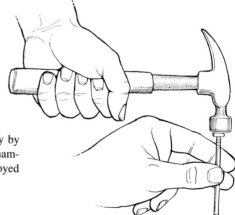

Fig. 1-32. Strong power grip imparted primarily by the thumb, ring, and small fingers around the hammer handle with delicate precision tip grip employed to hold the nail.

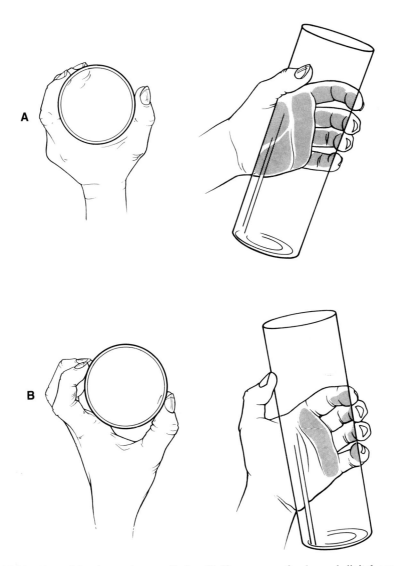

Fig. 1-33. A, Normal hand grasping a cylinder. Uniform areas of palm and digital contact are shaded. **B** Intrinsic minus (claw hand grasping the same cylinder). The area of contact is limited to the fingertips and the metacarpal heads. (From Brand, P.W.: Clinical mechanics of the hand, St. Louis, 1985, The C.V. Mosby Co.)

Certain activities may require combinations of power and precision grips, as seen in Fig. 1-34. Pinching between the thumb and the combined index and long fingers is a further refinement of precision grip and may be classified as either tip grip, palmar grip, or lateral grip, (Fig. 1-35), depending on the portions of the phalanges brought to bear on the object being handled. In these functions the strong contracture of the adductor pollicis brings the thumb into contact against the tip or sides of the index or index and long fingers with digital resistance imparted by the first and second dorsal interossei.

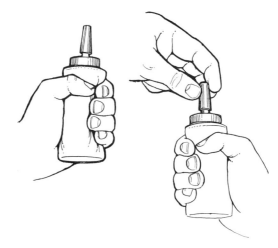

Fig. 1-34. Power grip used to hold the squeeze bottle with precision handling of the bottle top by the opposite hand.

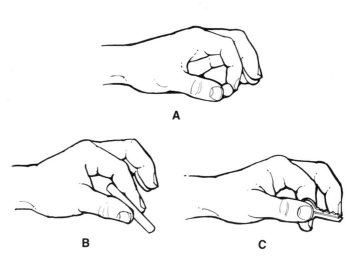

Fig. 1-35. Types of precision grip. **A,** Tip grip. **B,** Palmar grip. **C,** Lateral grip. (Modified from Flatt, A.E.: The care of the rheumatoid hand, ed. 3, St. Louis, 1974, The C.V. Mosby Co.)

The size of the object being handled dictates whether large thumb and digital surfaces, as in palmar grip, or smaller surfaces, as in lateral or tip grasp, are utilized. Flatt (1974) has pointed out that the dual importance of rotation and flexion of the thumb is often ignored in the preparation of splints, which permit only tip grip because the thumb cannot oppose the pulp of the fingers to produce palmar grip.

The patterns of action of the normal hand depend on the mobility of the skeletal arches, and alterations of the configuration of these arches is produced by the balanced function of the extrinsic and intrinsic muscles. Whereas the extrinsic contribution resulting from the large powerful forearm muscle groups is more important to hand strength, the fine precision action imparted by the intrinsic musculature gives the hand an enormous variety of capabilities. Although one need not specifically memorize the various patterns of pinch, grasp, and combined hand functions, it is important to understand the underlying contribution of the various muscle-tendon groups, both extrinsic and intrinsic, to these activities. Injuries or diseases that affect the integrity of the arch system or disrupt or paralyze the extrinsic or intrinsic muscles will have a profound impact on hand function.

It is hoped that this chapter will serve as a reference guide for the important anatomic and kinesiologic considerations presented in the ensuing chapters on hand splinting.

CHAPTER 2

Biologic basis for hand splinting

James W. Strickland

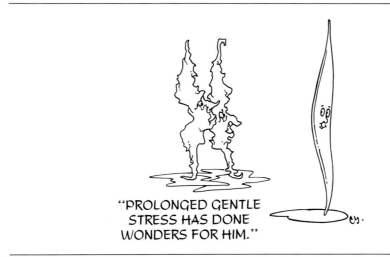

"PROLONGED GENTLE STRESS HAS DONE WONDERS FOR HIM."

Splints are used to put all or part of the hand at rest so that diseased, injured, or surgically violated tissues can undergo orderly, uninterrupted healing. They are also used to favorably influence tissue healing and minimize the development of restrictive scar tissue, which has a detrimental effect on normal joint and tendon movement. In many clinical situations there is an appropriate time for the use of both immobilizing and mobilizing splints to control the essential events of repair. A strong appreciation for the biologic state of the involved tissues will aid in making decisions as to whether the injured part should be managed by rest or stress and the best timing for the use of each type of splint. This chapter provides insight into the nature of normal and abnormal tissue healing in the human hand and the biologic basis for the use of splints as part of a treatment program designed to restore maximum functional recovery.

I am extremely grateful to Mr. Gary W. Schnitz for the excellent illustrations used in this chapter.

Whether secondary to intraarticular destruction, capsular fibrosis, tendon adhesion, or skin and soft tissue scarring, the reduction or cessation of function of the wrist or digital joints is profoundly detrimental to hand performance. To proceed with effective therapy to restore function in the involved joints, one must have a thorough understanding of the biologic basis for the underlying pathology. Why is the joint stiffened? Are the articular surfaces damaged? Are the capsular and ligamentous tissues thickened, scarred, or shortened? Are adherent flexor, extensor, or intrinsic tendons preventing motion by a tenodesis check-rein phenomenon? Is the skin, fascia, or subcutaneous tissue scarred or fibrotic? Are there many factors involved in combination to limit joint movement?

Armed with an understanding of the pertinent pathology, one must define the goals of splinting for a particular situation. Is the splint to be used to allow healing, to biologically modify contracted and scarred skin, subcutaneous tissue, fascia, or ligamentous tissues, or is it meant to lengthen tendon adhesions that have become fixed to bone or surrounding tissues? What dangers exist with regard to joint injury or tendon rupture?

Finally, when the pathologic process and the goals of splinting have been defined, consideration is given to the method of splinting that can most effectively impart the desired biologic alteration of the affected tissues. What is the most desirable vector for the application of force to a given joint? How much force should be imparted? For how long a period should the force be applied? Through how wide a surface? On what anatomical stuctures is the force being placed? What measurements will ensure the most effective application of the splint?

To answer these questions and proceed with the design, construction, and application of an effective splint, one must know the necessary sequence of biologic events involved in normal tissue healing and the aberrations in this process that may result in the loss of joint motion. Splinting methods can then be selected to alter and control these events to restore maximum function.

TISSUE HEALING

Normal hand function depends on the smooth, friction-free gliding of small cartilaginous articular surfaces and the excursion of stout collagenous tendons unimpeded by restrictive scars and adhesions. The biologic response of tissues to injury results in an alteration of their physical properties and the replacement of normal structures with scar tissue. Therefore a thorough understanding of wound healing and scar formation provides a foundation for the recognition and treatment of problems related to the successful restoration of function following hand injury and surgery.

It must be recognized that scar formation is nonspecific in the sense that the biologic processes and the sequence in which they occur are virtually identical in all organs and tissues. However, the final appearance of the healed scar and the effect it has on function may differ with respect to the specific organ or tissue involved. In the hand, any alteration in the physical characteristics or anatomic arrangement of tissues may prevent relative gliding and reduce function significantly. Although the functional effect varies, the common denominator for the healing of all tissues is scar tissue. The components of the process of tissue healing sequentially include inflammation, fibroplasia, scar maturation, and wound contracture (Fig. 2-1). In the hand, it is particularly relevant that the presence of scar in specialized tissues such as tendon, bone, and joint can result in severe impairment of function. It should also be remembered that the process of wound healing results not only from accidental injury, but also from surgical intervention.

Inflammation

Following wounding, the initial biologic response is inflammation (Fig. 2-1, *A-C*). The open wound containing injured tissues and hemorrhage is easily contaminated by bacteria and foreign substances. Inflammation is a vascular and cellular response that serves several purposes, including the removal of microorganisms, foreign material and, necrotic tissue in preparation for repair. This inflammatory response is the same regardless of the cause of the injury and is characterized by a transient vasoconstriction, which is followed by vasodilation of local small blood vessels resulting in increased blood flow to the injured area. This phenomenon is associated with local edema and the migration of white blood cells through the walls of the blood vessels.

The removal of dead tissue and foreign bodies, including bacteria, is carried out by phagocytic cells; when some of the white cells die, their intracellular enzymes and debris are released and become part of the wound exudate. Some of these enzymes facilitate the breakdown of necrotic debris and others dissolve connective tissue. The acute inflammatory response usually subsides within several days except in those wounds which become contaminated with bacteria or retain foreign material; in these cases the wounds continue to have a persistent inflammatory response and remain unhealed for quite some time. A wall of collagen may ultimately be laid down, resulting in the formation of a granuloma.

Fibroplasia

At the end of the inflammatory phase, migratory fibroblasts enter the wound depths and begin synthesizing scar tissue. This period of scar tissue formation is known as fibroplasia (Fig. 2-1, *D*). It usually begins at the wound site on the fourth or fifth day after injury and continues for 2 to 4 weeks. During this period the wound area becomes recognizable microscopically as granulation tissue with the formation of capillaries or endothelial budding, which results in a characteristic vascularity and redness of the involved tissues.

From the third to the sixth week after injury the number of fibroblasts and blood vessels within the wound slowly diminishes. As the cell population decreases, scar collagen fibers increase and the wound changes from a predominantly cellular structure to predominantly extracellular tissue. It is during this phase that fibroblasts manufacture collagen by a poorly understood mechanism. The collagen molecule is a complex helical structure whose mechanical properties are largely responsible for the strength and rigidity of scar tissue.

Tensile strength is defined as the load per cross-sectional area that can be supported by the wound, and it increases at a rate proportional to the rate of collagen synthesis. During the period of fibroplasia the tensile strength of the wound increases rapidly. As collagen is produced, the fibroblasts in the wound diminish. The disappearance of fibro-

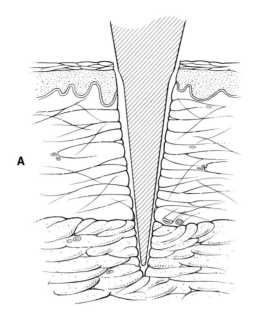

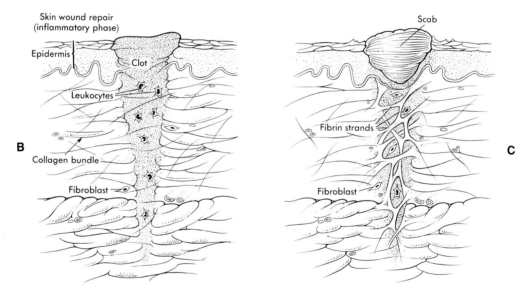

Fig. 2-1. Stages of wound healing. **A,** Initial injury: lacerating object producing injury to the epidermis, dermis, and subcutaneous tissues. **B,** Skin wound repair, inflammatory phase (early). The wound is filled with blood and cellular debris. Clotted blood unites the wound edges. Epithelial cells mobilize and begin migrating across the defect. Serum, plasma, proteins, and leukocytes escape from the venules and enter the wound area. Undifferentiated mesenchymal cells begin transformation to mature fibroblasts. **C,** Late migratory phase. Epithelial cells continue to migrate and proliferate. Debris is removed by leukocytes, and fibroblasts migrate into the wound area along fibrin strands. Capillaries begin regrowth by budding, and the open wound is recognizable as granulation tissue. (**A-E,** Modified from Bryant, M.W.: Ciba Clinical Symposium, vol. 29, no. 3, 1977.)

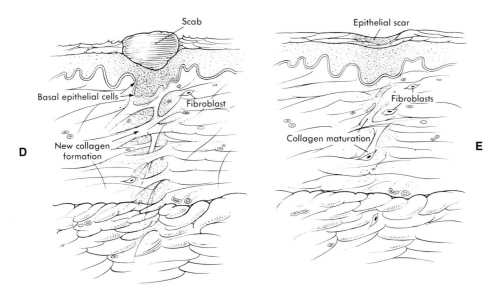

Fig. 2-1, cont'd. D, Fibroplasia (proliferative phase). Epithelium increases in thickness beneath the scab and forms irregular projections into the dermis. Collagen fibers are laid down in a random pattern. Capillaries continue to invade the wound and fibrin strands, debris, and leukocytes disappear. **E,** Maturation phase. Scab sloughs completely as epithelium resumes normal stratification. Collagen remodels in bulk and form and becomes organized. Wound strength increases and fibroblasts begin to disappear. Vascularity is restored.

blasts marks the end of the fibroblastic phase and the beginning of the maturation phase of wound healing.

Scar maturation

The scar tissue formed during the fibroblastic phase is a dense structure of randomly oriented collagen fibers. During the maturation phase of wound healing (Fig. 2-1, *E*), changes in the form, bulk and strength of the scar occur. Microscopically the weave or architecture of the collagen fibers changes to a more organized pattern, and the strength of the wound continues to increase despite the disappearance of fibroblasts and the reduction in the rate of collagen synthesis. Remodeling is a spontaneous process, and scars may remain metabolically active for years, slowly changing in size, shape, color, texture, and strength. It is during this phase that there is continuous and simultaneous collagen production and breakdown. If the rate of breakdown exceeds the rate of production, the scar becomes softer and less bulky. If the rate of production exceeds the rate of breakdown, then a keloid or hypertrophic scar may result.

Through an unknown mechanism, the surfaces against which scar tissue is deposited influence the nature of the remodeling process. Scar deposited in the presence of cut tendon ends remodels to mimic the organization of tendon bundles. Scar adjacent to an uninjured tendon surface tends to remodel to resemble peritendon. The rate and extent to which a scar remodels varies among individuals and also within the same individual depending on age at the time of injury. Younger animals have been shown to remodel scar tissues more effectively than older animals. In the young, remodeling is rapid and effective and this increased rate of metabolic turnover may be responsible for the excellent restoration of gliding seen in younger patients following injury to bone or tendon. The quantity of scar deposited is directly related to the amount of injured tissue; the larger the scar, the less likely the effective restoration of joint or tendon function.

Because wounds remain metabolically reactive for long periods of time, surgery or a second injury may further increase scar collagen synthesis and lead to more scarring. It may be many months before a wound is sufficiently healed to allow one to proceed with further reconstructive surgical procedures. The physical characteristics of the injured tissues may provide important clues as to the metabolic state of the wound. This prolonged period of metabolic activity may also explain the need for long-term splinting to prevent and overcome joint contractures resulting from wound scar formation.

Wound contracture

Open wounds with or without tissue loss undergo wound contraction with dramatic changes in size and shape. The process of contraction begins after a 2- or 3-day latent period, and by 2 to 3 weeks the wounds are often less than 20% of their original area. The forces of contraction will continue to close the wound until balanced by equal tension in the surrounding skin. In the hand this contraction may produce significant functional impairment. Contracture is, of course, beneficial to healing wounds but, in the hand, it may be functionally detrimental when it involves mobile tissues around or over joints. Splints appear to be an effective method of minimizing wound contracture.

Specific tissue healing

Although this general scheme is applicable to almost all tissues, hand injuries often involve complex wounding to the deep structures such as bone, joint, tendon, and nerve which must heal so that the unique function of each tissue will be restored. A brief discussion of the unique features of wound healing for each of these tissues is provided next.

Bone and cartilage healing. Unlike the healing by the scar formation of soft tissues, bone is capable of limited regeneration. As with the other tissues, the immediate response to injury includes inflammation and edema with associated bleeding in the marrow cavity and surrounding tissues (Fig. 2-2, *A*). Within a few days the fibroblastic phase of soft tissue healing begins and osteogenic cells from the periosteum and endosteum of the bone begin migration and proliferation at the wound site. These cells lay down callus and a fibrous matrix of collagen to form a bridge between two bony ends at the fracture site (Fig. 2-2, *B*). The osteogenic cells nearest the bone surface appear to transform directly into osteoblasts and lay down a collagen matrix that calcifies directly into bone (Fig. 2-2, *C*). The precise mechanism of calcification is not well known, but it appears that the collagen matrix, perhaps in interaction with the surrounding ground substance, initiates crystal formation and deposition.

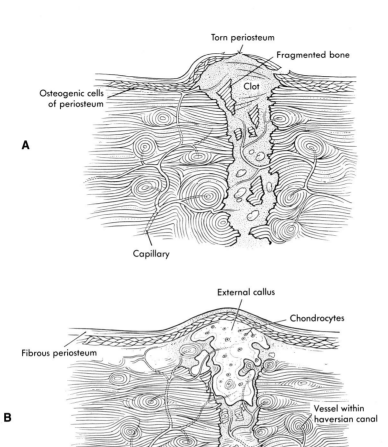

Fig. 2-2. Bone healing. **A,** Early stages of bone and fracture repair. Proliferation of osteogenic cells of the periosteum and of endosteal lining of haversian canals and marrow cavity. These cells differentiate into chondroblasts, which form cartilaginous callus. Osteoblasts, which form new bone, osteoclasts, which resorb dead bone and bone fragments, are present. Periosteal reaction extends beyond the fracture site. **B,** Intermediate phase of bone repair. An external callus of bone or cartilage is formed by osteogenic cells of the periosteum. Cells form bone in areas of high oxygen tension and form cartilage in areas of low oxygen tension. As new capillary growth proceeds, new bone replaces cartilaginous callus. Internal callus is formed by osteogenic cells of the endosteum and is primarily new bone. (**A-C,** Modified from Bryant, M.W.: Ciba Clinical Symposium, vol. 29, no. 3, 1977.) *Continued.*

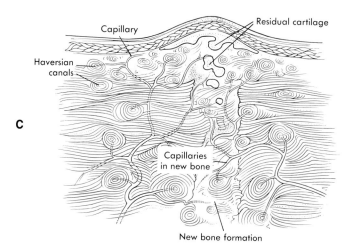

Fig. 2-2, cont'd. C, Late stage of bone repair. New bone of the external callus extends to join new bone of the internal callus and bridge the fracture defect. Bone is remodeled as osteoclasts resorb callus. Layers of bone laid down around blood vessels form new haversian systems.

Remodeling of bone occurs over a prolonged period and appears to be influenced by forces of stress in the healed bone. Although new cartilage formation occurs during bone repair, mature cartilage appears to be incapable of regenerating. Injuries to human articular cartilage appear to be repaired by fibrous union resulting from nonspecific inflammation and fibroplasia.

Tendon healing. The process of tendon healing (Fig. 2-3) is particularly important because the successful return of function following tendon interruption in the hand results not only from a union of severed tendon ends but also the restoration of gliding. These qualities would seem to be contradictory in that they require both a dense fibrous bond between the severed tendon ends and a free excursion of the tendon in the surrounding tissues. Unfortunately, adhesions resulting from the extrinsic contribution of surrounding tissues to tendon healing frequently restrict the ability of that tendon to glide.

Historically there has been considerable debate with regard to the mechanism of tendon healing, and investigators have been at odds as to whether a tendon has an intrinsic capability to heal itself or relies exclusively on the cellular response of the tendon sheath and the surrounding perisheath tissues for healing. Hand specialists are well aware that adhesions resulting from the healing process frequently limit tendon excursion, and historically these adhesions have been considered an essential source of reparative cells. Recent studies on the intrinsic healing capacity of tendons, however, suggest that adhesions may constitute a nonessential inflammatory response at the site of injury. Attention has been focused on attempts to alter the formation of adhesions following tendon repair by biomechanical, biochemical, and biophysical techniques. Until the mechanism of healing is more clearly defined, the restoration of tendon excur-

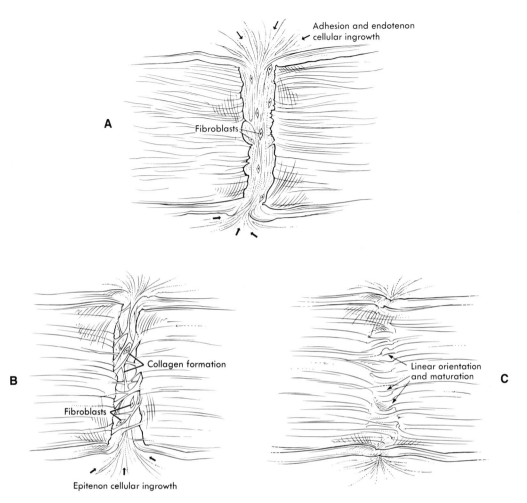

Fig. 2-3. Tendon healing. **A,** Two weeks. Following a cellular response of a tendon, tendon sheath, and surrounding perisheath tissues, fibroblasts and collagen fibers are present between the severed tendon ends and are oriented in a plane perpendicular to the long axis of the tendon. **B,** At 4 weeks the fibroblasts have started to become more longitudinally oriented and progressive organization and realignment of collagen fibers occur. **C,** At 8 weeks the collagen is mature and realigned in a linear fashion.

sion following interruption, repair, and healing will remain an inexact science and a frustrating clinical dilemma.

Nerve healing. Injury to peripheral nerves necessitates an entirely different type of tissue healing in that the severed nerve fiber must regenerate distally from the point of injury. The injury results in degeneration of the axon and myelin distal to the wound and, for a short distance, proximal to the wound (Fig. 2-4, *A*). Schwann cells in the distal stump grow toward the proximal stump, and macrophages clear cellular debris

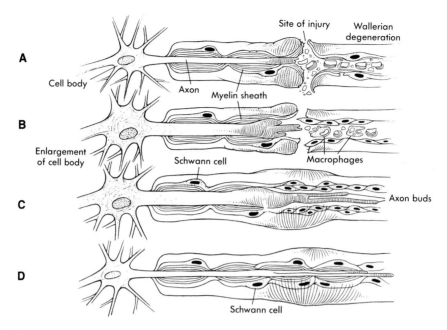

Fig. 2-4. Nerve healing. Axonal regeneration following peripheral nerve severance and repair. **A,** Injury results in degeneration of the axon and myelin distal to the wound and for a short distance proximal to the wound. **B,** A cell body and proximal stump of the axon enlarge as metabolic activity necessary for regeneration commences. The Schwann cells in the distal stump grow forward to the proximal stump and macrophages clear the debris. **C,** Proximal and distal stumps are united by Schwann cells and axonal buds migrate distally along the Schwann cell column in an endoneural tub. **D,** Schwann cells surround the axon and form a myelin sheath. (Modified from Bryant, M.W.: Ciba Clinical Symposium, vol. 29, no. 3, 1977.)

from the distal nerve. The cell body and proximal stump of the axon enlarge as the metabolic activity necessary for regeneration commences (Fig. 2-4, *B*). Ultimately, the proximal and distal stumps of the nerve are united, and axon buds migrate distally along the cell column in the endoneural tube (Fig. 2-4, *C*). Finally, Schwann cells envelop the axon and form a new myelin sheath (Fig. 2-4, *D*). The time required for this process varies depending on the nature of the injury, the time of repair, and the proximity of the nerve injury to the central cell.

Repair of a peripheral nerve therefore involves the regeneration of a portion of a highly specialized cell and not of a single tissue. By careful nerve repair the surgeon hopes to provide the optimum setting for successful axonal regrowth. Regenerating axons eventually reach one of several types of receptors or motor endplates, and despite the most careful microscopic repair, distribution of these axons is random. If a sensory axon terminates in a motor endplate or if a motor axon terminates in a sensory endplate, useful function is impossible. Unfortunately, the final performance of even the most meticulous microscopic nerve repair is subject to chance, and normal function is rarely achieved except in extremely young individuals.

JOINT STIFFNESS AND TENDON ADHESIONS

Loss of motion of the wrist or small joints of the hand may result from a combination of edema, scar formation, and muscle contracture. These conditions render the hand stiff by interfering with joint mobility or muscle-tendon excursion. Edema is the first and most obvious reaction of the hand to injury. Although it is reversible in its early stages, persistent edema may result in marked tissue scarring and fibrosis. The amount of edema formation is probably related to the severity of the injury to the involved tissues and results in an alteration in capillary permeability. The protein-rich edema fluid attracts water into the interstitial spaces until normal capillary permeability is reestablished. The fluid fills the interstices of the collateral ligaments and the soft tissue surrounding joints and tendons. Edema is usually most noticeable on the dorsum of the hand because the palmar tissues are fixed and nonyielding, whereas the dorsal skin is freely movable and lax. As edema collects on the dorsum of the hand, the metacarpophalangeal joints are forced into hyperextension and the proximal interphalangeal joints assume a flexed position. Collagen is then deposited about the collateral ligaments as well as the flexor and extensor tendons, which become bound to the surrounding immobile structures. Uncontrolled edema comes to involve all the tissues of the hand and results in restriction of both active and passive movement. The fluid is soon supplanted by scar tissue, which can lead to severe and often permanent contractures. Treatment of reversible edema must be prompt and aggressive because control of the resultant contractures is extremely difficult. Consequently, optimal management of the injured hand includes elevation and early mobilization of joints to minimize edema and limit restrictive scar formation.

Scar tissue can form in almost any area involved in the edema process (Fig. 2-5). This means that not only may the area of injury become the site of scar formation, but also that tissues distant from the injury site may also become involved because of the effects of chronic edema. In addition to the prejudicial effect scar tissue has on joint motion and tendon excursion, muscle tissue may become involved and undergo a process known as myostatic contracture. If the tension within a skeletal muscle is completely removed for a while, the muscle belly shortens at this retracted length. Early on, active and passive exercises or splinting can overcome this contracture; however, if the muscle is allowed to remain in a shortened position for a number of weeks, attempts to promptly restore it to its original length may be impossible or may lead to muscle damage. Denervated or paralyzed muscle does not develop myostatic contracture, which suggests that the normal reflex patterns must be present for the development of this condition. Myostatic contracture apparently involves a change in the compliance of the elastin elements within the muscle fibers and may result in shortening of the muscle's resting length by as much as 40%.

Joint stiffness

Digital joint stiffness may result from direct injury or may occur secondarily when afflictions of the skin, fascia, tendon, tendon sheath, muscle or retinacular ligaments prevent joint motion for a prolonged period (Fig. 2-6). This may result in secondary shortening of the joint capsule or collateral ligaments, which limits motion even after

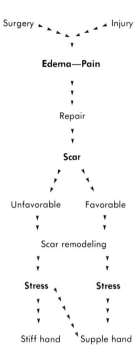

Surgery — Injury

Edema—Pain

Repair

Scar

Unfavorable   Favorable

Scar remodeling

Stress   **Stress**

Stiff hand   Supple hand

Fig. 2-5. Sequence chart depicting the events following surgery or injury that can terminate in either a stiff hand or a supple, functional hand. Scar that results from injury can be biologically unfavorable or favorable, and its final characteristics. can determine the ultimate functional result. (From Weeks, P.M., and Wray, R.C.: The management of acute hand injuries: a biological approach, ed. 2, St. Louis, 1973, The C.V. Mosby Co.)

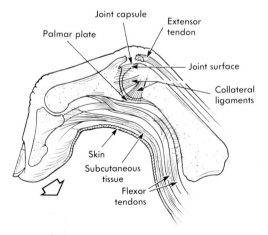

Fig. 2-6. Pathology involving various anatomic structures may result in digital joint stiffness or contracture. This flexion contracture of the proximal interphalangeal joint may result from one or more of the following: (1) disruption of the extensor tendon, (2) fibrosis of the joint capsule, (3) damage to or destruction of the articular surface, (4) injury or secondary shortening of the collateral ligaments, (5) injury or shortening of the palmar plate, (6) adhesions or shortening of the profundus or superficialis tendons, (7) scarring or contracture of the subcutaneous tissue or fascia, and (8) scarring or contracture of the skin.

the initiating factors have been removed. The vicious triad of injury, edema, and immobilization inevitably leads to restrictive scar tissue, adherent tendons, shortened ligaments, and myostatic muscle contracture. Crushing injuries, lacerations, and burns commonly result in sufficient tissue injury to produce diminished joint motion; various combinations of injury to skin, bone, joint, and tendon may also lead to stiffness. Factors unique to each injury, which will govern the rate of functional recovery and the possibility for permanent joint contracture, include hemorrhage, edema and prolonged immobilization of a joint in a position favorable to contracture. Infection may also contribute to the development of joint stiffness, and individual variations with respect to collagen maturation will produce different amounts of recovery in different patients with the same injury or surgical procedure.

Common digital contractures and their causes are discussed next. A characteristic combination of findings in the severely stiffened hand includes metacarpophalangeal joint extension, proximal interphalangeal joint flexion, and adduction contracture of the thumb web. A brief review of the factors contributing to the deformity at each joint level will be presented for six types of contracture.

Distal interphalangeal joint contracture. Because of its terminal position on the digit, the distal interphalangeal joint is most vulnerable to crushing injuries, which produce considerable damage to all of the periarticular tissues. Particularly, the joint capsule and collateral ligaments may be damaged by this type of injury, and the edema that results from crushing is often long lasting and results in substantial scarring and limitation of joint motion. Unfortunately, this stiffening is often at least partially permanent and does not respond well to exercise, splinting, or therapy. The degree of functional disability resulting from distal interphalangeal joint contracture is not great because function at the metacarpophalangeal joint and proximal interphalangeal joint is usually retained.

Proximal interphalangeal joint extension contracture. These contractures most frequently result from crushing injuries to the joint and involve scarring of the dorsal joint capsule and dorsalmost fibers of the cord portion of the collateral ligament. Adherence of the central extensor tendon with or without involvement of the intrinsic muscle tendons may also result in this deformity, and scarring of the dorsal skin or articular surface damage may also contribute. The outlook for overcoming this contracture by gentle exercise and splinting programs is favorable, although one must be careful not to cause further damage to the extensor tendon or joint.

Proximal interphalangeal joint flexion contracture. Flexion contractures of the proximal interphalangeal joint most frequently result from direct injury to the joint or from chronic edema and immobilization with the joint in a flexed attitude. Shortening of the palmar plate, with its proximal lateral check-rein extensions, and of the collateral ligaments is the most frequently implicated factor in this deformity, although scarring and adhesion of the palmar skin, flexor tendons, or flexor tendon sheath are often associated components of the contracture. Efforts in extension mobilization splinting may be quite disappointing when this contracture is marked and has become fixed.

Metacarpophalangeal joint extension contracture. The collateral ligaments at the metacarpophalangeal joint are eccentrically placed. Because of the cam configuration of the metacarpal head, the collateral ligaments are lax with the joint in full extension and tight with the joint in flexion. Injury or chronic edema around the joint can result in the deposition of new collagen around the collateral ligaments in their slack position and allow them to shorten. Flexion may rapidly become limited depending on the degree of ligamentous shortening. To a lesser extent, the extension contracture may result from injury or thickening of the dorsal capsule, adherence of the extensor tendon to the metacarpal, scarring of the dorsal skin, obliteration of the palmar synovial pouch, or direct articular damage. Efforts to mobilize this joint by exercise programs or splinting may be successful if initiated early.

Metacarpophalangeal joint flexion contracture. Flexion contractures of the metacarpophalangeal joint are the least frequent of the digital joint deformities and are most frequently associated with ischemic contracture of the intrinsic musculature. Disorders of the palmar skin or palmar fascia or scarring about the palmar synovial pouch may result in this deformity. Adherence or shortening of the flexor tendons or the overlying origin of the fibroosseous canal may also contribute. Efforts at improving function by exercise programs or splinting may not succeed in lengthening the offending structures, and surgical release may be required.

Thumb web contracture. Adduction deformity of the first web space can be an extremely disabling contracture and may result from simple scarring of the skin between the thumb and index finger. Scarring of the fascia or musculature of the first web space may also result from direct injury, ischemia, or chronic edema, and secondary stiffening of the carpometacarpal joint may result. Distention of the dorsal first web skin by edema will pull the thumb into adduction, and myostatic contracture of the first dorsal interosseous or adductor pollicis muscles results in further deformity. Efforts at serial web space widening may be successful if the scarring is not extensive, although surgical release of the offending tissues is frequently required.

Tendon adhesions

Limited excursion may result from direct injury to flexor, extensor, or intrinsic tendons, and the scar resulting from the healing of contiguous tissues may also result in excursion-limiting adhesions to these structures. In particular, fractures of the metacarpals or phalanges in areas where they have a close anatomic relationship to the digital tendons may result in the tendons becoming bound in a nonyielding fracture callus, which, in addition to reducing the amount of active motion possible, provides a check-rein restriction on the passive ability to flex or extend the involved joints (Fig. 2-7). These limitations of joint motion secondary to tendon adhesions are well recognized and can be determined by careful physical examination. For example, adhesions occurring between the extensor tendon and the metacarpal limit the distal excursion of the extensor mechanism and restrict composite flexion of the digital joints. Although one might be able to fully flex the metacarpophalangeal joint with the proximal interphalangeal joint in extension or fully flex the proximal interphalangeal joint with the metacarpophalangeal joint in full extension, the check-rein phenomenon produced by the diminished excursion of the extensor tendon does not permit composite flexion at both joints. Sim-

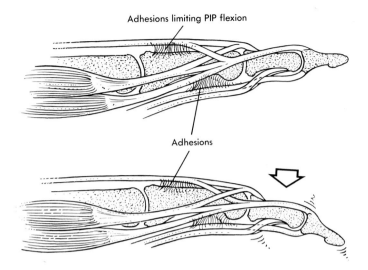

Fig. 2-7. Dorsal adhesions may form between the extensor mechanism and the proximal phalanx or palmarly between the flexor tendons and the proximal phalanx as a result of tendon injury, fracture, or crushing injury. The restricted excursion of the extensor mechanism can limit active extension or active and passive flexion of the proximal interphalangeal (PIP) joint. Flexor tendon adhesions can limit active flexion or active and passive extension.

ilar testing is possible on the palmar side of the involved digits, and this type of careful examination allows one to differentiate motion loss secondary to tendon adhesions from true joint stiffening.

Efforts at improving tendon excursion include early joint motion following fracture, crush injury, or tendon damage. Active and passive exercise programs have been designed to provide controlled tendon gliding and are felt to have added considerably to the final results following tendon interruption. In addition to providing a beneficial biologic effect on adhesion formation around healing tendons and their adjacent tissues, these motion programs diminish the likelihood of secondary joint stiffening and are probably effective in reducing edema formation.

BIOLOGIC RATIONALE FOR SPLINTING
Influence on scar remodeling

It is apparent that the scar formation and wound contracture that are an integral part of the orderly healing of hand tissues may have a great influence on tendon gliding and joint movement. Measures designed to prevent digital stiffness include elevation, positioning of joints to lessen the possibility of collateral ligament shortening, implementation of early motion programs, relief of pain, control of edema, elimination of hematoma formation, prevention of infection, and the use of mobilization splints. Although very little meaningful scientific information has been provided to indicate at which points during the healing process it is most appropriate to use immobilization or mobilization splints to favorably control the production and remodeling of scar tissue, a review of the biologic sequence of the reparative process may allow us to draw some reasonably sound conclusions.

There seems to be little benefit in using mobilizing splints that apply stress to the healing wound during the period of inflammation. Stress at this time might result in separation of repaired structures or a prolongation of the inflammatory phase by inflicting repeated injury to the involved tissues. Therefore it is probably appropriate to use splints that immobilize the involved part during the inflammatory phase and withhold the application of stress for 1 or more weeks depending on the specific injury or surgical procedure.

During the period of fibroplasia, which usually begins during the second week and continues for 6 weeks, it may be biologically suitable to institute the use of mobilization splinting designed to provide light stress with the hope of returning function as quickly as possible. The decision to apply stress to healing tissues during this phase is mitigated by the condition of injured or repaired structures. Unstable fractures, collateral ligament injuries, extensor tendon repairs, nerve repairs, skin grafts, and some flexor tendon repairs may be vulnerable to further damage or disruption with the premature application of stress. The use of mobilization splinting should be withheld until 3 to 6 weeks have elapsed. If there are no healing tissues that might be jeopardized by the early application of stress, then gentle mobilization efforts may be commenced within the first or second week. Careful observation of splinted areas and measurements of hand edema and motion changes in the involved joints indicate the efficacy of the use of splints on the biology of the healing tissues.

After the sixth week of wound healing, during the period of scar maturation and remodeling, it may be appropriate to increase the amount and duration of application of the force being imparted to the healing structures. Ideally, whatever joint stiffening and loss of tendon excursion may have developed during the inflammatory and fibroplastic stages will have resulted from immature scar that can still be favorably altered and modified by the judicious use of mechanical stress. Mobilization splints applied during this stage are designed to influence the remodeling collagen and ensure the maximum recovery of articular gliding and tendon excursion. The process of wound contracture may also be favorably modified by the use of splints that resist the contractile influence of wound healing on the movable parts of the injured hand.

Weeks (1973) has stated that the only acceptable clinical method we have of accelerating the modification of scar tissue is the application of stress to the scar. Splints may be implemented to assist the conversion of unfavorable scar to favorable scar by controlling the biologic process of synthesis and degradation of collagen. Mobilization splints must be designed to maximize the amount of stress applied to the offending scar while minimizing damage to normal hand tissues. The amount and direction of the force applied by a mobilization splint must be carefully monitored to prevent damage to the skin and subcutaneous tissues and to avoid undue compression or distraction of the involved joints. The force must not be applied too rapidly or the ligaments may not have the capacity to undergo the desired biologic alteration and may rupture.

An important concept emphasized by Brand (1984) is that stretch represents a passive action which results in elongation of the elastic elements of various tissues. Elongation that is accomplished by stretch inevitably shortens again when the force on the involved tissues is relaxed. If tissues are pulled to the point of rupture, a vicious process of inflammation and scar formation results, and the ultimate effect on healing is worse than if the stretching force had never been applied. Brand also suggests that true lengthening of any living tissue results from an alteration of the activity of living cells as they constantly take up and absorb old tissues and lay down new tissue components. Old collagen is absorbed and new collagen is laid down in new patterns that are responsive to specific tissue requirements. When applying a splint, one hopes to stimulate the living cells to provide the most favorable new tissue rather than to try to lengthen or break old tissues. This may be accomplished by keeping the tissues in a ''physiologic state'' that creates the appropriate demands on the new cells to make changes in the configuration of new tissues. Brand stresses that the best method to accomplish this is to keep the involved tissues in a prolonged state of mild tension.

This application of stress to injured hand tissues should be directed toward minimizing the reparative response and maximizing the biologic reorganizational response. Its application may be opposite to that which one normally considers when attempting to modify scar configuration. For instance, in an effort to mobilize an adherent tendon in the palm, stress from a splint must be applied distally rather than relying on the usual proximal stress resulting from muscle contracture. Application of a small constant force has been shown to be much more beneficial than the intermittent application of large forces (Fig. 2-8). Clinically useful information with regard to the behavior of hand scars can be made by observing the response of given tissues to their initial loading while the scar is still immature. Improvements in joint motion and a decrease in edema may indicate a favorable modification of the scar maturation process.

Hand splints implemented in an effort to provide the most favorable remodeling of scar and adhesions are most effective if they use the entire range of motion that is possible in the joints of the involved hand. Splints should be designed to hold tension on the restraining tissues and scar for a given period of time. As already pointed out, the tension need not be high, and the hand should be positioned so that joint or tendon scar and adhesions are the limiting factors for movement. Alternating the direction of splinting to gently pull the offending tissues in opposite directions is also important. When sufficient healing of injured or operated tissues has occurred, some increase in the tension of dynamic splints and their period of application can then be allowed, and active muscle contracture by the patient will be beneficial.

Unfortunately, the application of splints often involves little more than trial and error rather than a scientific process involving the direct application of methods for the careful measurement of the amount of force being applied by a particular splint and concerns for the mechanical aspects of force application. Consideration of the appropriate vector, moment arm, the amount of force applied, and the length of force application is very important and must be carefully correlated with the state of tissue healing in the affected part. Recently several investigators, including Brand (1985), Madden (1976), and Weeks (1973), have expressed the need for a more scientific approach to the application of external stress and have begun to provide information that will ultimately be useful

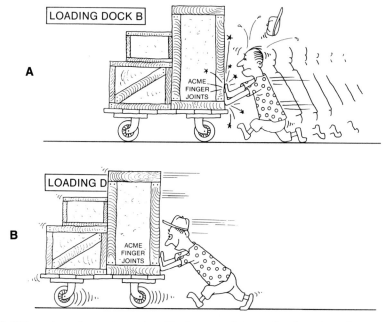

Fig. 2-8. This cartoon demonstrates the effectiveness of the application of small constant forces in an effort to move an object (or joint) **(B)** and the ineffectiveness of intermittent application of large forces **(A).** The same principles apply to the use of splints in an effort to produce a favorable biologic influence on scar tissue.

in the preparation and application of biologically effective splints. A great deal of additional study is necessary to better understand the exact effect of various stress forces being applied to specific areas of scarring, contracture, and adhesions. Data from the writings of Brand, Madden, and Weeks are included in the following discussion.

Splint biodynamics

It is important that those involved in the preparation and application of hand splints have an understanding of what tissues are the limiting factors in the diminished movement of a given joint. Is it periarticular scarring or adherent tendons or a combination of both which prevents joint rotation? The injured hand should be inspected for areas of wounding, edema, inflammation, infection, and the amount of active and passive motion loss. Alterations in joint movement produced by variations in the posture of adjacent joints can also point out which tissues are preventing normal motion. A reasonable assessment can then be made as to whether a particular scar has the biologic potential to undergo favorable remodeling.

Initial considerations for a splinting program should be directed toward determining the immediate mechanical effects of stress on scar tissue so that the clinician can best predict the subsequent biologic course that will follow splint application. As the splinting process proceeds, an observation of the changes in the motion of the involved joints gives an indication of the effectiveness of a particular splinting regimen on the mechanical properties of the remodeling scar. Then appropriate alterations in the splinting program can be made. Again, our clinical skills are directed at most favorably altering the biologic processes of collagen degradation, synthesis, and reorganization.

When applying forces in an effort to improve joint rotation, one must recognize that the direction and amount of force applied by the splint are critical to its biologic efficacy. There must be great concern for the mechanics involved in the various methods of force application and the effect of resultant forces on the injured part. Care must be taken to prevent undue traction or compression, and one must not confuse the manipulation of scar tissue that often leads to rupture with the gentle loading of injured tissues. Brand (1985) has pointed out the effectiveness of to-and-fro tension on adhesions and scar in an effort to alter their configuration and favorably produce tissue lengthening. This may be done either by exercise programs or by alternating flexion and extension splinting.

Force, area, and pressure determinations. The amount of force that can be applied to a given digit to improve joint rotation is limited by the ischemic effects produced by the splint, which is in contact with the finger. The pressure exerted on the skin cannot exceed the capillary pressure in the cutaneous vessels for a long time or ischemia will result. Capillary pressure averages about 30 to 35 mm Hg. To ensure perfusion, forces applied to the skin cannot be excessive. The pressure produced by a well-fitting splint is dissipated over its area of skin contact, and measurements of this area can be multiplied by measurements of the force imparted by the splint to determine the exact pressure applied to the contact surface. These simple measurements can be incorporated into the process of hand splint preparation and fitting to determine how much force they are generating over a given area of application. Because rubber bands are frequently employed to provide the force during mobilization splinting, it is important to determine their exact force. There is little uniformity in the elasticity of these simple rubber rings, which are manufactured without consideration for this exacting biologic use. The force generated by rubber bands can be measured with a simple spring-loaded scale, which determines the tension on the rubber band at the exact length that will be used in a given splint (Fig. 2-9). Combined with measurements of the area of application of the attached slings, one can make a reasonably accurate determination of the amount of pressure imparted to the offending scar tissue and its overlying skin (Fig. 2-10). Serial readings, of course, are necessary to determine changing forces in the rubber bands and altered areas of sling contact as the range of motion of the involved joint improves.

Weeks (1973) states that the average person can tolerate 6 oz of force for up to 4 hours and lesser amounts of force for much longer periods (Fig. 2-11). Fortunately, the excessive force that produces ischemia also causes pain, which will serve as an effective warning system. One must therefore be very careful about the use of splints in the anesthetic hand, where this alarm mechanism is not present. Many biologic variables, including the nature of the injury to skin and subcutaneous tissues, the stiffness of tissues that surround small blood vessels, and the temperature of the skin, can alter the veracity of pressure calculations to some extent.

Brand suggests a usful guide with regard to the amount of pressure that can be safely

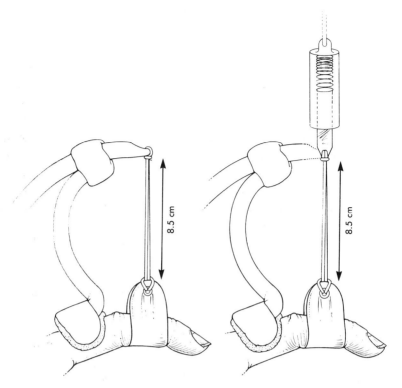

Fig. 2-9. A simple spring-loaded scale can measure the force generated by a rubber band and sling combination attached to an outrigger splint. It is important that the scale measure the force of the rubber band at the exact length it will be used in the splint.

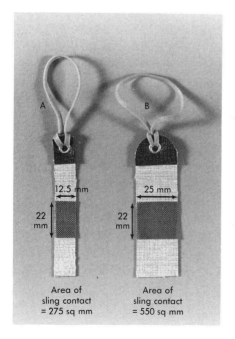

Fig. 2-10. Depicts the varied contact area on the palmar and lateral aspects of a digit created by two slings of varied width. The small sling (**A**) is 12.5 mm wide and has 22 mm of circumferential contact with the digit. It therefore has an area of sling contact of 275 mm. The wider sling (**B**) has 25 by 22 mm of contact with the digit, for an area of sling contact of 550 mm. The amount of force that can be tolerated using the wider sling is significantly greater.

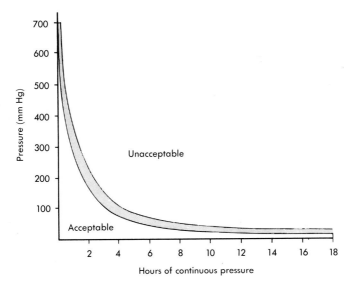

Fig. 2-11. Allowable pressure versus time of application for tissue over bony prominences. This curve gives general guidelines for the application of splinting force, but should not be taken to provide absolute values. (Redrawn from Reswick, J.B., et al., editors: Bedsore biomechanics, London, 1976, The McMillan Press, Ltd.)

applied by splinting (Table 2-1). He states that in short-term application (less than 2 hours) ischemia should not be a problem, and the numbers in Table 2-1 can be ignored. Actual pressure necrosis is likely only in insensate hands because a patient with normal sensation will discard a splint because of the discomfort produced by ischemia.

Brand condemns the use of typical slings to apply force in mobilization splints because changes in the posture of the finger result in a tilting of the sling and localization of the pressure to a smaller area of contact. He points out that when a sling is in good position with a 90–degree angle of approach, a contact area of 4 cm² applied with 200 gm of force results in $(200 \div 4)$ 50 gm/cm² pressure at the point of application. Changes in joint position that result from this tension alter the contact area of the sling and impart the same force on a much smaller surface area. At 70 degrees the sling takes the force on less than one third of the available sling surface, and the pressure then rises to 150 gm/cm², an unacceptable amount that could cause necrosis within a few hours. Because this amount of pressure is painful, the patient will almost certainly not use the splint, and consequently its effectiveness as an influence on scar remodeling is lost.

This observation indicates the need for a frequent review of the mechanics of each splint with modifications when necessary to ensure that the maximum amount of contact surface of a given sling is being used. Brand also points out that reaction bars such as the dorsal phalangeal bar of an outrigger splint can apply uneven pressure and are likely to cause ischemia and pain. Because of their reciprocal midposition in the three-point system, these bars apply force which is twice that of the proximal and distal ends of the splint. He further states that one must be wary of small tolerable stresses applied repet-

Table 2-1. Guide to duration of pressure application*

Short-term (less than 2 hrs)	Long-term (continuous for more than 8 hours)
50 mm Hg/mm^2	30 mm Hg/mm^2
75 gm/cm^2	50 gm/cm^2
1 lb/in^2	12 oz/in^2

*Modified from Brand, P.W.: Clinical mechanics of the hand, St. Louis, 1985, The C.V. Mosby Co.

itively, which result in shearing injuries to underlying tissues. The more the repetition of the stress applications, the more likely the unfavorable consequences.

We can see that, although we still lack many of the answers to the appropriate application of forces in modifying the biologic healing process and restoring maximum tendon excursion and joint motion, it is possible to provide some scientific measurement of exactly what forces are being imparted by a given splint. At the present time simple measurements of the forces imparted by a rubber band, the area of splint contact, and the mechanics of splint design and application can aid in the preparation of a physiologically safe and a biologically effective splint. Careful clinical monitoring, however, is still paramount, and a simple observation of the appearance of the skin underlying a sling can provide considerable information.

Blanching occurs when there is too much tension, and a good mobilization splint applies constant tolerable tension that can be maintained for long periods. Small increments of improvement of joint motion can be achieved in this manner and are preferable to methods that involve strong forces applied over short periods of time in an effort to make rapid gains. These techniques often rupture scar and underlying tissues and set up a vicious cycle of inflammation, further scarring, and contracture, which are detrimental rather than beneficial to the recovery of function.

Splinting for tendon adhesions. The high propensity for injured tendons to develop excursion-limiting adhesions following repair has resulted in a number of techniques designed to impart a controlled amount of tendon motion at an early stage of tendon healing. It is hoped that these methods will favorably modify the quantity, strength, and length of adhesions and permit the maximum recovery of tendon performance. Flexor tendon injuries in the digital canal are particularly prone to the development of adhesions, and programs designed to provide digital joint motion and tendon movement by means of active extension–passive flexion (rubberband) or passive flexion and extension have been employed to produce the desired biologic alteration of the tendon healing process. In some excellent animal studies, Gelberman and associates (1983) have demonstrated that these methods are effective in decreasing adhesion formation and increasing the tensile strength of repaired tendons.

Efforts to restore tendon gliding are designed to result in biologic modification of the scar around the tendon. At the present time the only effective clinical method for accomplishing this favorable scar remodeling is the application of stress to the offending tissue. Passive joint motion directed to provide stress on peritendinous adhesions may

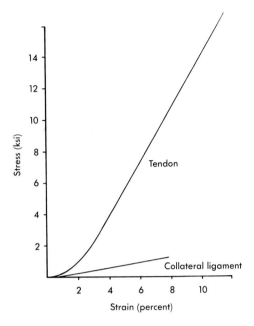

Fig. 2-12. Stress-strain curves for tendon and metacarpophalangeal joints are depicted. (From Weeks, P.M., and Wray, R.C.: The management of acute hand injuries: a biological approach, ed. 2, St. Louis, 1973, The C.V. Mosby Co.)

be effective, although it must be recognized that certain scars simply do not yield to stress. The favorable remodeling of the scar around a tendon is best accomplished by applying stress to the tendon, which in turn transmits the stress to the scar. Weeks (1973) has demonstrated that small loads impart significant elongation of tendons and that as the load increases, the percentage of elongation rapidly decreases. He plotted his results on a stress-strain curve, which demonstrated that as an initial small load was applied, a significant elongation of the tendon occurred. As the load was increased, the percent of elongation rapidly decreased until further loading resulted in tendon breakage (Fig. 2-12). He felt that these changes correlate with the physical alterations occurring in the tendon as the collagen fibers are changed from their normal wavy pattern to a straightened configuration. He concluded that we could assume that the strain recorded after the application of small forces to a tendon was the result of changes in the restricting scar.

The clinical importance of this information again lies in the need to provide small but continuous forces, whenever possible in opposite directions, in an effort to modify and elongate restrictive tendon adhesions. Overzealous efforts to achieve rapid gains by the application of large forces will not prove to be biologically effective and may result in tendon attenuation or rupture.

Splinting for joint contractures. When collateral ligaments are subjected to increasing load, their response may be somewhat different from that seen in the tendon. Weeks (1973) carried out experiments and determined the percentage of elongation of ligaments subjected to various loads. He plotted his information on a stress-strain curve (Fig. 2-12). Ligaments were found to exhibit a much greater elongation with a much smaller load than do flexor tendons. He further noted that when a ligament with predominantly elastic fibers was subjected to a small force, it reached a functional length quite rapidly.

Weeks made further observations regarding the phenomenon known as *creep,* which involves an elongation of a structure when a load is applied and maintained at a constant level over time. Although in human flexor tendon the amount of creep is very small, a ligament was found to demonstrate considerably more elongation. He does note, however, that when a ligament of predominantly elastic fibers is subjected to a small force, the creep cannot be measured accurately. It was his impression that when the load is applied to a finger, the elongation that occurs actually reflects creep in the scar around the ligament rather than the ligament itself. The load levels that can be applied and tolerated by a finger are far below those which cause tendon or ligament elongation, and changes that occur are probably the result of physical changes within the scar tissue.

There must be particular concern for the effect of excessive stress on a joint when it is applied for too long a period or with too great a mechanical advantage. The joint quickly reaches the maximum rotation permitted by the scar tissue, and at that point the joint can be forced open like a book. The ligaments do not have a chance to undergo

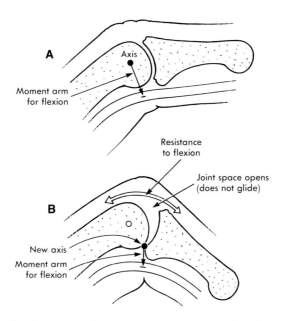

Fig. 2-13. A, When the functional axis is the same as the anatomic axis, the flexor tendon has good moment arm for flexion. **B,** When gliding is blocked at the joint surface, the functional axis for flexion moves to a point on the joint surface where the joint now tilts (not glides). The moment arm for flexion is now reduced to the point that the flexor tendon loses its ability to actively flex, and the joint opens like a book. (From Brand, P.W.: Clinical mechanics of the hand, St. Louis, 1985, The C.V. Mosby Co.)

biologic alteration. The forces the splint applies can tend to angulate the finger without true congruous articular gliding (Fig. 2-13). Articular surface destruction or joint sub-luxation may result. One must therefore have a realistic understanding that some short-ened collateral ligaments simply cannot be sufficiently elongated by splints to result in improved joint motion. Extension contractions at the metacarpophalangeal joint perhaps serve as the most appropriate clinical example of this problem.

Measurements of biologic activity

In an effort to determine the effectiveness of splinting programs in modifying the biologic processes involved in tissue healing and scar formation it is important to mea-sure the response of the affected tissues. Hand performance perhaps can best be deter-mined by serially measuring changes in the active and passive range of motion through-out the course of the splinting program (Fig. 2-14). Brand indicates that torque angle measurements are more objective for passive range of motion and use standard weights or springs applied to a given finger to determine changes in joint angles resulting from the application of these weights (Fig. 2-15). Measurements of skin temperature, sensa-tion, strength, and functional performance also describe the efficacy of a given program. Particularly important are tests that evaluate the range of motion of a given joint while changing the position of proximal joints such as the wrist or metacarpophalangeal joint.

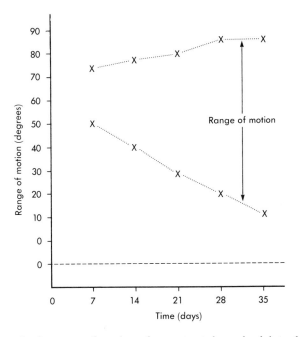

Fig. 2-14. Changes in the range of motion of a contracted proximal interphalangeal joint at standard torque resulting from serial measurements over 1 month. The graph depicts an improved range of motion caused mostly by an increase in the angle of extension. (From Brand, P.W.: Clinical mechanics of the hand, St. Louis, 1985, The C.V. Mosby Co.)

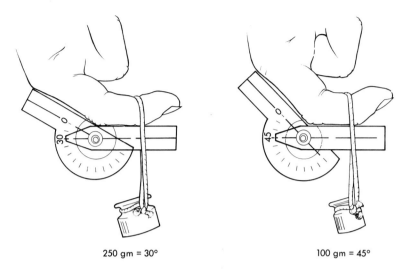

250 gm = 30°　　　　　　　　　100 gm = 45°

Fig. 2-15. Torque-angle measurements provide a more objective measurement of the passive range of motion. In this way, the passive position of a given joint can be consistently measured with the application of a constant force, and changes in the position of the joint resulting from the application of increased weight can also be observed. In this drawing a 100 gm weight applied to a digit results in a 45 degree flexed attitude to the proximal interphalangeal joint. Weight of 250 gm increases the extension to 30 degrees. (Modified from Brand, P.W.: Clinical mechanics of the hand, St. Louis, 1985, The C.V. Mosby Co.)

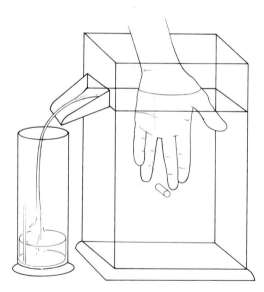

Fig. 2-16. Transparent hand volumeter to determine hand volume. The rim of the overflow spout is wide, level, and flat. The tank is filled to the overflow level, after which the hand is immersed in the tank. A transverse rod ensures immersion to the same level with each measurement. The overflow is measured and often compared with the volume on the opposite, uninjured side to give an indication of the amount of edema present. (Modified from Brand, P.W.: Clinical mechanics of the hand, St. Louis, 1985, The C.V. Mosby Co.)

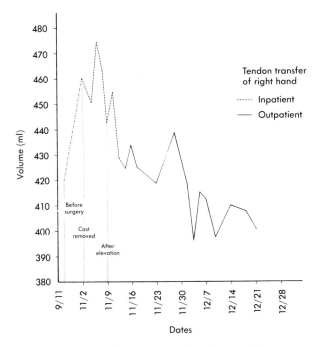

Fig. 2-17. An example of a record of hand volume based on serial measurements with a volumeter. These determinations were used after a tendon transfer. Note comments at different points in the patient's treatment program, such as ''before surgery,'' ''cast removed,'' and ''after elevation.'' (Modified from Brand, P.W.: Clinical mechanics of the hand, St. Louis, 1985, The C.V. Mosby Co.)

These tests can provide useful information as to whether the loss of joint motion results from diminished tendon excursion or is the primary result of periarticular fibrosis.

Brand states that, after the removal of compressive dressings, the hand will have been dependent on external support for several weeks and looks almost normal. Within 24 hours edema fluid fills the unsupported hand, particularly if it is allowed to be dependent. It then takes several days of vigorous range of motion exercises and elevation to get the normal pumping action of the hand restored and the hand volume improved. He recommends the regular use of a volumeter to provide measurements of upper extremity edema and feels that this measurement can be used as a rough determinant of the biologic state of the hand (Fig. 2-16). A volume graph based on serial measurements can indicate when the therapeutic effects may have been too vigorous, resulting in tissue strain and inflammation (Fig. 2-17). He emphasizes that exercises for mobilizing the hand and reducing excessive fluid should be simple, frequent, light, and repetitive.

SUMMARY

This chapter emphasizes the importance of a thorough understanding of the biologic changes in the hand as a response to disease, injury, or surgery. Unfortunately, scar tissue is an inevitable and necessary ingredient of the normal healing process, and its presence may be extremely prejudicial to hand function, where it may limit tendon excursion and small joint gliding. Carefully conceived, constructed, and applied hand splints can rest injured tissues or apply gentle stress to the restrictive scar tissue surrounding the normal elastic and gliding tissues and maximize joint performance. One must, however, have an appreciation for the biologic events necessary to satisfactory tissue healing and the effect the application of stress will have on this process. The concept that little is accomplished by the mechanical lengthening of scarred tissues and that by applying a mobilizing splint one hopes to stimulate living cells to provide more favorable new tissue is critical. The application of too much stress over too short a period of time or embarking on ill-conceived or ill-constructed splinting programs may prove to be far more detrimental to the overall performance of the involved joints than if no splinting program had been initiated at all.

Although we are still lacking in good scientific evidence to indicate the most appropriate timing for the application of stress to the injured hand and to date have very little understanding as to the appropriate amounts of force to apply to a given joint and for what period of time, it appears that the application of small loads over a sustained period, utilizing the most advantageous mechanics of application, will lead to the most effective biologic remodeling of restrictive scar and the best long-term performance of the hand.

CHAPTER 3

Classification and nomenclature of splints and splint components

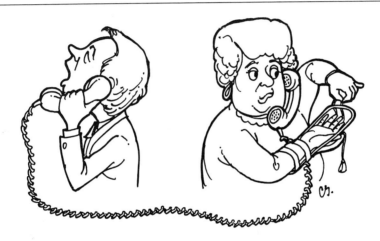

"NO, NO, MRS. SMITHSON, THE LITTLE THING-A-MA-JIG
GOES ON THE END JOINT OF YOUR PINKY FINGER."

Because hand splinting encompasses a profusion of devices and terminology, and because similar splints may be used for dissimilar purposes, description and classification of various splints are often fraught with confusion, redundancy, and omission. Historically, there has been a variety of splint classifications. These include groupings according to purpose, configuration, mechanical properties, power source, material, and anatomic site. Each method has advantages and disadvantages, and, although some classification systems are more precise than others, none effectively provides a clear description and separation of individual splints and components. The need for common descriptive splint terminology has been apparent to clinicians, students, and patients for years.

The purpose of this chapter is threefold: (1) to familiarize the reader with basic historical concepts that comprise the foundation of current splinting techniques by reviewing six established methods of splint classification; (2) to introduce a new method

71

of splint classification based on force complexity, joints involved, and kinematic purpose; and (3) to provide a common vocabulary of splint component terminology to facilitate further discussion and communication.

ESTABLISHED SPLINT CLASSIFICATIONS

Despite discrepancies, familiarity with the various methods of splint categorization provides a basis for understanding the origins of current hand splinting methods and general splinting nomenclature. As has been noted, splints may be classified according to the intent or purpose of application.

Purpose of application

Splints may be designed to *prevent deformity* by substituting for weak or absent muscle strength as in peripheral nerve injuries, spinal cord injuries, and neuromuscular diseases. They may be used to *support, protect, or immobilize joints,* allowing healing to occur after tendon, vascular, nerve, joint, or soft tissue injury or inflammation. *Correction of existing deformity* represents another commonly encountered reason for splint application. To achieve the full potential of active joint motion of the hand, the remodeling of joint and tendon adhesions often requires the prolonged slow, gentle, passive traction that can best be provided by splinting. Splints also may provide directional *control* for coordination problems and serve as a basis for the *attachment* of specialized devices that may facilitate and enhance hand function.

External configuration

External configuration has often served as a basis for the categorization of hand splints. This method includes the subcategories of bar splints, spring splints, contoured splints, and combinations thereof.

Bar splints. Bar splints, because of the narrowness of design, must be fabricated in strong inelastic materials such as stainless steel, aluminum, and the thicker high-temperature plastics. Historically, two major forms of bar splints have evolved (Fig. 3-1) from which most other splints derive their design concepts.

Spring splints. Spring splints, as exemplified by many of the LMB, Bunnell, Capener, and Wynn Parry splints, rely on three-point pressure and spring-action forces to provide dynamic mobilization (Fig. 3-2).

Contoured splints. Because of their ease of fabrication with low-temperature materials that may be fitted directly to the patients, contoured splints have revolutionized hand splinting techniques, moving them out of the realm of the orthotist and into therapy clinics and physician's offices (Fig. 3-3). Since the low-temperature materials lack the rigidity required, splint designs of necessity have become wider. Fortuitously, this has resulted in greater patient comfort because of decreased splint pressure from an increased area of force application.

Combinations. Combinations of bar, spring, and contoured splints comprise the fourth subcategory. Engen, Bailor, and the Wire-foam splints (Fig. 3-4) are examples of how the strength of metal may be coalesced with the close-fitting capabilities of plastics.

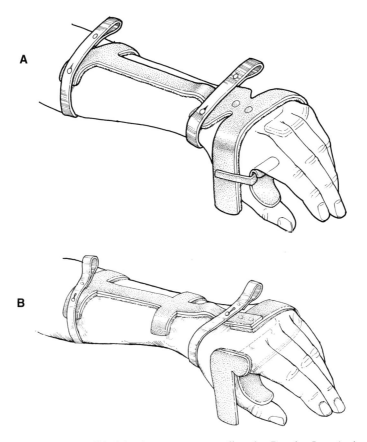

Fig. 3-1. Bar splints, exemplified by long opponens splints by Rancho Los Amigos **(A)** and Bennett (Warm Springs) **(B)** differ in placement of the uninterrupted metacarpal bar.

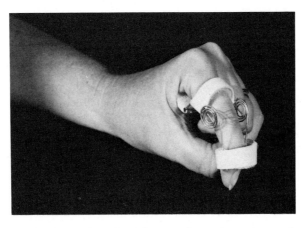

Fig. 3-2. The Capener splint provides dynamic extension assist to the proximal interphalangeal joint through forces generated by bilateral springs and a three-point pressure system.

Mechanical characteristics

Hand splints may also be grouped according to inherent mechanical characteristics,resulting in two major subdivisions: static splints and dynamic splints. *Static splints* have no moving parts and are used to provide support and immobilization, while *dynamic splints* employ traction devices such as rubber bands, springs, cords, or Velcro strips to alter the range of passive motion of a joint or joints. Confusion arises with this method of classification, since some splints possess static properties but are used to improve the motion of stiff joints. This is accomplished by serially altering the splint or by fitting new splints every 2 or 3 days to maintain slight tension on the joint(s) being

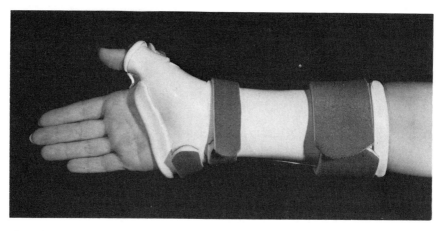

Fig. 3-3. Contoured splints are often more comfortable to wear because of increased surface contact of the splint with the extremity.

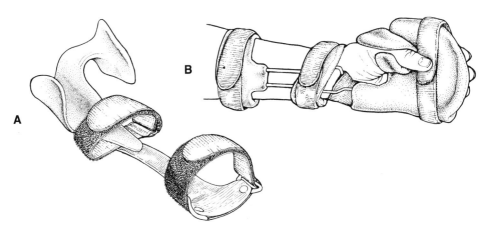

Fig. 3-4. The Engen (**A**) and Wire-foam (**B**) splints combine metal and plastic to produce a durable, close-fitting, adjustable splint.

mobilized as range of motion increases. Examples of static splints that are used to mobilize joints through serial adjustments include cylinder casts and thumb web spacers.

Source of power

The source of power is another categoric method that divides control splints into those which utilize internal power and those which provide external power. These splints are often more complicated to fabricate than are some of the more temporary splints and therefore require more durable materials, mechanical joints, and tension-adjusting systems. These are frequently used in cases of severe upper extremity paralysis. *Internally powered splints* rely on the use of the patient's residual muscle power at a given joint to produce motion of nonfunctional joints following various paralytic conditions (Fig. 3-5). *Externally powered splints* are driven by an external source such as

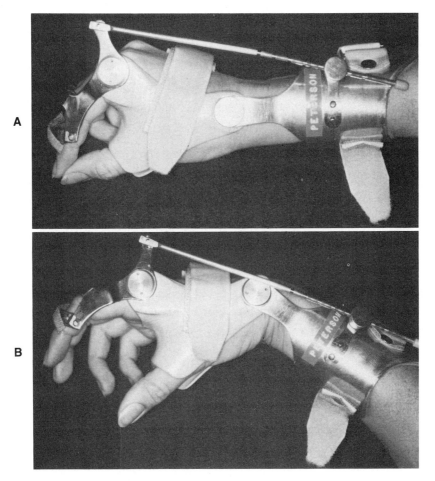

Fig. 3-5. Digital grasp and release patterns are controlled by active wrist extension (**A**) and gravity-assisted flexion (**B**) in this tenodesis splint.

a battery or carbon dioxide artificial muscle. Generally, both the internal and external power splints are designed to permit gross grasp through wrist extension, or tenodesis effect.

Materials

A fifth means of classification is based on the materials from which splints are fabricated. Categories include *metal, plaster,* and *plastic;* subcategories within this classification system change as technology advances and new products are introduced. This is especially true of the plastics, where newer or improved substances frequently make established materials obsolete.

Anatomic part

The final classification system relates to the anatomic part splinted, as in *wrist splints, finger splints,* or *thumb splints*. These subcategories are grouped according to the primary intent of a given splint but do not describe the existence of secondary joints that may also be affected by the splint.

• • •

This retrospective consideration of splint classifications is important because it encompasses a cumulative framework of splinting knowledge. In studying newer splinting techniques it must be recognized that pathologic conditions of the hand have not been altered; neither have the principles of mechanics, design, construction, and fit. Only the materials have changed, permitting modern clinicians to use splint components that are similar in function to those used by their predecessors but which are more easily contoured and fabricated.

DESCRIPTIVE CLASSIFICATION SYSTEM

The primary objective of any classification system is to facilitate understanding and communication through organization of subject matter into a systematic arrangement of similar characteristics. Previous splint classifications failed to be useful because they either did not limit adequately or they were too confining. To be relevant, a splint classification system must meet certain criteria. It should be practical, easy to use, flexible enough to allow options, but structured sufficiently to provide definitive guidelines. Ideally, for a postoperative patient, the surgeon would request a specific class splint based on purpose and anatomic and surgical considerations; the choice of design and materials would be left to the discretion of the hand therapist responsible for constructing and fitting the splint. This method allows both individuals to fully utilize their own highly specialized levels of expertise to prepare a uniquely integrated treatment approach.

The intent of introducing a new method of splint classification is to provide a more definitive means of grouping splints based on three criteria: (1) the types of splinting forces employed and the spatial planes in which they occur, (2) the anatomic site of emphasis, and (3) the primary kinematic goal of the splint. When describing a given splint, one uses three adverbs to delineate the ''how,'' ''where,'' and ''why'' of the splint. This results in such descriptive phases as ''long wrist extension splint,'' ''compound finger flexion splint,'' or ''simple proximal interphalangeal immobilization splint.''

How?

The first descriptive category, the ''how'' of a splint, is divided into three subcategories that allow grouping according to the complexity of the splinting forces and the planes in which they affect motion. Utilizing a single-direction force, a *simple splint* affects motion at one or multiple joints within a segment in a similar manner (Fig. 3-6). A *compound splint* affects motion at two or more joints within a segment in a dissimilar manner through opposing force systems (Fig. 3-7). Splints designated as *long*, the third and final option, are those designed to influence the amplitude of the long extrinsic tendons on a given joint or joints. By incorporating the wrist in a splint acting on the digits it is possible to negate or control extrinsic muscle forces (Fig. 3-8). Similarly, two-part long splints may be utilized to improve motion at the wrist by immobilizing the digits in a favorable position.

Where?

The anatomic site of emphasis defines the ''where'' of the splint. If all joints of a digital ray are similarly affected, the term *finger* or *thumb* is applied. If, however, the emphasis of the splint is more specific, the individual joint level(s) involved should be named. For example, a splint affecting both the proximal interphalangeal and distal interphalangeal joints would be labeled interphalangeal, whereas one whose forces are directed to the proximal interphalangeal joint alone would be referred to specifically as proximal interphalangeal.

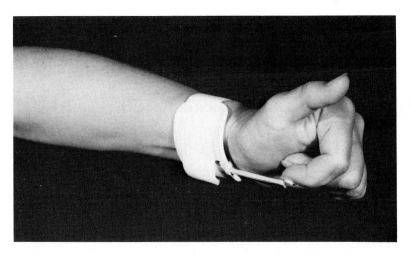

Fig. 3-6. A simple finger flexion splint exerts a similar force on all joints of the digit.

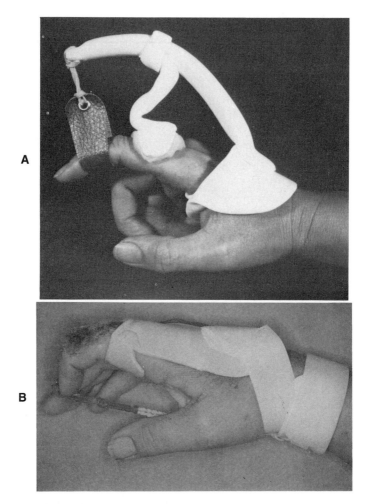

Fig. 3-7. These compound proximal interphalangeal joint extension (**A**) and flexion (**B**) splints differ in force direction but mechanically function alike.

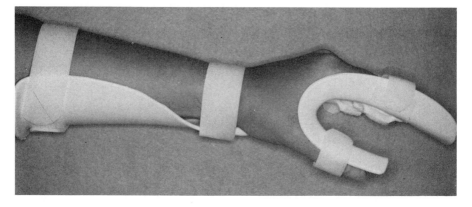

Fig. 3-8. The resting pan splint is an example of a long finger/thumb immobilization splint.

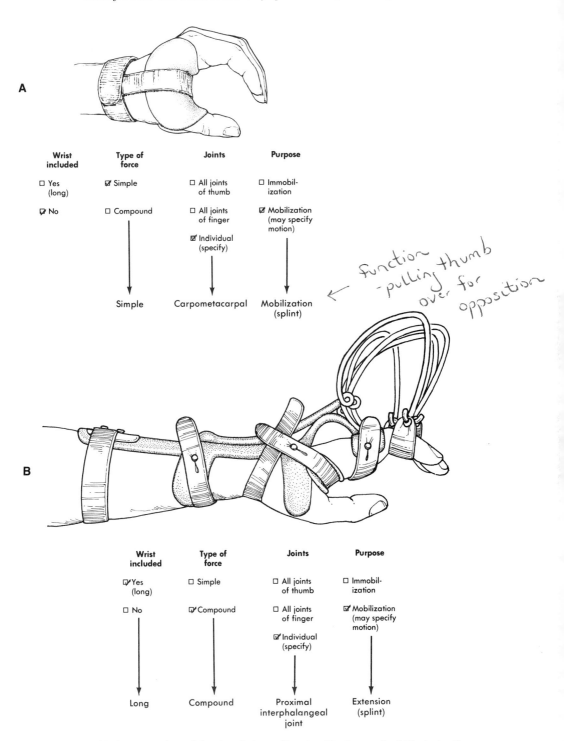

Fig. 3-9. This graphic interpretation of the descriptive splint classification method illustrates the fundamental concepts involved. **A,** Simple carpometacarpal (CMC) mobilization splint. **B,** Long compound proximal interphalangeal (PIP) extension splint.

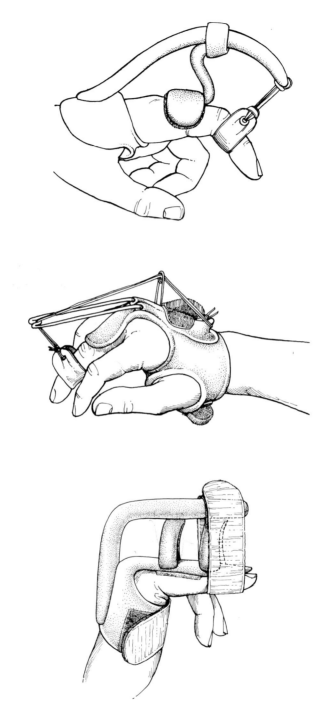

Fig. 3-10. Although their configurations and types of traction differ, these three splints have the same classification: compound PIP extension splint.

Why?

The third and final adverb refers to the "why" of the splint and is defined by kinematic terminology. What is the intent of the splint? Does it flex, rotate, or abduct, or is its primary purpose to immobilize? The addition of this functional purpose completes the descriptive triad and provides an immediate conceptualization of a given splint type (Fig. 3-9).

Posing and answering these three questions results in a descriptive splint classification based on well-defined categories that are large enough to include an array of splints but small enough to clearly delineate specific force, site, and purpose characteristics (Fig. 3-10).

SPLINT COMPONENT TERMINOLOGY

A splint is no more than a series of specialized parts that perform specific functions. Some of these parts directly affect the position of the hand, whereas others maintain the alignment and spatial interrelationships between the various splint components. When assessing a hand with the intent of applying a splint, one should not think of the splint as a whole, but rather as interconnected parts, each meeting a specific need for a given clinical hand problem. There is no standard splint that can be prescribed for a given pathologic situation. No one has decreed that similarly functioning splint parts must look alike or can be used only with certain diagnoses. Each patient presents different problems, even though the specific injury or disease may be similar to those of others. The patient must be approached without preconceived ideas, to allow for the creation of a splint, part by part, that meets not only physical but emotional and environmental requirements. An inability to accommodate to these individual factors is the main cause for failure of many commercial splints. Remember, patients and their hands do not come in small, medium, and large!

To effectively accomplish component splint designing, a sound knowledge of the basic splint parts and their purposes is essential. As was noted earlier in this chapter, each splint part has a task for which it has been designed. It may vary in shape from splint to splint, but its purpose will remain constant. Some parts mobilize, some support, others stabilize, and still others provide attachment sites. Following is an alphabetic listing of splint parts, their purposes, and pertinent information concerning each component. This list is meant to provide a basic foundation of common language for further communication. It should not be viewed as definitive, but rather should be added to, elaborated upon, and deleted from as the splint maker accumulates experience and expertise.

C bar (Fig. 3-11)

This bar is fitted in the first web space for the purpose of maintaining or increasing the distance between the first and second metacarpal bones. Its presence affects motion at the carpometacarpal joint of the thumb. The C bar is frequently elongated to incorporate a thumb post or an index palmar phalangeal bar. Its width should not impede the movement of the mobile fourth and fifth metacarpals. Because the extension of this component in the form of a phalangeal bar blocks metacarpophalangeal flexion, care should be taken to maintain through exercise full metacarpophalangeal flexion of the index finger.

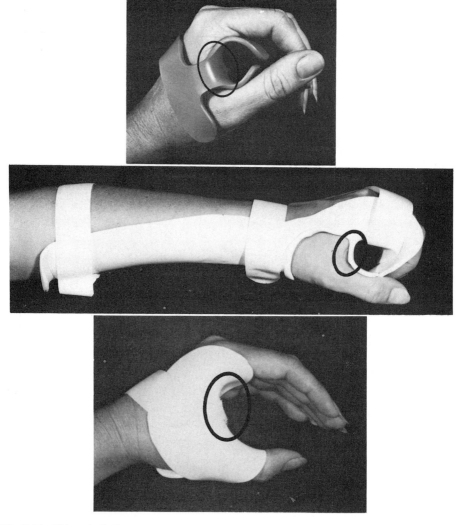

Fig. 3-11. Although dissimilar in appearance, all three of these splints employ C bars to maintain the first web space and thumb CMC motion.

Connector bar (Fig. 3-12)

This component is responsible for maintaining the alignment and position of other splint parts. Depending on specific location and purpose in regard to the overall splint design, connector bars may or may not be constructed of materials homologous to the splint.

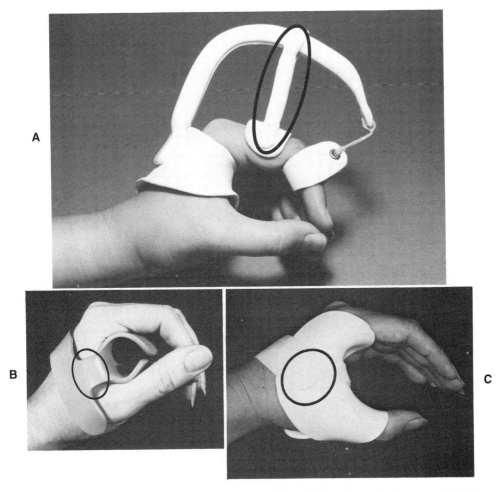

Fig. 3-12. A connector bar can be a separate piece **(A and B),** or it can be integrated into the body of the splint **(C).** (**A** courtesy Erica Stern, M.S., O.T.R., Lawrence, KS and Mary Jo Rinke, O.T. Orthotics Assistant, Kansas City, MO)

Crossbar (Fig. 3-13)

This transverse medial or lateral extension, in combination with similar bars, provides splint stability on the forearm and hand. Crossbars may be used in pairs, singly in three-point configuration with the most distal point often serving as a wrist deviation bar, or in the case of a highly contoured splint, with the proximal and distal bars molded together to form the continuous lateral aspects of a forearm trough.

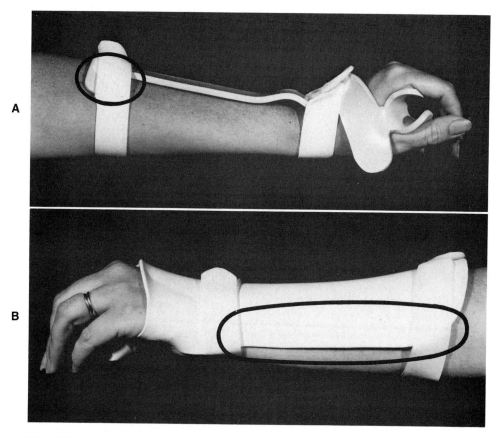

Fig. 3-13. A, Crossbars often provide the basis for strap attachment. **B,** Fused crossbars increase splint strength in contour designs.

Cuff or strap (Fig. 3-14)

This splint part is usually constructed of a softer, more pliable material and holds the splint in place on the extremity. Cuffs are frequently wider than straps and disperse pressure over half the lateral width of the segment in addition to increasing the area of force application on the dorsal or palmar surface. This results in greater patient comfort (see also discussion of finger cuff).

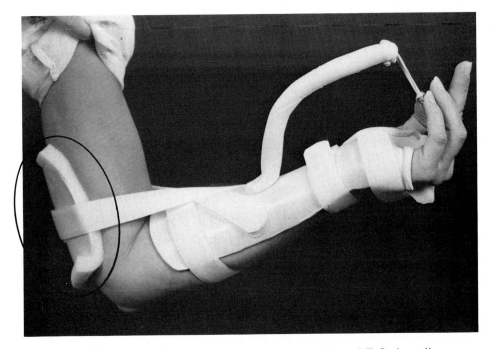

Fig. 3-14. A triceps cuff prevents distal migration of this long MP flexion splint.

Deviation bar (Fig. 3-15)

A deviation bar is an immobile component that positions the wrist or fingers in the coronal plane. It controls abduction/adduction movements of the fingers or wrist. To be fully effective, the height of this ulnarly or radially based bar should be no less than half the thickness of the segment to which it is fitted and no greater than the full segment thickness. These bars are usually continuations of the splint itself, thus providing contoured strength in addition to positioning.

Dynamic assist or traction device (Fig. 3-16)

This splint part creates a mobilizing force on a segment, resulting in passive or passive-assistive motion of a joint or successive joints. Dynamic traction devices may be made of self-adjusting resilient or elastic materials such as rubber or spring wire, or they may consist of more rigid materials such as Velcro, cording, or leather. The latter often rely on the wearer for adjustment.

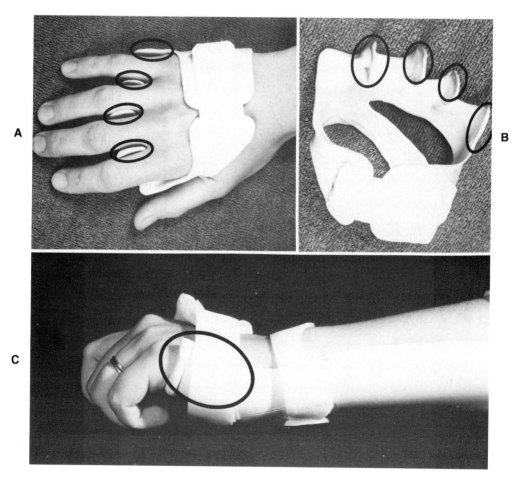

Fig. 3-15. Deviation bars prevent coronal plane motion of the fingers (**A** and **B**) or wrist (**C**). (**A** and **B** courtesy K.P. MacBain, O.T.R., Vancouver, BC.)

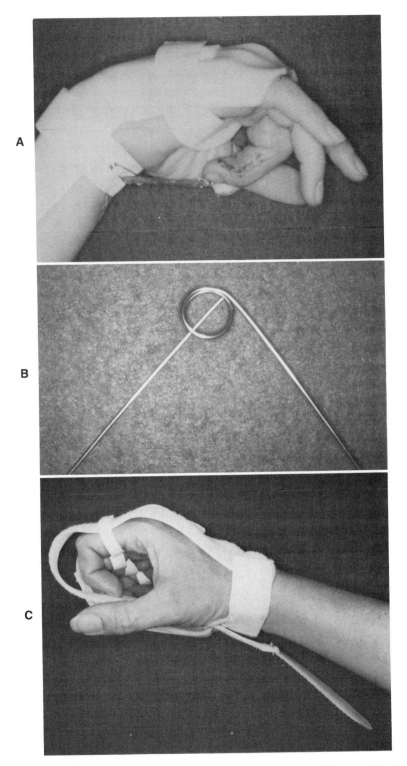

Fig. 3-16. Dynamic assists may differ considerably in inherent tensile properties. **A,** Rubber band. **B,** Spring wire. **C,** Velcro strap.

Finger cuff (Fig. 3-17)

This splint component circumferentially attaches a dynamic assist to the finger. Finger cuffs are most often made of a flexible but inelastic material; in the case of extension traction, they must be cut to allow full flexion of proximal and distal finger joints *(A)*. Designed by Paul Brand, M.D., cuffs made of plaster provide a very contiguous fit and are ideal for use with insensitive hands *(B)*.

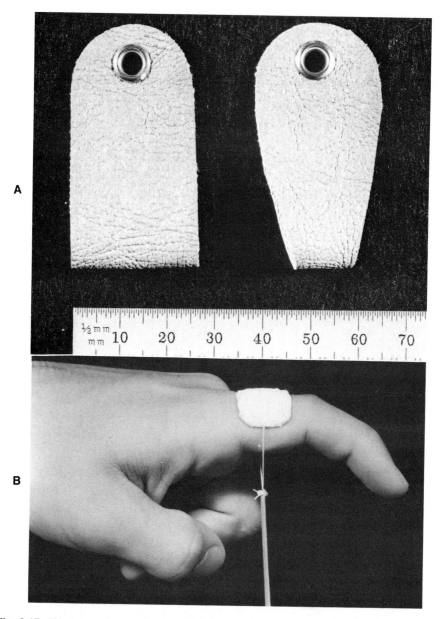

Fig. 3-17. (A) Trimmed properly, extension finger cuffs should not impede digital flexion. **(B)** A contiguous fit of this cuff on the dorsum of the finger is provided even in the absence of a 90° angle of approach of the dynamic assist.

Fingernail attachment (Fig. 3-18)

A fingernail attachment is any device or material that, when fastened to the finger-nail, provides an attachment site for a dynamic assist or traction. It may be adhered to the nail with a fast-setting ethyl cyanoacrylate glue or, in the case of a suture loop, tied through the distal free edge of the nail body. The idea of gluing dress hooks to finger-nails was originated by Carolina F. deLeeuw, M.A., O.T.R., while working on the burn unit of Brooke Army Hospital in the early 1960s.

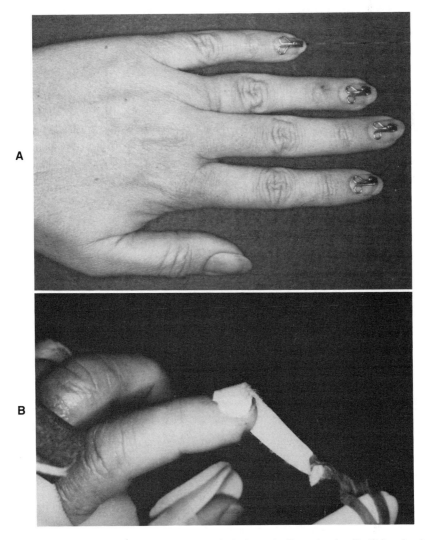

Fig. 3-18. Frequently used fingernail attachment devices. **A,** Dress hooks. **B,** Velcro hook tabs.

Forearm bar or trough (Fig. 3-19)

This longitudinal splint part rests proximal to the wrist on one or more surfaces of the forearm. The forearm bar provides the leverage to support the weight of the hand and, for maximum efficiency and comfort, should be at least two thirds the length of the forearm to minimize resultant pressure.

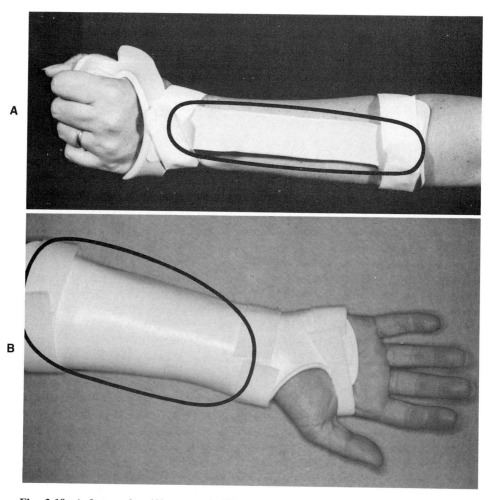

Fig. 3-19. A forearm bar (**A**) or trough (**B**) must be long enough to comfortably support the proximally transferred weight of the hand.

Hypothenar bar (Fig. 3-20)

The bar that palmarly supports the ulnar aspect of the transverse metacarpal arch is called a hypothenar bar and is frequently the continuation of an ulnar deviation bar or a portion of a palmar metacarpal bar. It should not inhibit flexion of the ring and small metacarpophalangeal joints and should be contoured carefully to provide a contiguous fit. Poor molding of the hypothenar bar may result in excessive pressure as the hand is used.

Joint

The mechanical overlapping of splint components results in either an axis of rotation (one rivet) or a solid immobile joint (provided by two or more rivets or by the cohesion or bonding of involved surfaces).

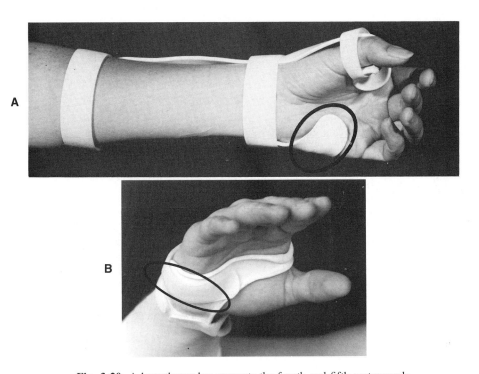

Fig. 3-20. A hypothenar bar supports the fourth and fifth metacarpals.

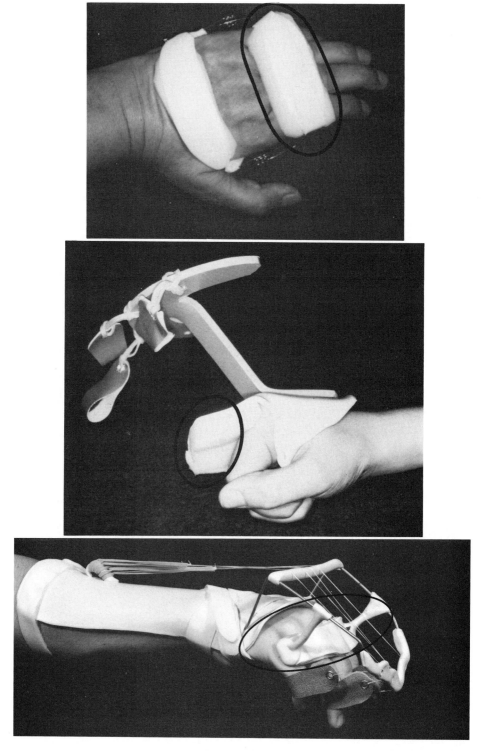

Fig. 3-21. Although dissimilar in appearance, these lumbrical bars all control the degree of metacarpophalangeal extension.

Dorsal phalangeal bar or lumbrical bar (Fig. 3-21)

This bar extends over the dorsal aspect of one or more proximal phalanges and prevents a predetermined amount of metacarpophalangeal extension or hyperextension. In the case of multiple fingers, the dorsal phalangeal bar also maintains the transverse arch at the phalangeal level. Because of the fragility of the dorsal skin and the magnified forces of a dynamic splint, padding is often required for pressure dissemination. The radial and ulnar sides of this bar should curve palmarly to half the width of the proximal phalanx to prevent lateral displacement of the finger or fingers from under the bar. Longitudinally a lumbrical bar should extend a minimum of two thirds the length of the proximal phalanx.

Metacarpal bar (Fig. 3-22)

This splint component supports the transverse metacarpal arch dorsally or palmarly. A correctly fitted metacarpal bar should allow full motion of the second through fifth metacarpophalangeal joints. The ulnar and radial extensions of a metacarpal bar frequently include a hypothenar bar or an opponens bar, respectively.

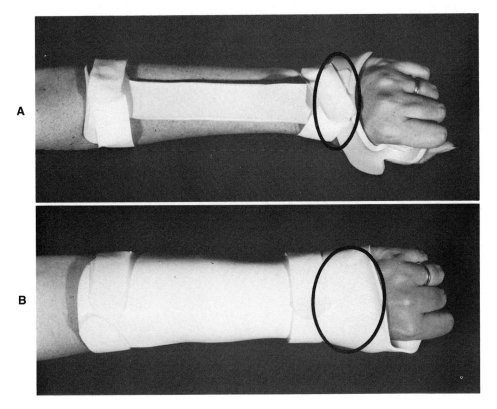

A

B

Fig. 3-22. Longitudinal measurements of dorsal metacarpal bars may vary from narrow (**A**) to those which incorporate or nearly incorporate the full length of the metacarpal(s) (**B**).

Opponens bar (Fig. 3-23)

This component, usually in conjunction with a C bar, positions the first metacarpal in various degrees of abduction and opposition while preventing radiodorsal motion of the first metacarpal. It should be long enough to fully control the first metacarpal bone but should not be so long that it interferes with placement of the hand.

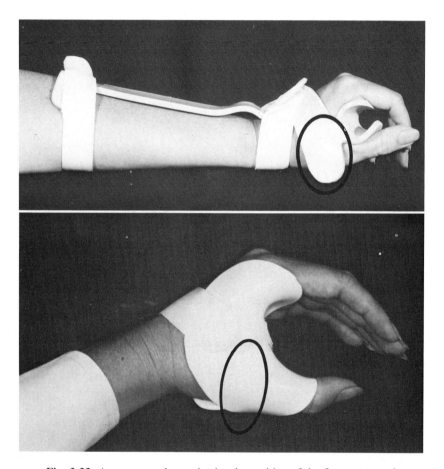

Fig. 3-23. An opponens bar maintains the position of the first metacarpal.

Outrigger (Fig. 3-24)

This splint part is extended out from the main body of the splint for the purpose of positioning dynamic assists or traction devices. To maintain correct alignment of the traction devices, the length of an outrigger must be adjusted as change occurs in passive range of motion of the joint(s) being mobilized. Because the magnitude of the traction will be lessened with instability or material weakness, an outrigger should furnish a rigid or near-rigid foundation or fulcrum for the dynamic assists.

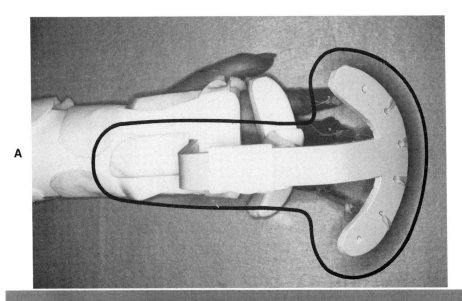

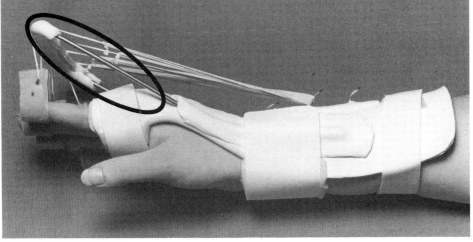

Fig. 3-24. The configuration of an outrigger varies according to purpose and material from which it is constructed. (**B** courtesy Lisa Dennys, B.Sc., O.T., London, Ont.; **C** from Hollis, I.: Innovative splinting ideas. In Hunter, J.M., et al., editors: Rehabilitation of the hand, St. Louis, 1978, The C.V. Mosby Co.; **D** from Leonard, J., Swanson, A., and Swanson, G.: Postoperative care for patients with Silastic finger joint implants [Swanson design], Orthopaedic Reconstructive Surgeons P.C. of Grand Rapids, MI, 1984.)   *Continued.*

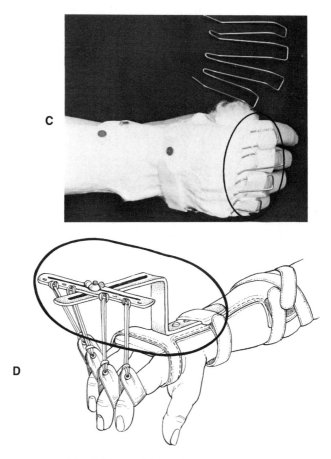

Fig. 3-24, cont'd. For legend see p. 95.

Palmar phalangeal bar or finger pan (Fig. 3-25)

The finger pan or palmar phalangeal bar maintains the transverse and longitudinal arches distally by providing palmar support to the phalanges. If the palmar phalangeal bar immobilizes only a portion of a segment, care should be taken not to inhibit the motion of adjacent more distal joints. The medial and lateral continuations of this bar frequently end in deviation bars, providing coronal plane control and splint durability through contour.

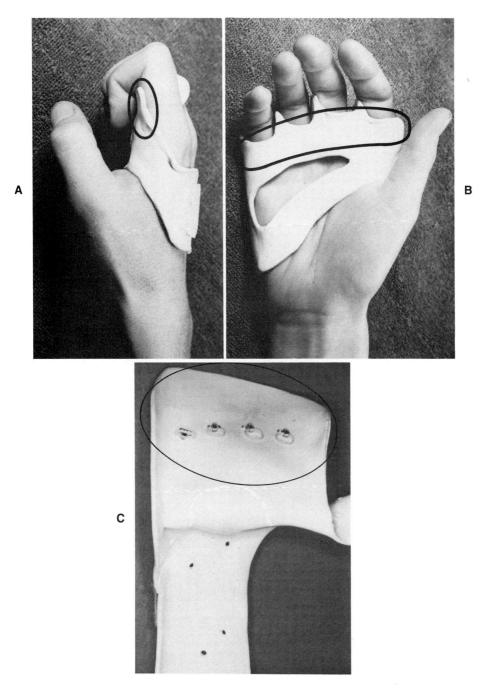

Fig. 3-25. A palmar phalangeal bar or finger pan may support one (**A**) or multiple (**B** and **C**) finger segments. (**A** and **B** courtesy K.P. MacBain, O.T.R., Vancouver, BC.)

Prop (Fig. 3-26)

A prop is an attachment that places the splinted extremity away from a supporting surface to prevent pressure from prolonged resting of the hand on a rigid or semirigid surface.

Reinforcement bar (Fig. 3-27)

This adjunctive splint component increases the strength and durability of the splint. Although an occasional reinforcement bar might be appropriate, the zealous use of reinforcement bars is frequently indicative of poor splint design or material choice. Correctly contoured material and the incorporation of sound mechanical principles is far more effective in providing splint strength than is the retrospective trussing with layers of material.

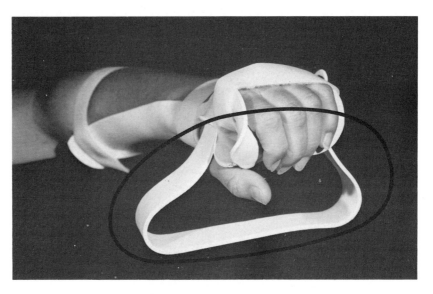

Fig. 3-26. A prop may be of assistance in preventing pressure breakdown in severe upper extremity paralysis.

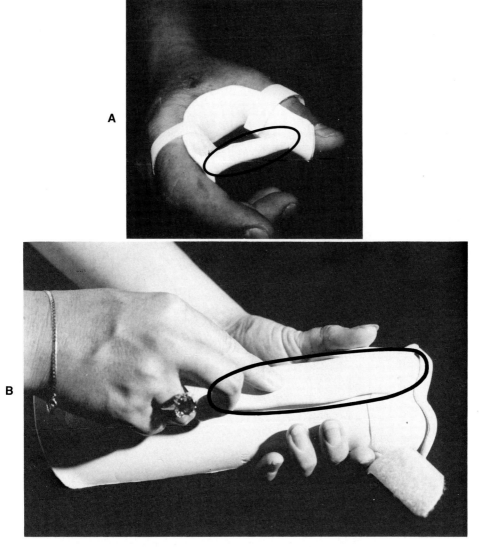

Fig. 3-27. A contoured reinforcement bar may be used to provide additional strength to a splint. (**A** courtesy Cynthia Philips, M.A.O.T.R., Boston, MA.)

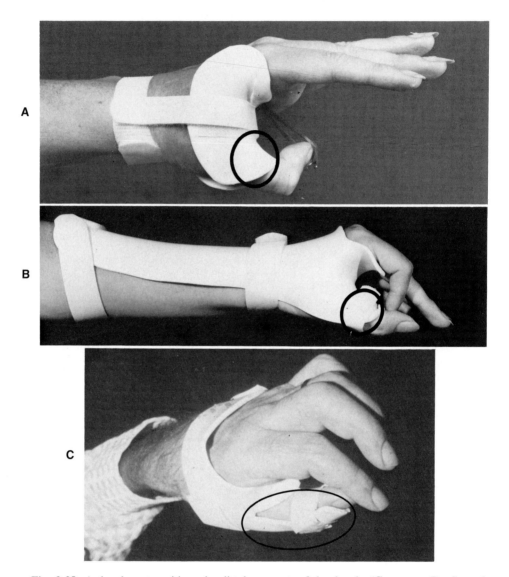

Fig. 3-28. A thumb post positions the distal segments of the thumb. (**C** courtesy Pat Samuels, O.T.R., Indianapolis.)

Thumb post (Fig. 3-28)

This splint part positions the proximal and distal phalanges of the thumb and is usually a distal extension of a **C** bar. When only the proximal phalanx is immobilized, full interphalangeal joint motion should not be inhibited by overextension of the thumb post distally. Since the configuration of this bar is often long and narrow, contouring of the material to half of the thickness of the splinted segment will allow for increased stability. When the immobile thumb is to be used in functional activities, it is preferable to design the thumb post to fit dorsally to allow the sensory areas of this thumb to be free for grasping.

Wrist bar (Fig. 3-29)

Whether fitted palmarly, dorsally, ulnarly, or on the radial aspect of the wrist, any splint part that supports the carpal area of the extremity may be considered a wrist bar. This bar frequently connects to the forearm bar proximally and the metacarpal bar distally. The positional attitude of this bar in the sagittal plane exerts substantial influence on the kinetic interrelationships of anatomic structures. As a result, the wrist bar must be positioned advantageously and with deliberation.

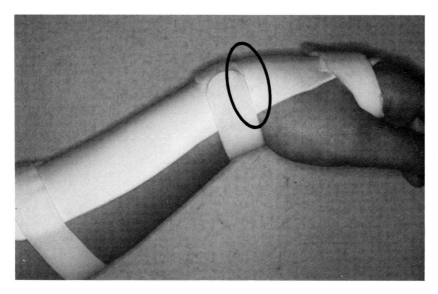

Fig. 3-29. A wrist bar placed in flexion will augment extrinsic finger extension.

SUMMARY

Although one must be cognizant of the various classification systems that have been offered for hand splints, it is important to avoid the confusion that will result from the redundancy of these systems. More important, the clinician involved in splint preparation should have a thorough knowledge of the nomenclature of the entire spectrum of splint parts, their capabilities, and indications. A creative flexibility must be developed that allows the experienced splint maker to draw from a large assortment of splint components in the preparation of a splint that will best suit the requirements of a particular hand problem. Adherence to a limited classification system may narrow these fabrication options and fail to adequately respond to the almost unlimited assortment of individual situations that exist in the diseased or injured hand. This chapter introduces a classification system that integrates force complexity, joints influenced, and kinematic purpose in an effort to provide a simple splint description terminology. We hope that this type of approach will best allow for a more accurate description of a given splint, thereby aiding therapists and physicians in the difficult area of communication.

CHAPTER 4

Hand assessment and splinting

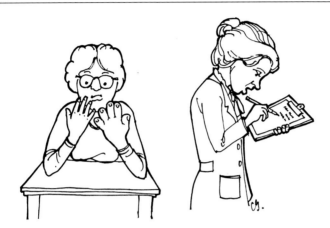

"NO NEED TO MEASURE, MRS. TIMBLY. I CAN TELL
YOUR HAND IS GETTING BETTER JUST BY LOOKING."

Thorough and unbiased assessment procedures furnish essential foundations for splinting programs by delineating baseline pathology from which splint designs may be created and patient progress and splinting methods may be evaluated. Assessment information also assists in predicting the rehabilitation potential of the diseased or injured hand and provides data to which subsequent measurements may be compared. Conclusions gained from evaluation procedures aid in ordering treatment priorities, promote both patient and staff incentive, and define functional capacity when rehabilitative efforts culminate. Through analysis and integration, assessment also serves as the vehicle of professional communication, eventually affecting the comprehensive body of hand rehabilitation knowledge.

Significantly influencing the design and configuration of hand splints, the evaluation process involves gathering and integrating data derived from various sources, including physician referral, direct observation,and precise measurements. A finished splint must not only meet the more obvious requirements of physical condition, it should also reflect

103

the patient's psychologic and socioeconomic capacities. Additionally, experience, preference, and philosophy of the members of the hand rehabilitation team are important factors in dictating splinting programs and, as such, must be considered in the overall assessment process. The purpose of this chapter is to review upper extremity assessment theory and techniques as applied to hand splinting concepts.

INSTRUMENT CRITERIA

A splinting assessment involves the use of a variety of evaluation techniques and instruments whose resultant data may be integrated to produce a clearly defined picture of composite hand function. Assessment tools range in sophistication from simple observational methods to highly complex standardized tests. While observational skills provide the initial basis for identifying pathology, specific measurements provide concrete numerical information about specialized components of hand function such as motion, strength, sensibility, temperature, mass, coordination, and dexterity. Both observation and measurement play vital roles in evaluating a diseased or injured hand for application of a splint.

Much of the initial impression of disease and dysfunction may be gleaned from astute interrogation, observation, and careful inspection and palpation of the extremity. A detailed history; observation of posturing and use of the hand; identification of skin and soft tissue condition, skeletal and joint stability, composite motion, general strength, musculotendinous continuity, pain, and neurovascular status; and a subjective appraisal of the patient's attitude toward his disability provide the examiner with the source and general parameters of the problem.

Once the patient's overall condition is understood, specific measurements should be taken to further delineate the problem. Directly influencing the interpretation and understanding of upper extremity dysfunction, both the quality of the instruments and the effects of the procedures used in the assessment process must be identified.

Because the caliber of information in a splinting assessment is dictated by the sophistication, predictability and accuracy of the measurement instruments used, it is critical to choose evaluation tools with care and forethought. Dependable, precise instruments provide data that is minimally skewed by extraneous factors or biases, thereby diminishing subjective error and facilitating objective and accurate definition. Additionally, instruments that measure diffusely produce undelineated and nonspecific data, and those proven to measure with precision yield more reliable and selective information. In an age of consumer awareness and accountability it is no longer sufficient to rely on "homemade" nonvalidated evaluation tools, which almost universally produce meaningless splinter data.

Equally important to the identification of instrument reliability and validity is understanding how the testing process can affect resultant data. Position of the extremity, fatigue, physiologic adaptation, length of the test, and motivation are but a few of the factors that can influence test results. Also, instruments that are used to measure hand dysfunction should not have been used as practice tools in therapy. Evaluation tools that have been used in the training process produce skewed data and render consequent information invalid and meaningless. Selection criteria must therefore reflect under-standing of testing protocol as well as instrumentation requirements.

Standardized tests, the most sophisticated of measurement instruments, have statis-tically proven to be both valid and reliable. They measure what they purport to measure (validity) and they measure consistently between examiners and from trial to trial (reli-ability). To date, the few truly standardized tests available for measuring upper extrem-ity dysfunction are limited to instruments that evaluate hand coordination, dexterity, and work tolerance. Surprisingly, most of the currently used assessment instruments lack many of the primary elements characteristic of standardized tests. When choosing in-struments for measuring upper extremity dysfunction, selection should be guided ac-cording to how closely inherent properties of the instrument coincide with those of standardized tools.

To qualify as a standardized test, an instrument must have all of the following elements: (1) a statement that defines the purpose or intent of the test, (2) correlation statistics or other appropriate measure of instrument validity (not mean or average val-ues), (3) correlation statistics or other appropriate measure of instrument reliability (not mean or average values), (4) detailed descriptions of the equipment used in the test, (5) normative data, drawn from a large population sample, which is divided into subcate-gories according to appropriate variables such as hand dominance, age, sex, or occu-pation, and (6) specific instructions for administering, scoring, and interpreting the test. Since relatively few upper extremity evaluation tools fully meet standardization criteria, instrument selection should be predicated on satisfying as many of the standardization requisites as possible, ensuring an identifiable level of quality control.

To be complete, a splinting assessment should address the total spectrum of upper extremity and hand performance and condition, including physical, psychologic, and socioeconomic factors. Since a universal upper extremity assessment instrument is non-existent, a variety of tools is needed to measure the various parameters of condition and performance. Both the American Society for Surgery of the Hand (ASSH) and the American Society of Hand Therapists (ASHT) have established guidelines for clinical assessment of the upper extremity, which include recommendations for measurement of range of motion, strength, sensation (ASSH), volume (ASHT), dexterity and coordina-tion (ASHT), and vascular status (ASSH).

RECORDING AND TIMING OF ASSESSMENT EXAMINATIONS

Not all patients who are evaluated for splints require all of the tests within an upper extremity assessment battery. Most hand specialists use a few quick tests to check hand function initially and add the more sophisticated testing procedures as dictated by the patient's condition. Generally, initial and final evaluations are more comprehensive, whereas intervening evaluations are less formal, concentrating on assessing progress in specific areas, such as active and passive range of motion, volume, and muscle strength. The frequency of reevaluation depends on diagnosis, physiologic timing, and the pa-tient's response to the application of the splint. For example, because they often respond quickly to splinting measures, early postoperative patients require more frequent measurements than do those individuals who have been splinted to correct longstanding deformities.

The actual recording of assessment data varies according to the specific test and to the amount of change observed. Motion values may be recorded on a daily, three times a week, or weekly basis, while strength measurements may require notation each month. The important concept is that change in status is documented with objective measurements at appropriate intervals.

Although evaluation data dictate the design of a splint, knowledge obtained from reevaluation sessions directs alterations in splint configuration and wearing schedule. Splinting a hand is a dynamic, ever-changing process that is intimately interwoven with and directed by information gleaned from assessment procedures. With the designing, constructing, and fitting of a splint comes the all-important responsibility of maintaining and updating its efficacy. This is done through vigilant reassessment of the hand and constant reevaluation of the exercise routine, wearing schedule, and the splint itself. Failure to attain anticipated goals in a diseased or injured hand is indicative of an immediate need for reassessment of the splinting and exercise programs.

CLINICAL EXAMINATION OF THE HAND
Referral information

The information provided in the initial referral is paramount because it directly influences the ultimate splint design and subsequent treatment. In addition to the patient's name, age, sex, hand dominance, hospital number, and designation of involved extremity, the signed referral should include diagnosis, date and reason for onset or injury, pertinent medical and/or history (with dates), purpose and timing of splint application, and specific instructions and precautions. Without this minimum baseline information the initiation of a splinting program should not be undertaken; unfortunately, in this age of litigation it is preferable to have this information in writing. Operative notes, radiographic reports, including arteriographic studies, and the results of pertinent testing procedures such as nerve conduction velocity studies (NCVs), electromyograms (EMGs), and Doppler scans are also essential for evaluating and treating upper extremity dysfunction.

Identification of the etiology, diagnosis, rehabilitation potential, physiologic timing, and physician's treatment philosophy allows early triage of possible therapy and splinting options. Since splinting theories differ considerably, it is important to differentiate initially between upper motor neuron lesions, and those organic or systemic diseases which follow chronic courses, from the often more acute peripheral lesions associated with upper extremity trauma. For example, a proximal interphalangeal joint hyperextension deformity is treated differently in a spastic hand, a rheumatoid arthritic hand, and a young athlete's hand. When dealing with postoperative patients it is essential to know which structures were involved, which structures were repaired, and the specific method of repair. Postoperative timing is also critical. A splint that is appropriate 8 weeks after repair might be detrimental at an earlier time because wound tensile strength could be insufficient to withstand splinting forces. Differing philosophies as to when and how certain injuries may be splinted during the early postoperative phase also make it imperative to know the preferences of the referring physician before embarking upon a course of splinting and therapy. A surgeon who prefers to immobilize tendons for 3 weeks postoperatively would be more than alarmed to discover that an early passive mobilization splinting and exercise program had been initiated for a patient with newly repaired flexor tendons!

Posture

The normal hand at rest assumes a consistent posture with the wrist in 10 to 15 degrees of dorsiflexion, the thumb in slight extension/abduction with the metacarpophalangeal and interphalangeal joints flexed approximately 15 to 20 degrees, and the fingers exhibiting progressively greater composite flexion to the ulnar side of the hand. The thumbnail lies in a plane perpendicular to that of the index finger, and at rest, the extended longitudinal attitudes of the four fingers converge on a small area at the base of the thumb near the opponens crease. When the wrist is brought into full extension, finger adduction and flexion increase, the transverse metacarpal arch flattens slightly, the extended longitudinal point of convergence moves proximally onto the forearm, and the thumb pad approximates the lateral aspect of the proximal phalanx of the index finger. Conversely, wrist flexion produces a passive attitude of finger abduction and extension, and although the thumb metacarpophalangeal and interphalangeal joints assume a nearly full extension posture, the thumb web space narrows as passive tension on the extensor pollicis longus tendon increases and the first metacarpal is adducted. Changes from the normal resting posture or from normal tenodesis effect are strong indicators of pathology and merit further investigation before splint design can commence.

Skin and subcutaneous tissue

A thorough examination of the surface condition and contours of the extremity helps define pathology and influences splint configuration. Closely correlated with neurovascular status, tissue viability, and the inflammatory process are skin color, temperature, texture, and moisture. These should be carefully noted. Alterations from normal extremity size and contour should also be identified, including areas of atrophy, tissue deficit, scarring, swelling, edema, and abnormal masses or prominences. Absence of wrinkles at or near joints may indicate loss of motion or inflammation, and callus formation and embedded surface grime are excellent clues as to how the hand is used. Since the application of any splinting device, no matter how well fitted, produces pressure and friction to the underlying cutaneous surface, tissue friability, especially in scarred or grafted areas, must be carefully evaluated. Splints should be designed such that they do not in any way place normal structures, healing structures, or tissue of questionable viability in jeopardy. In borderline cases circumferential or narrow components should be avoided, and whenever possible pressure should be minimized by increasing the area of application of strategic splint parts.

Bone

When splinting patients who have sustained injury to the skeletal structures of the forearm or hand, the clinician will find operative notes to be essential. In addition to identifying the site and type of fracture, it is critical to know how stable the reduction is, the method used to obtain and maintain good alignment, other related injuries and repairs, and the amount of time elapsed since the reduction. Complications, including rotational deformity, delayed union, pseudoarthrosis, and malunion, must be assessed, and the presence of fixation devices such as K-wires, compression plates, and screws should be noted. Portions of a splint may be designed to support and protect the fracture site and others to mobilize stiffened adjacent joints. If pins or wires are positioned such that pressure from the splint causes discomfort, components must be adapted to avoid encroaching upon these areas. Splinting should be knowledgeably integrated with the pace of physiologic healing and should not unduly stress the mending fracture site. Wound healing principles and how they are affected by the application of external forces must be clearly understood. A splint that may be appropriate 6 to 8 weeks after reduction could actually be ineffective or detrimental if applied at an earlier time. Although fixation devices often allow early motion to those joints of the hand which do not require immobilization to stabilize the fracture, it is important to understand the inherent forces involved and their physiologic repercussions before splint application may begin. Incorrect splinting or timing of splinting may result in further deformity and pain. Close communication between members of the rehabilitation team is therefore essential to obtain optimal functional results.

Joint

Joint stability, passive motion, etiology, and elapsed time since injury and repair are important when evaluating articular function. With the exception of the five-ligament complex of the thumb carpometacarpal joint, each digital articulation achieves stability through a consistent configuration of three ligaments. A pair of collateral ligaments provides lateral stability, and a dense palmar plate allows a full arc of flexion while preventing excessive hyperextension of each joint. Continuity, relative length, and glide of these ligaments must be carefully assessed, since unstable joints, subluxation, dislocation, and limited passive motion directly influence the purpose of splint application, resulting in numerous splint designs, each created to meet specific requirements. Immobilization or blocking splints depend upon physiologic timing and are often utilized to protect healing ligamentous structures and limit motion until tensile strength is sufficient to tolerate normal motion and resistance. Joints whose supporting ligaments have been attenuated by disease or trauma may be improved functionally through the application of control splints. Mobilization splints that apply gentle, prolonged forces are used to correct passive joint deformity.

Differentiating pathology at the capsular or articular level from pathology involving the musculotendinous system is imperative in achieving efficacious splint design. A hand-based splint that does not incorporate the wrist may be used for joint motion limitations resulting from shortened or fibrosed periarticular structures or intraarticular adhesions. The presence of extrinsic musculotendinous pathology requires a splint design that controls the wrist in addition to providing corrective forces to more distal digital joints. Both the tenodesis effect on passive joint motion (Fig. 4-1) and the relative tightness of the intrinsic muscles (Fig. 4-2) must be identified before the final splint configuration may be reached.

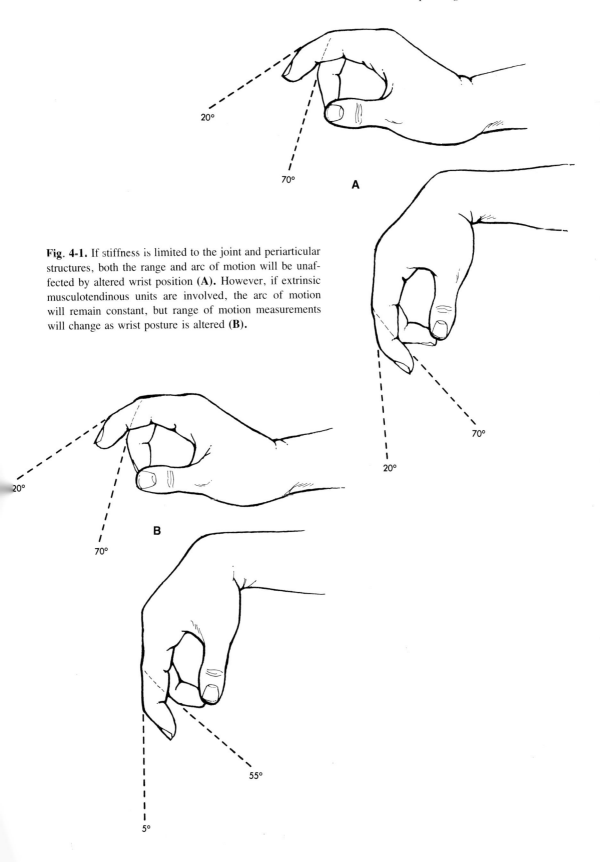

Fig. 4-1. If stiffness is limited to the joint and periarticular structures, both the range and arc of motion will be unaffected by altered wrist position (**A**). However, if extrinsic musculotendinous units are involved, the arc of motion will remain constant, but range of motion measurements will change as wrist posture is altered (**B**).

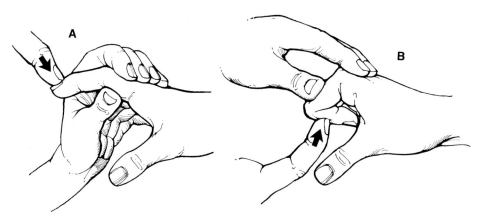

Fig. 4-2. If the intrinsic muscles have become tight, full passive flexion of the proximal interphalangeal joint will be absent when the metacarpophalangeal joint is held in extension (**A**); full passive proximal interphalangeal flexion is possible with the metacarpophalangeal joint in flexion (**B**).

Muscle and tendon

Diminished or absent active motion in the presence of normal passive articular motion may indicate loss of muscle tendon continuity, impaired contractile capacity, or limitation in tendon glide. The effect is observable in the resting hand when the normal cascading posture of the digits is altered, and pathology can be assessed through measurement of active motion of those joints spanned by the involved musclotendinous units and through manual muscle testing procedures. Again, relating diagnosis, surgical intervention, and physiologic timing is critical to designing splints that affect muscle tendon function. Tensile strength dictates splinting and exercise routines, and regardless of whether the purpose of application is for protection, substitution, or mobilization, if extrinsic muscle tendon units are involved, wrist position is a significant factor. Not only is the influence of tenodesis effect on distal joints important, the point at which involved tendons cross the wrist should also be identified. At this point tension on specific tendons can be altered by manipulating the attitude of the wrist. Especially significant during early wound healing, the effect wrist posture has on injured or healing structures influences the selection of splint components and determines splint length and configuration. This is also true when splinting to increase tendon excursion and active joint range of motion. As just noted, the underlying cause for limitation in joint range of motion must be carefully analyzed. Capsular or articular pathology often requires less complicated splint designs, whereas involvement of extrinsic tendons usually necessitates longer splints that control the wrist in addition to the digits.

Nerve

Both motor and sensory aspects of nerve function must be evaluated when assessing the hand for a splint. Motor nerves have predictable patterns of innervation, and disruption of these patterns indicates pathology or anomalous innervation, each of which must

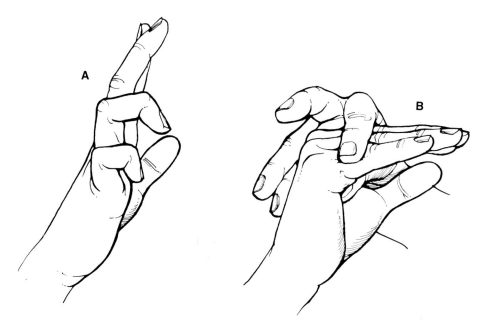

Fig. 4-3. Lack of innervation of the intrinsic muscles results in an inability to actively extend the interphalangeal joints of the ring and small fingers in ulnar nerve paralysis (**A**). This is due, however, to loss of intrinsic flexion at the metacarpophalangeal joint and concomitant zigzag collapse, rather than pathology of the extrinsic extensor muscle group (**B**).

be identified and analyzed before a splinting program may begin (Fig. 4-3). Intimately integrated with muscle function, the motor capacity of a nerve may be evaluated through NCVs, EMGs, and manual muscle testing procedures. Identifying areas of diminished or absent sensibility is also important to the design and fitting of hand splints, for these areas are especially vulnerable to damage from pressure and friction. Although a splint may be fitted correctly, the lack of sensory feedback from the extremity often results in an absence of the frequent unconscious adjustments normally made by the patient. This leads to tissue breakdown through pressure necrosis, rendering the splint unwearable and useless. Forewarned, the hand specialist may incorporate into the design of the splint wider and longer components, thereby distributing splinting forces over a greater area and decreasing the potential for pressure and friction. The Semmes-Weinstein calibrated monofilaments and the two-point discrimination test are useful tools for identifying areas of sensibility dysfunction (Fig. 4-4). Areas of pain, dysesthesia, and hyperesthesia also should be noted and recorded.

Vascular status

In addition to Doppler and arteriographic studies, monitoring skin temperature and color and composite mass of the extremity are essential to understanding the vascular status of a diseased or injured hand. Areas with questionable tissue viability should be carefully defined, and splints should be adapted to prevent obstruction of venous return

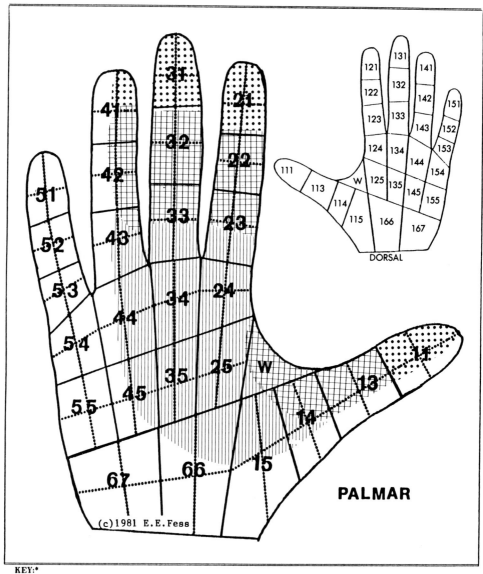

KEY:*

		Filament	Pressure (gm/mm2)
☐	Normal	1.65 - 2.83	1.45 - 4.86
▦	Dimished light touch	3.22 - 3.61	11.1 - 17.7
▤	Diminished protective sensation	3.84 - 4.31	19.3 - 33.1
⦂	Loss of protective sensation	4.56 - 6.65	47.3 - 439.0
▨	Untestable	6.65	439.0

*Levine, S., Pearsall, G., & Ruderman, R.: J Hand Surg., 3:211, 1978.

Name _____

Number _____

Hand _____ *RIGHT* _____ *9·3·86*

Fig. 4-4. Areas of sensibility disruption should be identified before a splinting program is initiated.

and arterial flow. By increasing the area of force application of splint components and achieving a contiguous fit, the specialist may reduce pressure. Additionally, factors that could affect splint fit, such as local swelling or generalized edema, should be noted and recorded. Splint designs that employ circumferential components or forces that may jeopardize tissue viability should be avoided in hands that exhibit signs of vascular instability. Areas that depend on newly established collateral circulation and lymphatic drainage should be treated with extreme caution, and splinting measures should be undertaken only after close consultation with the referring physician. As time progresses the sensitivity of these areas to pressure decreases, and splinting and exercise routines may be gradually graded in intensity. Once a splint is fitted, an increase from baseline temperature or volume readings may indicate that too much force is being utilized and an inflammatory reaction is taking place. Conscientious monitoring of alterations in hand size, temperature, and color provides guidelines as to the physiologic response of the hand to treatment methods, allowing timely intervention and manipulation of splinting and exercise techniques.

Function

Careful observation of the patient during evaluation sessions assists the examiner in discovering how the patient views his disabiity and how he uses the extremity. Is the hand protected or guarded by the patient? Is there reluctance to remove it from a pocket, glove, or dressing? Does he willingly allow examination and touching of the hand? Is the extremity used spontaneously? Are normal use patterns apparent or are certain parts of the hand avoided as objects are grasped and released? Are proximal joints of the extremity used to substitute for lost or limited distal joint range? Is the manner in which the hand is used altered when vision is occluded? Are callus formations and embedded surface grime noticeable? Does pain seem to be a limiting factor? Are motions smooth and coordinated?

Queries about difficulties encountered during activities of daily living, or during vocational and avocational tasks may also be illuminating during assessment of general extremity function. Is the patient independent in self-care? Is he employed? Are there tasks he can no longer accomplish at work or at home?

Information gleaned from observation and interrogation help form a general concept of how the extremity is used and the patient's attitude toward the disability. Dexterity and coordination tests further refine understanding through generation of numerical data, which may be compared to that of normal subjects.

UPPER EXTREMITY ASSESSMENT INSTRUMENTS

Upper extremity evaluation instruments are divided into four basic categories: condition, motion, sensibility, and function.

Condition assessment instruments

Condition involves the neurovascular system as it pertains to tissue viability, nutrition, inflammation, patency of vessels, and arterial, venous and lymphatic flow. By noninvasive monitoring of extremity volume, skin temperature, and arterial pulses, the status of the skin, subcutaneous tissues, and neurovascular function is more clearly defined.

Volume. Based on the principle of water displacement, commercially available volumeters may measure composite extremity mass (Fig. 4-5). In 1981 Waylett and Seibly reported the commercial hand volumeter to be accurate to within 10 ml when used according to the manufacturer's specifications. Circumferential measurements may also be taken at predetermined levels using a tape measure or calipers. Although the accuracy of this technique depends on consistency of placement and tension of the tape or calipers, it provides a quick means of assessment that is especially applicable in situations where immersion in water is inappropriate. Normal comparison values for either volumetric or circumferential measurements may be obtained from the contralateral extremity.

Vessel patency. The Doppler scanner may be used to map arterial flow through audible ultrasonic response to arterial pulsing; and because of its direct relationship to digital vessel patency, skin temperature may be used to assess tissue viability in the distal extremity.

Motion assessment instruments

The measurement of motion involves muscle/tendon continuity, contractile and gliding capacity, neuromuscular communication, and voluntary control. Techniques for evaluating upper extremity motion include goniometric measurements and the determination of isolated muscle strength.

Range of motion. Goniometric evaluation of the upper extremity is essential to monitoring articular motion and musculotendinous function. Both passive and active motion should be recorded using an appropriate size goniometer and, as recommended by the American Academy of Orthopaedic Surgeons (AAOS), with 0 degrees as neutral starting position. Digital motion is measured on either the lateral or dorsal aspect of the joint, provided that consistency of placement is maintained throughout the examination and during subsequent tests (Fig. 4-6). Normal motion values are obtained from measurement of the contralateral extremity or from norms developed by the AAOS. Although goniometric measurement is not technically a standardized assessment tool, it does provide consistent and accurate information for which norms have been established.

Composite digital motion values may be computed as total active motion and total passive motion. Total active motion equals the summation of active flexion measurements of the metacarpophalangeal, proximal interphalangeal, and distal interphalangeal joints of a digit, minus the active extension deficits of the same three joints. Total passive motion is computed in a similar manner using passive motion values. Expressed as a single numeric value, total motion reflects both the extension and flexion capacities of a single digit (see Appendix E).

Brand's technique of torque range of motion refines passive range of motion measurement by applying predetermined, consistent amounts of force to stiffened joints. Once measured, a torque/length curve may be constructed for each joint by plotting

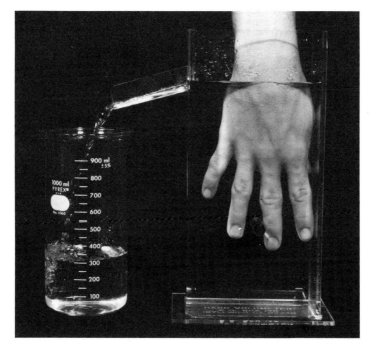

Fig. 4-5. The volumeter measures composite hand mass and has been shown to be accurate to within 10 ml when used according to specifications.

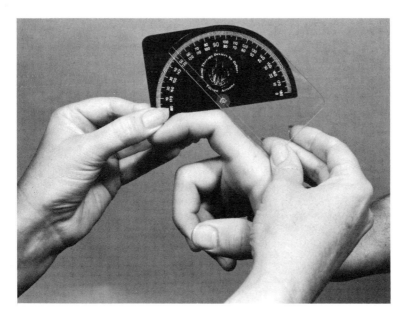

Fig. 4-6. Either lateral or dorsal placement of the goniometer is appropriate, provided that consistency is maintained for subsequent examinations.

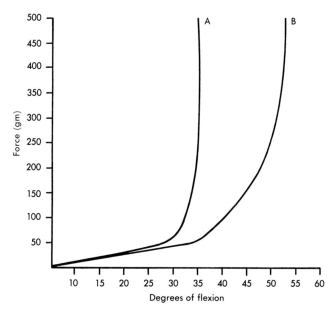

Fig. 4-7. This torque range of motion graph indicates that the proximal interphalangeal joint of the long finger *(B)* has more passive "give" than that of the index finger *(A)* indicating that the long finger may respond more readily to mobilization splinting.

coordinates on a graph, and the relative degree of stiffness of the joints may be visualized (Fig. 4-7).

Muscle strength. The determination of isolated muscle strength through manual muscle testing may be used to define the effects of peripheral nerve or musculotendinous dysfunction in the upper extremity. Although criteria for grading muscle strength have been improved, portions of the test are subject to examiner interpretation. To enhance inter-rater reliability, it is important that all members of the team use the same method of conducting and interpreting manual muscle examinations. Currently numerous grading systems exist, but the two most frequently used are Seddon's numerical system of 0 through 5 and the ratings of zero, trace, poor, fair, good, and normal recommended by the Committee on After-Effects, National Foundation for Infantile Paralysis, Inc. The latter is further refined by a plus-minus system for accomplishment of partial ranges.

Sensibility assessment instruments

Sensibility relies on neural continuity, impulse transmission, receptor acuity, and cortical perception. Assessment of sensibility may be divided into sudomotor/sympathetic response and the abilities to detect, discriminate, quantify, and recognize stimuli.

Sympathetic response. Both Moberg's ninhydrin test and O'Rain's wrinkle test identify areas of disturbance of sweat secretion after peripheral nerve disruption. The involvement of sympathetic fibers in a peripheral nerve injury results in areas of dry denervated skin that do not react to environmental warmth (dry or wet) by sweating or

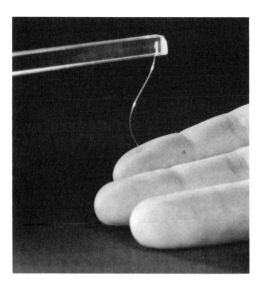

Fig. 4-8. Depending on the diameter of the filament, the Semmes-Weinstein calibrated monofilaments control the amount of force applied as light touch/pressure.

wrinkling. The ninhydrin and wrinkle tests measure physiologic reactions that cannot be controlled by the patient and are therefore objective. Onne (1962) and Phelps and Walker (1977) have shown that these sympathetic responses correlate positively with sensibility return only in early, completely transected peripheral nerves. This significantly reduces the validity and reliability of these tests. While inclusion of a sympathetic response test in an assessment battery for use with specific patients is helpful, it should not be relied on as a primary sensibility assessment instrument.

Detection. Detection, the most fundamental level on the sensibility continuum, requires the patient to perceive a single-point stimulus from normally occurring atmospheric background stimuli. A result of von Frey's work in the late 1800s, the Semmes-Weinstein calibrated monofilaments consist of 20 nylon monofilaments that are graded in diameter and individually attached to handles. The amount of force transmitted by each monofilament is directly related to its diameter (Fig. 4-8). As gradually increasing pressure is applied, each filament bends at a specific force, thereby controlling or limiting the magnitude of the touch/pressure stimulus. This results in a spectrum of calibrated light to heavy forces that may be used to assess cutaneous touch capabilities in patients who exhibit peripheral sensory dysfunction. The smallest diameter filament perceived by the patient within a designated area of the hand is recorded. As testing instruments the monofilaments are unique in their ability to actually control the amount of force applied.

Discrimination. Discrimination, the second level in the sensibility assessment continuum, assesses the patient's capacity to perceive stimulus *A* from stimulus *B*. This requires detection of each stimulus as a separate entity and the ability to distinguish between the two. Discrimination requires finer reception acuity and more judgment on the part of the patient than does first-level detection.

Weber's two-point discrimination test is the most commonly used method of assessing sensibility of the hand. Affording better accuracy and consistency, blunt tip calibrated calipers have replaced the traditional unfolded paperclip as the instrument of choice. Relying on absence of skin blanching to control the amount of force applied, and with the caliper tips oriented longitudinally on the digit, the examiner randomly applies one or two points to the hand. Following each stimulus, the patient reports whether he feels one or two points. The narrowest caliper width at which the patient makes 8 of 10 correct responses is the distance reported. (NOTE: The number of correct responses required may vary slightly from examiner to examiner.) Bell and Buford (1982) reported that, even with experienced examiners, the amount of force applied between one and two points easily exceeds the resolution or sensitivity threshold for normal sensation. They also noted that the tremendous variance in pressures applied resulted in poor levels of inter-rater reliability. This perhaps explains some of the lack of agreement in reporting discriminatory function.

Quantification. Requiring tactile stimuli to be organized into gradients, quantification is the third level on the sensory capacity hierarchy. A patient might be asked which of several alternatives is roughest, most irregular, or smoothest; or he might be required to rank the items from smoothest to roughest. Although there are no tests specific to this area currently available, some of the sensory reeducation techniques incorporate the basic concepts of quantification. For example, representing an important initial step toward standardization of sensibility instruments, Barber's dowel textures have reliability studies done on normal subjects.

Recognition. Recognition, the final and most complicated sensibility level, is based on the patient's ability to identify objects. Seddon's coin test and Porter's letter test are examples of instruments that use identification of items or shapes to assess functional sensibility. The picking-up test described by Moberg may also be adapted to include identification of picked-up objects when vision is occluded.

Function assessment instruments

Hand function reflects the integration of all systems and is measured in terms of grip/pinch, coordination and dexterity, and ability to participate in activities of daily living and vocational and avocational tasks.

Grip strength. A commercially available hydraulic dynamometer (Fig. 4-9) may be used to measure grip strength. In a study of reliability of grip assessment instruments by the California Medical Association, the Jaymar dynamometer was recommended because of its consistency of measurement. Proportional correlations between grip strength and height, weight, and age have been reported by Schmidt and Toews (1970), who also found that the minor hand was equal to or stronger than the dominant hand in 28% of the normal population. Studying the effect of wrist position on grip, Pryce (1980) reported the strongest grip measurements occurred with the wrist in 0 to 15 degrees extension. The American Society for Surgery of the Hand (1978) recommends that the second handle position be used in determining grip strength and that the average of three trials be recorded. Fess (1982) found that the problem of fatigue is eliminated in protocols using the three-trial system for five consecutive handle readings if a 5-minute

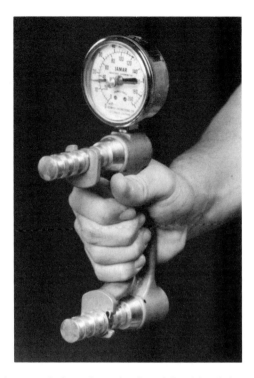

Fig. 4-9. Maximum grip strength depends on the size of the object being grasped. Normal values for the five handle positions form a bell-shaped curve.

rest is provided after each handle setting. Normal adult grip strength changes according to the size of the object being grasped, and grip scores for the five consecutive Jaymar handle positions create a bell curve, with the first position being the least advantageous for strong grip, followed by the fifth and fourth positions. Strongest grip values occur at the third and second handle positions. It is important to understand that inconsistent handle position could be erroneously interpreted as advances or declines in patient progress.

Pinch strength. Using a commercially available pinchometer, three types of pinch may be assessed, including (1) prehension of the thumb pulp to the lateral aspect of the index middle phalanx (key, lateral, or pulp-to-side); (2) pulp of the thumb to pulps of the index and long fingers (three-jaw chuck, three-point chuck); and (3) thumb tip to tip of index finger (tip-to-tip). The mean value of three trials is recorded as recommended by the American Society for Surgery of the Hand, and comparisons may be made with scores from the opposite hand.

Coordination and dexterity. Standardized tests that measure upper extremity dexterity and coordination are available in several levels of difficulty.

The Jebson hand function test requires gross coordination and dexterity and is inexpensive to assemble and easy to administer and score. It consists of seven subtests: (1) writing, (2) card turning, (3) picking up small objects, (4) stimulated feeding, (5) stacking, (6) picking up large lightweight objects, and (7) picking up large heavy objects. Jebson norms are categorized according to maximum time, hand dominance, age, and sex.

Another example of a standardized tests that measures gross coordination and dexterity is the Minnesota rate of manipulation test (MRPT). Five functions are included in the MRPT: (1) placing, (2) turning, (3) displacing, (4) one-handed turning and placing, and (5) two-handed turning and placing. Norms of this instrument are based on more than 11,000 subjects.

The Purdue pegboard evaluates finer coordination than the previously discussed instruments. It requires prehension of small pins, washers, and collars. Measurement categories are divided into (1) right hand, (2) left hand, (3) both hands, (4) right, left, and both, and (5) assembly. Normative data are defined according to gender and type of job.

The Crawford small parts dexterity test adds a more difficult dimension to measurement of upper extremity coordination and dexterity. This test requires subjects to control not only their hands but also small tools, such as tweezers and a screwdriver, and correlates positively with vocational activities that demand very fine coordination skills.

Other hand coordination and dexterity tests are available. These should be carefully evaluated according to the criteria for standardized tests discussed earlier in this chapter to ensure that they measure accurately and consistently. Although many tests claim to be standardized, few actually meet the requisites.

Activities of daily living, vocation, and avocation. Based on observation and interviews, activities of daily living, vocational, and avocational assessments identify specific tasks the patient is unable to perform without difficulty or independently. Once identified, each task must be carefully analyzed to discover why the patient is experiencing problems. Is range of motion sufficient? Does lack of strength influence performance, or is there a problem with coordination? Eventually a pattern of deficit becomes apparent, and the direction and emphasis of a treatment program begin to emerge. According to individual patient requirements, splints can be designed to increase range of motion, to provide control, to substitute for absent muscle power, or to serve as a base of attachment for adapted equipment.

OTHER CONSIDERATIONS

Additional factors that must be evaluated to create splint designs that meet the unique requirements of each individual include the patient's age, motivation, ability to understand and carry out directions, response to injury, and probable response to the application and wearing of a splint. For example, splinting materials or designs for adult patients may not be appropriate for a thumb-sucking toddler whose hand is frequently moist. A complicated splint could further confuse a forgetful geriatric patient, and a shy teenager may not comply with a schedule that requires wearing a splint to school.

Because splinting materials and procedures are often expensive, economic variables should also be taken into consideration. Is the patient able to bear the burden of these expenses? Are there less costly alternatives? Will the patient be able to schedule return visits for splint adjustments around family and occupational responsibilities?

Finally, the preferences and philosophic orientation of the members of the hand rehabilitation team significantly influence splint design. Although often taken for granted and overlooked, these factors must also be identified and evaluated. Why is a given splint design "traditionally" applied? Can a more efficacious splint be designed? Does this splint really meet the needs of this patient, or is it simply more expedient for those involved in the construction and fitting process?

SUMMARY

Formal assessment procedures provide the data upon which splinting and exercise programs are created and adapted to meet the unique requirements of individual patients. Assessment also identifies and directs the need for adjustments as changes occur and assigns numerical value to treatment results. Without the use of evaluation tools that measure consistently and accurately, a definition of pathology and identification of change are often nebulous and indistinct, and splint application may be more harmful than beneficial to the patient. Splint designs should not only reflect the physical requirements of a diseased or injured hand, they should also satisfy individual patient variables. Assessment data are the foundation on which splints are created and used; without this essential information splints should not be designed, constructed, or fitted.

PART TWO

Principles

CHAPTER 5

Mechanical principles

Reduce pressure by increasing the area of force application.
Control parallel force systems by increasing the mechanical advantage.
Use optimum rotational force when mobilizing a joint by dynamic traction.
Consider the torque effect on a joint.
Consider the relative degree of passive mobility of successive joints within the
     longitudinal segmental kinetic chain.
Consider the effects of reciprocal parallel forces when designing splints and
     placing straps.
Increase material strength by providing contour.
Eliminate friction.
Avoid high shear stress.

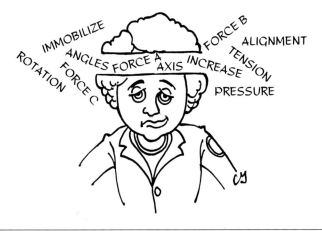

Splinting requires the application of external forces to the extremity; therefore it is essential to understand the basic mechanical principles involved in the design, construction, and fitting of all hand splints. Many therapists have learned the basic concepts of mechanics through trial and error, deductively choosing an approach that yields the most favorable result. Few, however, have the opportunity, expertise, or time to specifically analyze the differences among the available methods. Physicians, although usually possessing a more formal understanding of biomechanics, frequently do not apply this knowledge to splinting in clinical situations, accepting without question a poorly functioning splint that will ultimately produce less favorable results.

The purpose of this chapter is to integrate material from the field of mechanical engineering with the fundamental knowledge of the medical specialist as it pertains to splinting. To clarify the mechanical concepts involved, scale diagrams, red force arrows, and simple formulas illustrate the basic principles. For a more in-depth explanation, additional mathematic equations are presented in Appendix A. Gravitational forces have not been included in the examples in this chapter so that the specific principles can be emphasized and further clarified.

PRINCIPLES

Increase the area of force application. Since splinting materials are, to varying degrees, rigid, their improper application to the extremity may cause damage to the cutaneous surface and underlying soft tissue as a result of excessive pressure. This often occurs in areas where there is minimal subcutaneous tissue to disperse pressure, such as over bony prominences or in areas where the inherent structure of the splint predisposes to increased pressure of mechanical counterforces.

The formula

$$\text{Pressure} = \frac{\text{Total force}}{\text{Area of force application}}$$

indicates that a force of 25 gm applied over an area of 1 cm by 1 cm would result in a pressure of 0.25 gm per square millimeter. If, however, the same 25 gm of force were distributed over an area of 5 cm by 5 cm, the pressure per square millimeter would be decreased to 0.01 gm, or $\frac{1}{25}$ the pressure per square millimeter. In other words, increasing the area of force application will decrease the pressure.

Clinically this has the following implications: (1) wider, longer splints are more comfortable than short, narrow splints (Fig. 5-1); (2) rolled edges on the proximal and distal aspect of a palmar splint and the distal aspect of a dorsal splint cause less pressure than do straight edges (Fig. 5-2); (3) continuous uniform pressure over a bony prominence is preferable to unequal pressure on the prominence (Fig. 5-3); and (4) because some splint components must be narrow and the resultant force great, a contiguous fit is paramount (Fig. 5-4). Generally, a continuous force applied to the extremity should not exceed 50 gm per square centimeter.

The addition of an elastomer lining to a splint helps to provide a close-fitting support surface for the hand (Fig. 5-5). Padded materials such as heavy felt or foam rubber also give uniform pressure distribution because of their inherent properties and are valuable in reducing pressure in areas where the forces are great and the splint is narrow. Padding may be appropriate in such instances, but the zealous use of padding should not substitute for care in designing, fabricating, and fitting the splint.

Using an increased area of application to disperse the forces causing pressure is also important in the construction of a splint. Rounded internal corners diminish the effects of force on the splint material (Fig. 5-6), as do continuously smooth edges (Fig. 5-7).

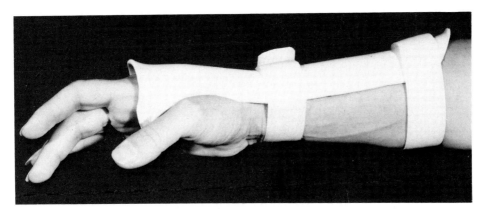

Fig. 5-1. Because of minimized pressure forces and improved mechanical factors, patient comfort is enhanced by splints with greater contact area.

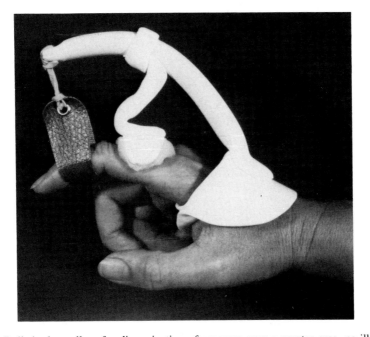

Fig. 5-2. Rolled edges allow for dissemination of pressure over a greater area, as illustrated in the C bar of this splint.

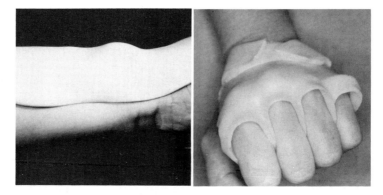

Fig. 5-3. A congruous fit over bony prominences will reduce the possibility of soft tissue damage by evenly dispersing pressure forces over a larger area.

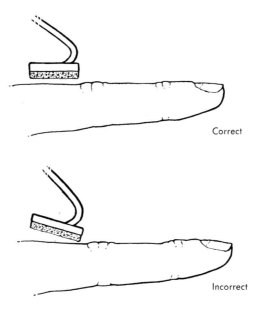

Correct

Incorrect

Fig. 5-4. To reduce pressure, the full surface area of a dorsal phalangeal bar should contact the dorsum of the proximal phalanx. This is one of the few components where padding is almost manditory.

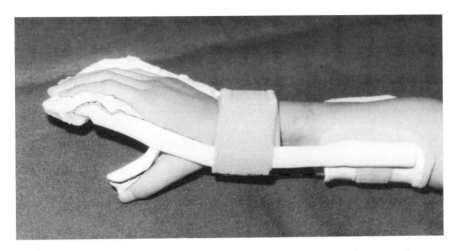

Fig. 5-5. Providing a contiguous fit, an Elastomere lining may be used to decrease splint pressure in a difficult-to-fit extremity. (Courtesy Kimiko Shiina, O.T.R., Tokyo, Japan.)

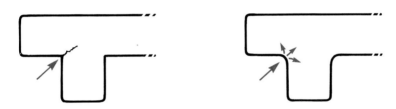

Fig. 5-6. Rounded internal corners increase splint durability by dissipating forces.

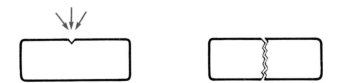

Fig. 5-7. An edge imperfection creates convergence and increases the chances for material fracture.

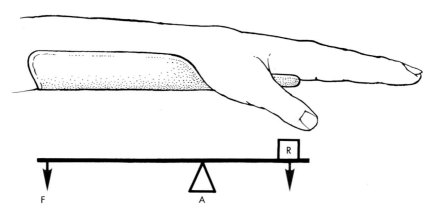

Fig. 5-8. Many splints may be functionally classified as first-class levers. *F,* Force; *A,* axis; *R,* resistance.

In addition, rounded external corners and edges decrease the possibility of excessive pressure on underlying skin.

Increase the mechanical advantage. The design and construction of splints should be adapted to include use of favorable force systems. Many splints fail because of patient discomfort or because of fractured components. These problems may result from inattention to the lever systems at play between the splint and the extremity or between the individual splint parts.

If the splinted forearm, wrist, and hand are viewed as a parallel force system with the wrist being the axis (A), the hand being the weight or resistance (R), and the forearm providing the counterforce to the force (F) of the proximal end of the forearm trough of the splint, the splint itself may be considered a first-class lever (Fig. 5-8) and may be further analyzed as to force lines of action, moment arms, and resultant forces. When the wrist is in neutral position, the forearm trough works as a force arm (FA), the perpendicular distance between the axis and the force line of action (FLA). The palmar metacarpal bar functions as the resistance arm (RA), the perpendicular distance between the axis and resistance line of action (RLA) (Fig. 5-9). If the weight of the average hand is approximately 0.9 pound, and if lengths of the forearm trough and palmar support are 8 inches and 2½ inches, respectively, the resultant force at the proximal end of the splint may be computed according to the formula

$$F \times FA = RA \times R$$

or

$$F = \frac{R \times RA}{FA}$$
$$= \frac{0.9 \times 2.5}{8}$$
$$= \frac{2.25}{8}$$
$$= 0.28 \text{ pound}$$

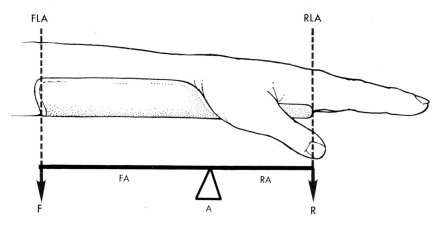

Fig. 5-9. Identification of mechanical terminology as it relates to a first-class lever system expedites subsequent force analysis. *FLA*, Force line of action; *FA*, force arm (perpendicular between axis and FLA); *A*, axis; *RA*, resistance arm (perpendicular between axis and RLA); *RLA*, resistance line of action.

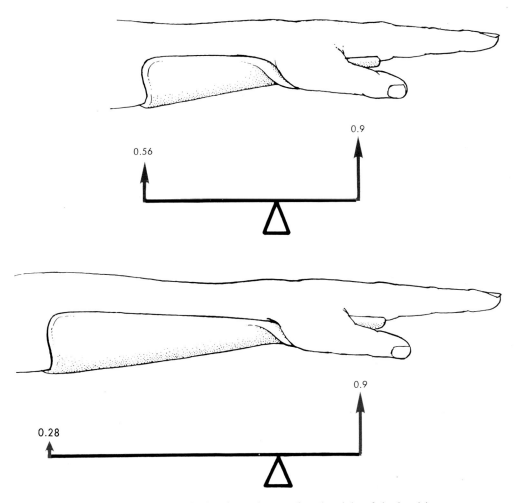

Fig. 5-10. As shown in these scale drawings, the transferred weight of the hand is more comfortably supported by the leverage of a long forearm bar.

If, however, the forearm trough (FA) were only 4 inches in length and the palmar support and resistance remained unchanged, the force at the proximal end of the splint would be twice as great (Fig. 5-10), resulting in patient discomfort and considerably magnifying the chances for pressure problems of the underlying soft tissue:

$$F = \frac{R \times RA}{FA}$$
$$= \frac{0.9 \times 2.5}{4}$$
$$= 0.56 \text{ pound}$$

To simplify the concepts of parallel forces, the splints in Figs. 5-8 to 5-10 are shown in neutral position. Similar concepts apply to any rigid support regardless of shape (Fig. 5-11). If the weight of the hand, its direction of force, and the length of the palmar support are constant, the resulting force at the end of the splint may be decreased by lengthening the forearm trough. This concept may be further generalized to include other types of splints and splint components. Given a constant resistance, resistance line of action, and resistance arm, the amount of force at the opposite end of the first-class lever may be decreased by increasing the length of the force arm (Fig. 5-12).

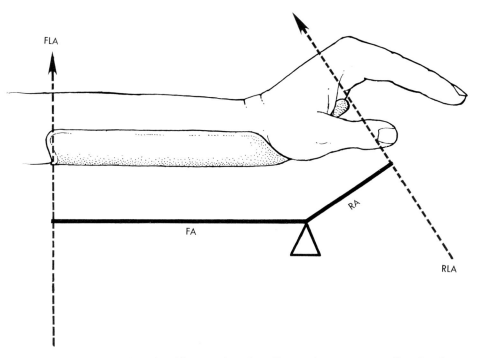

Fig. 5-11. With the wrist bar placed in extension, the splint continues to act as a first-class lever, but the direction of the resistance line of action is altered. *FLA,* Force line of action; *FA,* force arm; *RA,* resistance arm; *RLA,* resistance line of action.

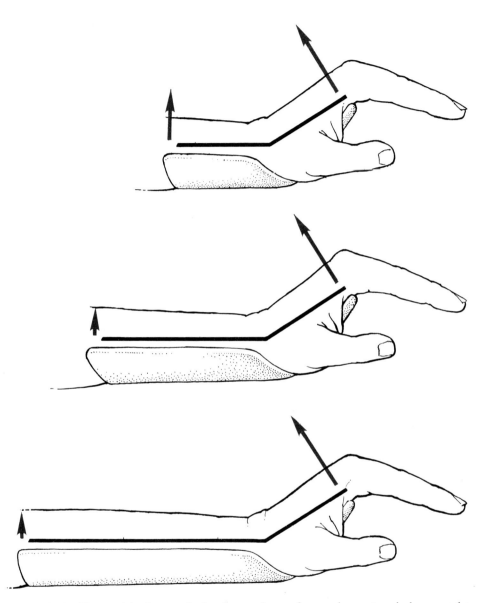

Fig. 5-12. As illustrated in these scale drawings, a longer forearm bar or trough decreases the resultant pressure caused by the proximally transferred weight of the hand to the anterior forearm.

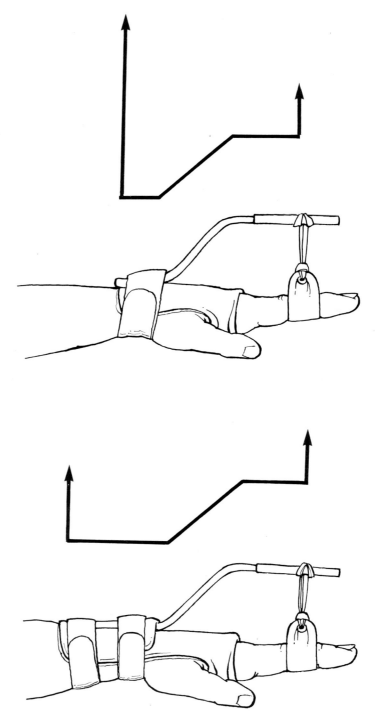

Fig. 5-13. An extended outrigger attachment length produces less leverage on the proximal bond or rivet (drawings to scale).

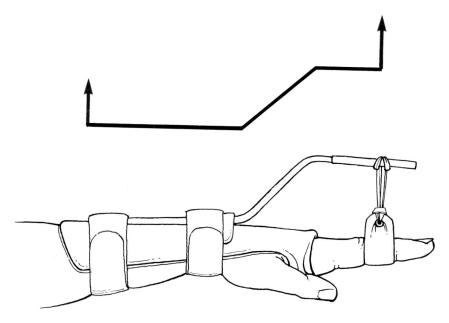

Fig. 5-13 cont'd. For legend see opposite page.

The preceding examples indicate the relative relationship between the length of the force arm and the length of the resistance arm, which is designated mechanical advantage (MA):

$$MA = \frac{\text{Force arm}}{\text{Resistance arm}}$$

In the previous examples, when the force arm was 8 inches, the mechanical advantage was 3.2, but the mechanical advantage was decreased to 1.6 when the forearm trough was shortened to 4 inches. Splints with greater mechanical advantage will produce less proximal force, resulting in diminished pressure and increased comfort.

Careful control of the force system between splint components will also augment the durability of splints. For example, consider the lever action of an outrigger on the proximal bond or rivet attaching the outrigger to the forearm trough. If the outrigger is viewed as a rigid first-class lever system, the amount of force generated on the proximal attachment may be computed for progressively increased attachment lengths when the resistance, resistance line of action, and resistance arm remain unchanged (Fig. 5-13). A longer force arm will result in a longer attachment bar and increased mechanical advantage, producing less force on the proximal bond and a stronger, more durable union of the two splint parts.

The combination of the first two mechanical principles supports the common experiential findings that long, wide splints are more comfortable and more durable than are short, narrow ones. When a segment is being splinted, the splint should extend approximately two thirds its length and be contoured to half its width.

Use optimum rotational force. The mobilization of stiffened joints through traction requires a thorough understanding of the resolution of forces to obtain optimum splint effectiveness without producing patient frustration or increased damage through joint compression or separation.

Theoretically any force applied to a bony segment to mobilize a joint may be resolved into a pair of concurrent rectangular components acting in definite directions. These two components consist of a rotational element producing joint rotation and a translational element producing joint distraction or compression (Fig. 5-14). As a force approximates a perpendicular angle to the segment being mobilized, the translational element is lessened and the rotational component increases until at 90 degrees the full magnitude of the force is applied in a rotational direction (Fig. 5-15). In practical terms this means that dynamic traction should be applied at a 90-degree angle to harness the force potential of the traction device without producing an unwanted pushing or pulling force on the articular surfaces of the involved joint. This also means that, as the passive range of motion of the joint begins to improve, the outrigger to which the traction device is attached must be adjusted to maintain the 90-degree angle (Fig. 5-16). In the case of multiple joint splinting, when motion limitations may not be the same, it may be necessary to provide one or more outrigger extensions for adjacent fingers to maintain the required 90-degree angle of pull (Fig. 5-17). Careful attention to the patient's complaints about the splint provide useful clues as to its mechanical function. If the patient observes that the finger cuffs tend to migrate distally or proximally on the fingers, a 90-degree angle probably has not been achieved or maintained.

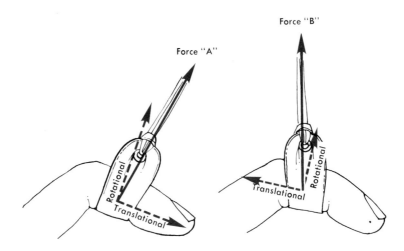

Fig. 5-14. Any force may be analyzed according to rotary and nonrotary components.

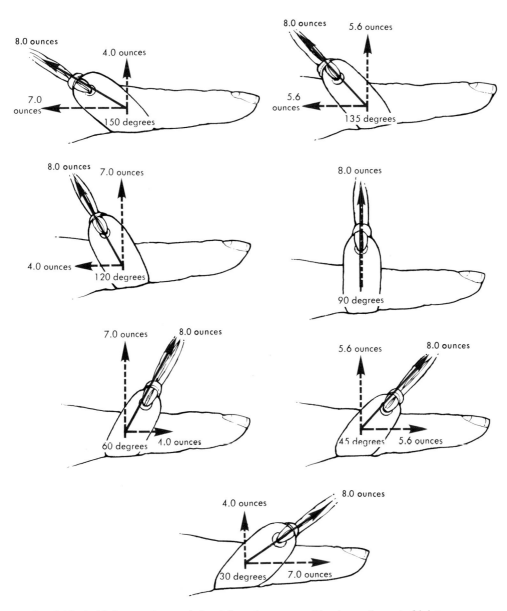

Fig. 5-15. At 90 degrees the translational force is zero, resulting in no element of joint compression or distraction. *Dotted lines,* Rotational force; *dashed lines,* translational force; *solid arrows,* traction assist force.

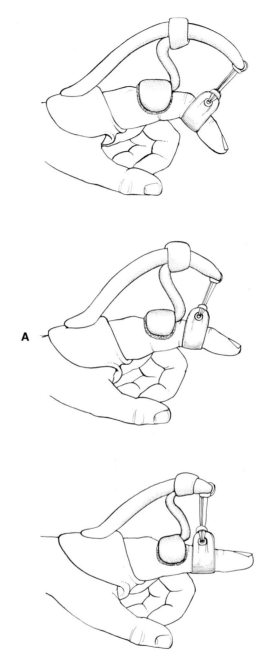

Fig. 5-16. A 90-degree angle of the dynamic assist to the mobilized segment must be maintained as passive joint motion changes. **A,** High profile. **B,** Low profile.

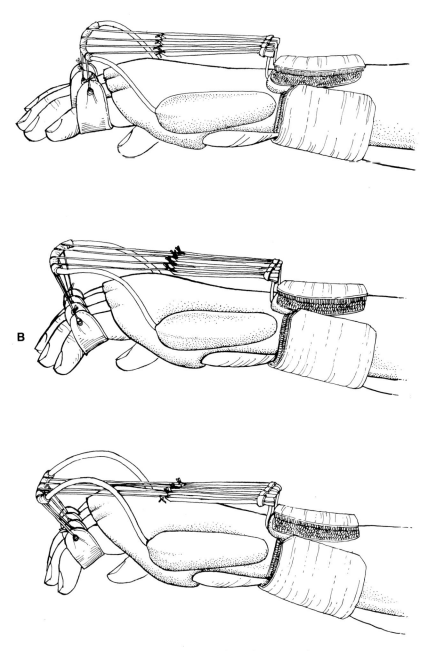

Fig. 5-16, cont'd. For legend see opposite page.

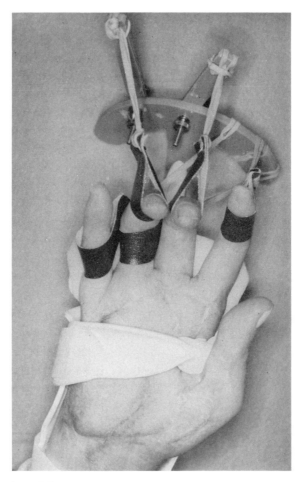

Fig. 5-17. Adaptation of the outrigger is often necessary to maintain a perpendicular pull on segments whose passive joint motions are dissimilar.

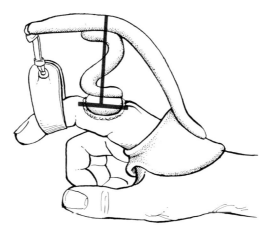

Fig. 5-18. A 90-degree angle of approach of a dorsal phalangeal bar to the proximal phalanx prevents proximal or distal migration of the bar.

In compound splint designs two rotational forces affect digital joint motion. While the dynamic assist applies force in one direction, the dorsal phalangeal bar (lumbrical bar) applies force in an opposite direction. Just as the dynamic assist must have a 90-degree angle of approach to the segment being mobilized, so must the dorsal phalangeal bar, but its force is instead directed to the proximal segment. Providing inelastic traction, the connector bar/dorsal phalangeal bar unit must have a 90-degree angle of approach to the segment being stabilized to be fully effective (Fig. 5-18). If a 90-degree angle of approach is not present, the dorsal phalangeal bar moves distally or proximally when the dynamic assist is attached to the finger and the patient uses his hand.

An analysis of the interaction between rotational and translational elements may also provide insight as to why some three-point pressure splints such as safety pins and joint jacks become clinically less effective as the flexion angle of the joint is increased (Fig. 5-19). Once again, clinical experience is verified by mechanical force assessment. Since the proximal and distal translational elements produce joint compression with resulting abatement of the rotational components, joint jacks and safety pin splints are more appropriately employed for flexion contractures of 35 degrees or less.

Consider the torque effect. Torque equals the product of the force times the length of the arm on which it acts ($T = F \times FA$). This concept is important in splinting because the amount of pull from a dynamic assist is not equal to the amount of rotational force or torque at the joint. The amount of torque depends on the distance between the joint axis and the point of attachment of the dynamic assist. The torque increases as the distance between the two increases if the applied force is held constant (Fig. 5-20). This explains why a patient may be able to tolerate a given amount of traction at one location

	A	**B**
	Parallel force system	Resolution of distal force

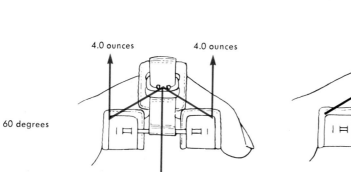

0 degrees

A: 4.0 ounces — 4.0 ounces — 8.0 ounces

B: 4.0 ounces

30 degrees

A: 4.0 ounces — 4.0 ounces — 8.0 ounces

B: 4.0 ounces — 3.99 ounces — 1.37 ounces

45 degrees

A: 4.0 ounces — 4.0 ounces — 8.0 ounces

B: 4.0 ounces — 3.63 ounces — 1.69 ounces

60 degrees

A: 4.0 ounces — 4.0 ounces — 8.0 ounces

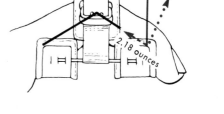

B: 4.0 ounces — 3.35 ounces — 2.18 ounces

Fig. 5-19. For legend see opposite page.

Fig. 5-19. While the magnitude of the parallel forces of a three-point pressure splint remain constant with the proximal interphalangeal joint in various degrees of flexion **(A),** the rotational and translational components of the proximal and distal forces (only distal end illustrated for simplicity) change until at 60 degrees the compression force (translational) on the joint is nearly two thirds that of the rotational force **(B).** Clinically this means that the greater the flexion deformity the less effective the splint becomes in its ability to correct the deficit. (Key: Dotted arrow = rotational force; dashed arrow = translational force; solid arrow = traction force.) (Special recognition to Kenneth Dunipace, Ph.D., Chairman of the Division of Engineering, Purdue University School of Engineering and Technology at Indianapolis for his assistance with the analysis of this splint.)

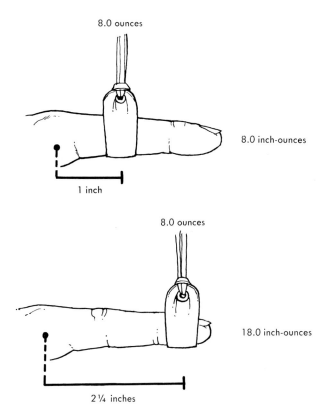

Fig. 5-20. As the distance between the joint axis and the point of attachment of the dynamic assist increases, the amount of torque on the joint increases.

but cannot tolerate the same amount when the attachment device is moved distally. Patients may be taught to use the torque phenomenon advantageously by advancing their finger cuffs distally as their pain tolerance permits. This must be done judiciously, however, since too much distal advancement may result in an inferior angle of the traction device or in attenuation of ligamentous structures.

Consider the relative degree of passive mobility of successive joints. When a force is exerted on a proximally based, multiarticular segment, all parts of the segment are moved in the direction of the force if motion of the successive joints is unimpaired. When motion is limited or stopped at a given articulation, the remaining mobile joints are moved in the direction of the force with minimal motion occurring at the restricted joint. In other words, when all joints within a longitudinal ray exhibit stiffness, they may be dynamically splinted in unison (Fig. 5-21). If an inequality of passive motion exists, the splint must be adapted to stabilize the normal joints within the segment, allowing the full magnitude of the traction to be directed toward the less mobile joints (Fig. 5-22). If these changes are not made, the rotational force is dissipated in unwanted motion at the mobile joints, resulting in potential damage to the normal joints and ineffective traction on the stiffened joints.

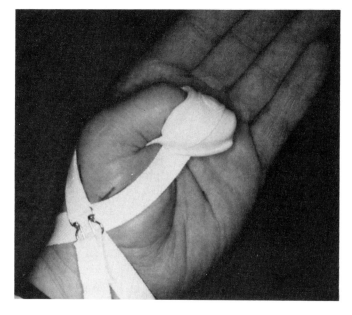

Fig. 5-21. A simple classification splint is appropriate when all joints involved have a similar passive range of motion.

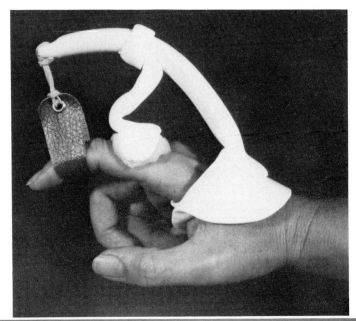

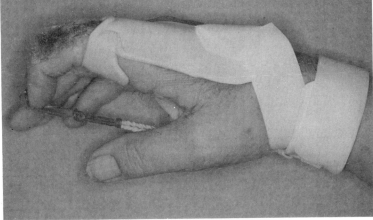

Fig. 5-22. A compound splint allows optimum mechanical purchase when joint motion is unequal within the longitudinal ray. The proximal segment is stabilized and the distal segment(s) receives the mobilizing force.

Consider the effects of reciprocal parallel forces. The use of three parallel forces in equilibrium as exemplified by a first-class lever system is basic to splinting of the hand, with the splint acting as the proximal and distal counterforces to the forces of the hand and forearm and a strap at the axis of the splinted segment providing the reciprocal middle force. In an analysis of the interrelationships of forces in a first-class lever system in equilibrium, the combined downward weights must be opposed by an equal upward force at the axis: A + B = C (Fig. 5-23). This means that the middle opposing force is of greater magnitude than the force at either the proximal or distal end of the splint. These reciprocal parallel forces form the basis for what is frequently termed *three-point fixation*. Since the middle force in splinting is frequently placed over a joint (Fig. 5-24), care should be taken to minimize the amount of pressure exerted on the underlying soft tissue. This can be accomplished by widening the area of force application.

Understanding parallel force systems also allows the accurate prediction of high-stress areas within the splint itself. Because the summation of the proximal and distal forces equals the middle opposite direction force, it becomes readily apparent why splints with wrist bars frequently become fatigued and fracture at the wrist, and outriggers break at the level of the proximal bend (Fig. 5-25). When the mechanical advantage (MA) is increased, the middle opposing force is decreased (Fig. 5-26). Anticipation of the greater magnitude of the middle force allows preventive measures to be taken during the design and construction phases. The forearm bar may be lengthened to decrease the force and the vulnerable area may be contoured or reinforced to increase the mechanical strength of the material.

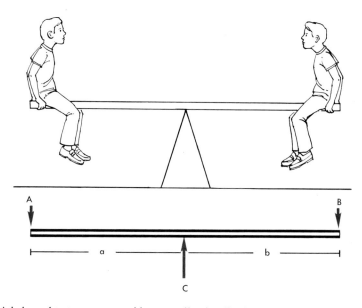

Fig. 5-23. A balanced teeter-totter provides an easily visualized representation of a first-class lever in equilibrium. The combined downward weights (*A* and *B*) must be opposed by an equal opposite force *(C)*.

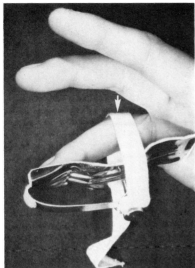

Fig. 5-24. If not monitored carefully, excessive pressure at the site of the middle opposing force *(arrow)* may cause soft tissue damage.

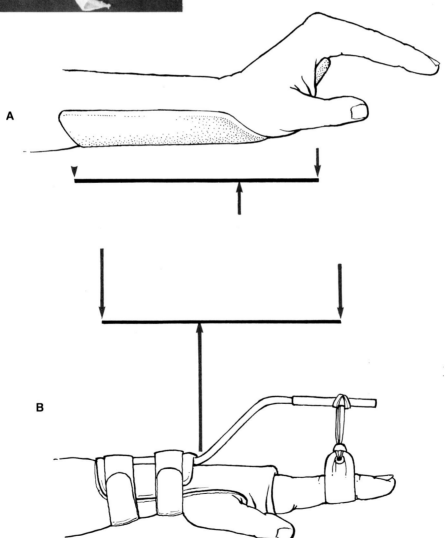

Fig. 5-25. Analyses of the parallel force systems present in a simple wrist extension splint **(A)** and a long finger extension splint **(B)** indicate the areas of greatest stress to be at the wrist and the proximal bend of the outrigger, respectively.

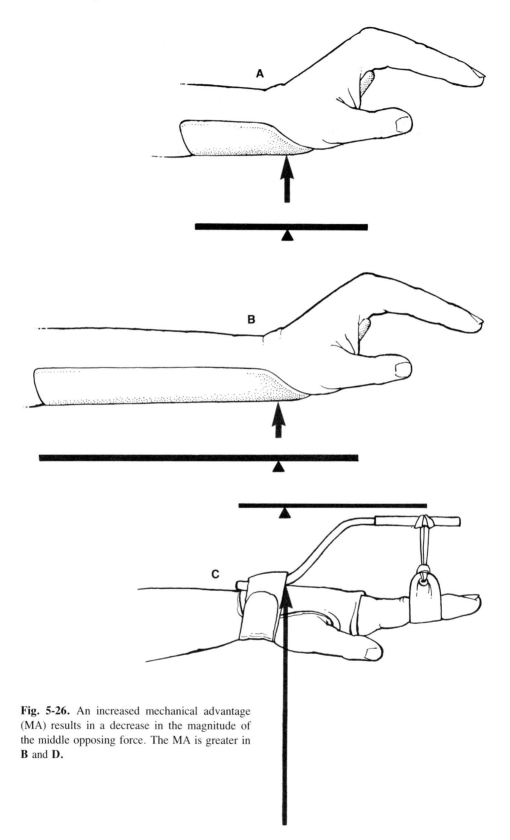

Fig. 5-26. An increased mechanical advantage (MA) results in a decrease in the magnitude of the middle opposing force. The MA is greater in **B** and **D.**

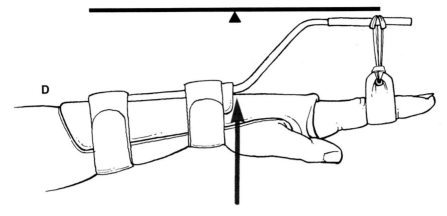

Fig. 5-26, cont'd. For legend see opposite page.

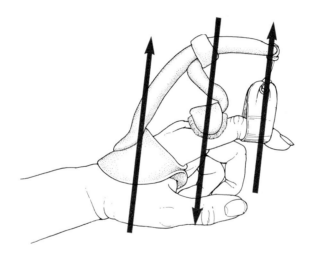

Fig. 5-27. Reciprocal parallel forces may be identified in this compound proximal interphalangeal extension splint.

Another example of reciprocal parallel forces is the force interrelationships within a dorsal outrigger with a dorsal phalangeal bar. The dorsal phalangeal bar provides a reciprocal middle force to the upward force at the proximal and distal ends of the splint (Fig. 5-27). The resulting downward force at the dorsal phalangeal bar is greater than the forces at either end of the splint, further explaining the clinical finding that pressure is consistently a problem under dorsal phalangeal bars and must be dealt with by good fit and dissemination of pressure through padding.

The concept of three-point reciprocal forces may be of further assistance in attempts to eliminate splint pressure over a given area. For example, the middle opposing force on a dorsal outrigger without a dorsal phalangeal bar occurs at the distal aspect of the dorsal metacarpal bar, resulting in downward force on the back of the hand. If splint pressure in this area were contraindicated due to edema, poor skin quality, or underlying

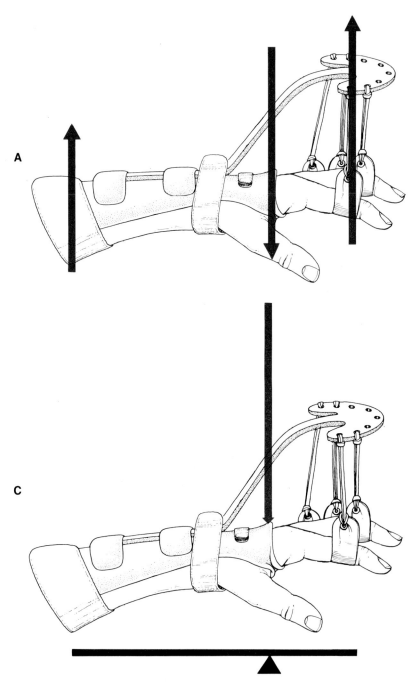

Fig. 5-28. Addition of a dorsal phalangeal bar changes the site of application of the middle opposing force **(A** and **B).** Because of an increased mechanical advantage, the force at the dorsal phalangeal bar is less than the force at the dorsal metacarpal bar **(C** and **D).**

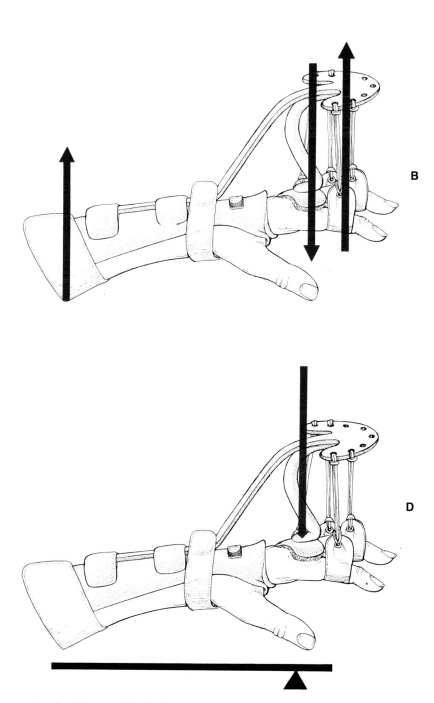

Fig. 5-28, cont'd. For legend see opposite page.

metacarpal fractures, the addition of a dorsal phalangeal bar would change the position of the middle reciprocal force to the dorsum of the proximal phalanx, resulting in rotation upward, away from the back of the hand by the dorsal metacarpal bar (Fig. 5-28, *A* and *B*). The addition of a dorsal phalangeal bar also increases the mechanical advantage of the splint and decreases the magnitude of the middle opposing force (Fig. 5-28, *C* and *D*).

Provide contour. The time-honored engineering principle of strength through contour is directly applicable to the design and construction of hand splints and is in many instances a concept that is concomitant with the previous consideration of force dissemination and use of leverage.

When a large force is placed on a flat, thin piece of material, the counterforce produced by the material is insufficient, and the material bends. If, however, the material is contoured into a half-cylinder shape, the material has, in mechanical terms, become stiffer (Fig. 5-29) and produces a greater counterforce, enabling the material to withstand greater forces without bending (Fig. 5-30).

In considering the design of a splint and the materials to be used, one must take care to match the design to the material properties. The low-temperature materials commonly used in physicians' offices and therapy departments for splint fabrication are easily bendable in sheet form, requiring splint designs that provide strength through contour. The thicker high-temperature plastics and specific metals conversely do not need the additional strength attained through material contour and are appropriate for the narrower bar type of splints. Outriggers may be constructed of either kind of material, but, if a low-temperature plastic substance is chosen, mechanical thickness is essential for strength in the form of either a hollow tube or solid coil (Fig. 5-31).

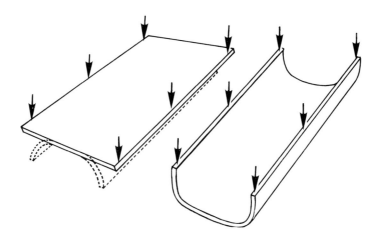

Fig. 5-29. Contour mechanically increases material strength.

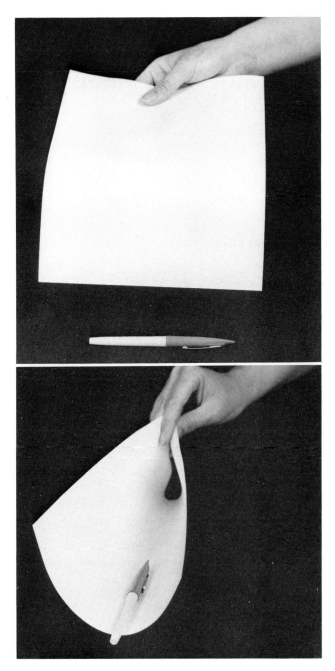

Fig. 5-30. A flat sheet of paper cannot hold the weight of a pen, but, when the paper is contoured into a partial cylinder shape, the pen is supported.

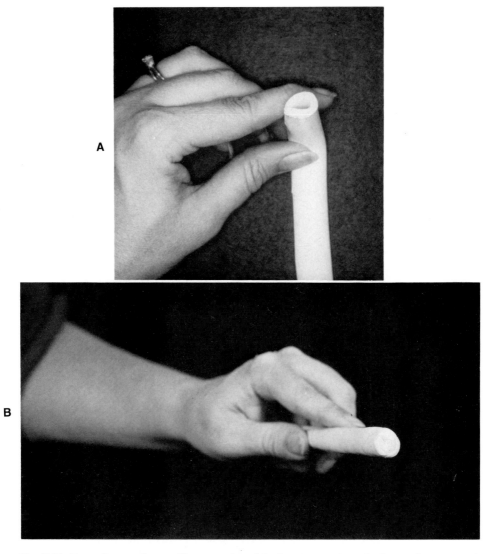

Fig. 5-31. Depending on the specific properties of the low-temperature plastic, outrigger strength may be increased by forming a tube (**A**) or solid coil (**B**).

Eliminate friction. Kinetic friction occurs when surfaces in contact with each other move relative to one another. If a difference in density exists between the surfaces, the harder surface may begin to erode the softer, less dense surface. If the surfaces are similar, damage may occur on either side or on both sides.

Clinically kinetic friction may occur between the splint and the extremity or between contiguous cutaneous surfaces. In either case it may result in skin irritation, blistering, and eventual breakdown. Friction caused by a splint usually indicates poor fit, improper joint alignment, or inefficient fastening devices. Friction between cutaneous surfaces such as adjacent digits may often be abated by interposing a layer of gauze bandage between the two surfaces. Steps should be taken to alleviate the frictional problem at the first sign of cutaneous embarrassment, since, if the device is left unattended, prolonged trauma to the skin may render the extremity refractory to further splinting efforts until healing occurs.

Avoid high shear stress.* To begin, it is necessary to define a few important terms that describe the material behavior of soft tissues.

1. *Force* is a vector and therefore has a magnitude, direction, and point of application. It changes the direction and/or velocity of objects, and when applied to a surface, forces result in deformation of solid or semisolid substances.

2. *Strain* is a measure of the deformation of a material. It is defined as a ratio of the change in a reference length (gauge length) to the original length. Overall, or average, strain can be measured as can local strain (Fig. 5-32). These two are equal only in special circumstances. If the two points defining the gauge length are extremely close, strain can be thought of as varying from point to point within a material. Because it is a ratio, it is used instead of absolute displacement.

---

*Written and researched by David E. Thompson, Ph.D., Professor of Mechanical Engineering, Louisiana State University, Baton Rouge.

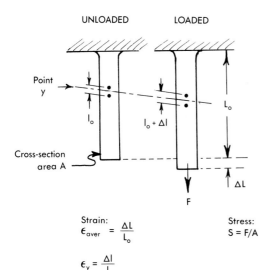

Fig. 5-32. Pictorial definition of stain in materials.

Strain:
$$\epsilon_{aver} = \frac{\Delta L}{L_o}$$

$$\epsilon_y = \frac{\Delta l}{l}$$

Stress:
$$S = F/A$$

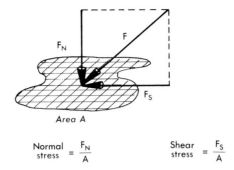

Normal stress $= \dfrac{F_N}{A}$ Shear stress $= \dfrac{F_S}{A}$

Fig. 5-33. Pictorial definition of normal and shear stress at a surface.

3. *Stress* describes the distribution of forces on the surface or within a material (Fig. 5-33). Force can be thought of as having both a normal component (perpendicular to the surface) and a shear component (parallel to or tangent to the surface). If these components are divided by the area over which they act, the ratios define normal and shear stresses. Although stress is defined at the surface of an object, stresses can be thought of as existing within the material as well.

Stress is a more meaningful term than just force. For example, if one pushes a finger onto the point of a tack with a force of 5 pounds, it will puncture the skin. However, the same force applied over one square inch will cause only a small indentation.

Normal stresses are usually termed pressure or tensile stresses. At a point within a substance, these stresses act equally in all directions. In a simple diagram of stress applied to a rectangular element (Fig. 5-34), the elements remain rectangular, even though they deform. High normal stresses are required to cause damage to soft tissues. Brand (1975) states that pressures in excess of 200 psi are required for single loads to cause damage to soft tissues, but in all probability the real damage to the tissues comes from shear and not pressure effects.

Modulus of elasticity. By plotting the normal stress within a test sample (Fig. 5-35) versus the resulting overall strain, engineers learn a great deal about the test material. For materials like steel, the slope of this curve is termed its modulus of elasticity. It is a measure of the stiffness of the material. Other materials, like aluminum, collagen fibers, and skin, have no linear relationship and may or may not be so simply characterized. In this case, engineers use the term *apparent modulus of elasticity* defined as the stress divided by the total strain. For soft tissues, there is a large region where the material deforms readily at very low stresses (Markenscoff, 1979; Sakata, 1972). The apparent elastic modulus is very low in this region. As the tissues reach high strains, however, the stress required to achieve additional strain rises markedly, and the apparent elastic modulus rises concomitantly.

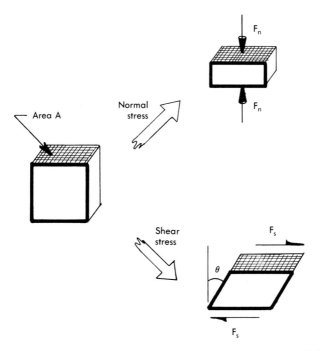

Fig. 5-34. The effects of normal and shear stress on an internal element within a material.

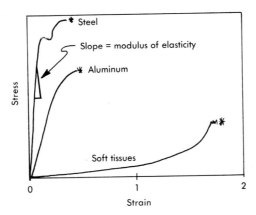

Fig. 5-35. Stress-strain relationships for steel, aluminum, and soft tissues. The vertical scale for the steel and aluminum curves has been altered to allow them to be included. Typical maximum stresses for steel are around 150,000 psi, compared with 300 psi for soft tissues.

Shear stresses, unlike normal stresses, are directional. Within a two-dimensional slice of material, their direction of action is defined in terms of the rotational direction of an element. As shown in Fig. 5-34, the rectangular elements have deformed in a clockwise manner into diamond shapes, and the resulting forces within the material are high. For soft tissues, this results in damage at much lower stress levels than for pure normal stress acting alone.

Shear modulus. There is an equivalent modulus to the elastic modulus, which defines a material's ability to resist shear stress instead of normal stress. This is the shear modulus, defined in terms of the shear stress divided by the angle of deformation of the rectangular elements (Fig. 5-34).

Stress concentrations (scar, changes in elastic modulus). A critical factor that is often overlooked in managing soft tissues relates to the mechanical properties of the tissues and any factors that cause dramatic variations in these properties. Scar tissue is extremely rigid and noncompliant in comparison with normal, healthy soft tissue. When tissue is loaded in the presence of either an internal or external scar, property variation results in a concentration of stresses where there are dramatic *spatial variations* in the strain or deformation in the region of the scar. An identical effect occurs where the applied loads change rapidly across a surface and large strain gradients result. Murphy (1971) discusses these and other effects.

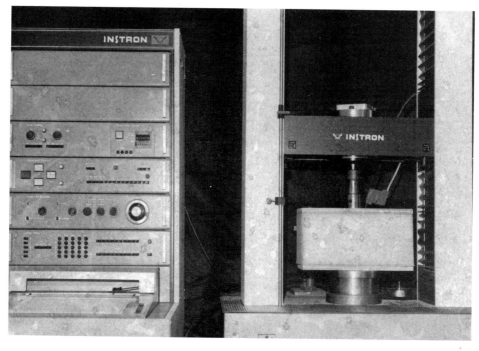

Fig. 5-36. The experimental setup showing the Instron testing machine with the foam test specimen in place.

An experimental demonstration. To illustrate the behavior of soft tissues, three simple experiments are included here. They use a 5 × 12 × 2-inch foam test sample mounted in an Instron materials testing machine. A sample was ruled with horizontal and vertical lines spaced ¼ inch apart to produce a grid of squares on the entire face. A piece of ¾-inch plywood was glued to the bottom of the specimen to distribute the loading uniformly along this edge (Fig. 5-36).

In the first test a smaller piece of wood was placed on the top surface, and the sample was loaded as shown in Fig. 5-37. At high loads the resulting strains and the distribution of shear and normal stresses are depicted graphically in their effects on the small squares on the specimen. In region *A*, the deformation of the squares is due to pure normal stress. The diamond-shaped squares in region *B* attest to the high shear produced in this region. It must be noted that this region is below the surface of the specimen and even outside of the area beneath the upper plywood loading bar. The shear in this region is due to the sudden change in the pressure at the surface of the specimen. Bennett (1971) demonstrated this edge effect mathematically.

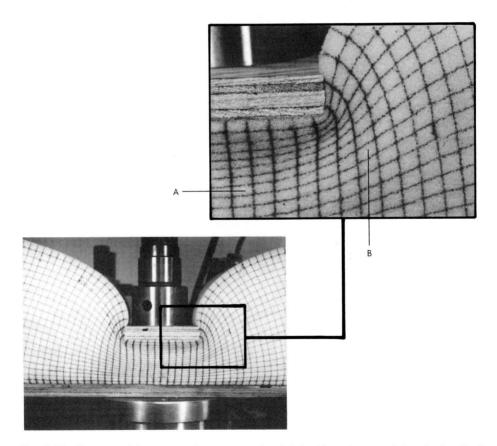

Fig. 5-37. Close-up of the test specimen at a strain of 0.5 with an inset depicting the localized effects of shear stress resulting in diamond-shaped elements.

When loaded uniformly in a second test (Fig. 5-38), no shear is produced anywhere within the specimen.

In the third test a small piece of harder rubber was inserted into the foam (Fig. 5-39). This was done to simulate a scar deep within the tissues. When the load was applied, the elements nearer the surface deformed more than the deeper structures. This is characteristic of soft tissues because of their nonlinear stress-strain relationship. Shear production can be seen around the edge of the loading bar and also around the edges of the simulated scar.

Discussion. According to Brand (1975), the human body responds to mechanical stress in one of three ways. If the stress is within acceptable limits, the tissues hypertrophy and become more robust in tolerating additional stress. If the stresses are very low,

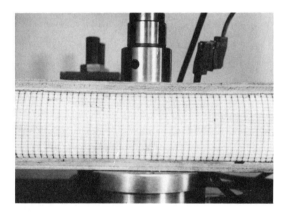

Fig. 5-38. Close-up of the test specimen with uniform loading at the same strain as in Fig. 5-37.

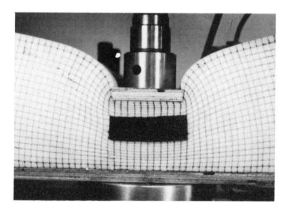

Fig. 5-39. Close-up of the test specimen with a simulated scar consisting of a hard rubber insert located deep within the specimen. The overall strain is the same as in the two previous figures.

the tissues atrophy and become more fragile. If the loads are excessive, however, the tissues break down and may ulcerate. If the tissues are then rested so they can heal, scarring results. Scar tissues create an environment where stresses are concentrated and further breakdown is more likely. It is therefore more appropriate to prevent scar altogether than to attempt to protect tissues after they have failed (Brand, 1975; Hampton, 1979).

If one examines the skin around the border of the heel and great toe, it is possible to see the body's response to shear stress resulting from a sudden change in normal stress. The pressures arising during gait are high in the regions immediately under the heel and great toe (Bauman, 1963), but they fall to zero as one moves around and out from under the weight-bearing areas. This rapid variation in pressure gives rise to shear, much the same as in the test shown in region *B* of Fig. 5-37. The buildup of callus in these regions is a direct response to shear stress and underscores its importance in the care and management of soft tissues.

The general principles of the application of mechanical stress to soft tissues are summarized as follows:

1. Avoid high pressure areas by spreading the stresses in space. This involves large surface areas. In all cases, the splint and/or padding should conform as closely as possible to the contours of the surface of the hand to afford the greatest possible contact area.

2. Avoid high shear effects by rounding sharp edges and keeping pressures low. In Fig. 5-4 the "incorrect" method shown not only produces large pressures, it creates extremely large shear stresses. The shear effects are amplified by any motion of the bar relative to the finger. The rolled edges of the splint shown in Fig. 5-2 reduce the shear effects caused by the sudden change in pressure at the edge of the splint.

3. Reduce the peak levels by spreading them out in time. Using protective materials has the effect of ameliorating pressure peaks caused by accidental bumping of splints on solid immovable objects. Increasing the thickness of the protective material will continue to spread the stresses in both space and time, but above a certain thickness this is impractical because it also causes instability and allows misalignment of the splint.

4. Beware of the effects of repetitive stresses. The damage to soft tissues is cumulative, and breakdown will occur more readily in regions already involved in an inflammatory response to mechanical trauma (Thompson, 1983).

• • •

The experimental work for this section on shear was done at the National Hansen's Disease Center, Carville, La., and the analysis of the results was accomplished in the Computer Graphics Research and Applications Laboratory at Louisiana State University, Baton Rouge. The funding for this research was provided by the U.S. Public Health Service, Department of Health and Human Services, under research contract 240-83-0060.

SUMMARY

Initially the clinician engaged in the preparation of hand splints may consider the mechanical principles of splinting to be technically difficult and not truly germane to the clinical situation. Nonetheless, it is extremely important that the general principles be learned and reviewed to ensure that the finished product is more than an accumulation of the splint maker's experience through numerous inefficient, nonproductive trials. The mathematic details of mechanical engineering or bioengineering are not essential to the basic conceptual understanding of the mechanics of splint design and preparation. A concentrated effort to understand the principles described in this chapter combined with periodic review as experience is gained will pay large dividends in the ultimate performance of a splint.

CHAPTER 6

Principles of using dynamic assists for mobilization

Identify optimum force magnitude parameters.
Identify optimum torque parameters.
Correlate physical properties of the dynamic assist with patient requirements.
Correlate physical properties of the dynamic assist with the design of the splint.
Consider the principles of mechanics and fit.
Control and maintain force magnitude.

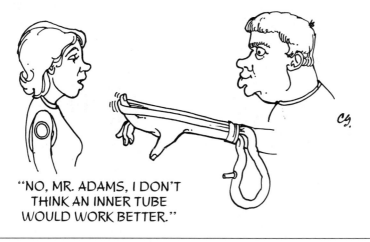

"NO, MR. ADAMS, I DON'T THINK AN INNER TUBE WOULD WORK BETTER."

Hand splints that are designed to increase or substitute for motion use carefully directed forces to correct or control joints limited by stiffness or loss of active power. Regardless of their external configuration, these splints must have a means of generating forces sufficient to apply prolonged gentle pull to stiffened joints in order to influence collagen alignment or to move passively supple joints through arcs of functional motion. Excluding serial splints, which rely on frequent alterations or replacements to improve

163

articular motion, mobilizing forces in splinting are produced by specialized components called *dynamic assists*. Providing elastic, inelastic, or spring traction, dynamic assists may be constructed of a variety of materials possessing considerably different physical properties (Fig. 6-1). A well-functioning dynamic assist should generate a consistent and controlled force, should conform to the splint design, and should be adapted to meet the unique requirements of the patient. Mechanical and fit principles, including angle of approach, torque, pressure, friction, and ligamentous stress must also be considered when fitting these components to a disabled hand. Dynamic assists are the fuel or power for mobilization splints; therefore it is essential that the criteria for and ramifications of using these components be thoroughly understood by all those involved in the rehabilitation process. Lack of knowledge may result in either an ineffective splint or a splint that actually causes damage to the hand. Too much force, torque, or pressure may cause additional inflammation, scarring, and deformity, and too little force or a poorly chosen material or design may actually prevent the patient from reaching full rehabilitative potential.

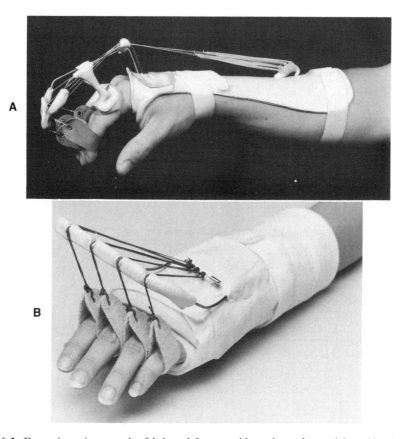

Fig. 6-1. Dynamic assists may be fabricated from a wide variety of materials: rubber band **(A)**, and elastic thread **(B)**. **(B** courtesy Barbara Allen, O.T.R./L., Oklahoma City.)

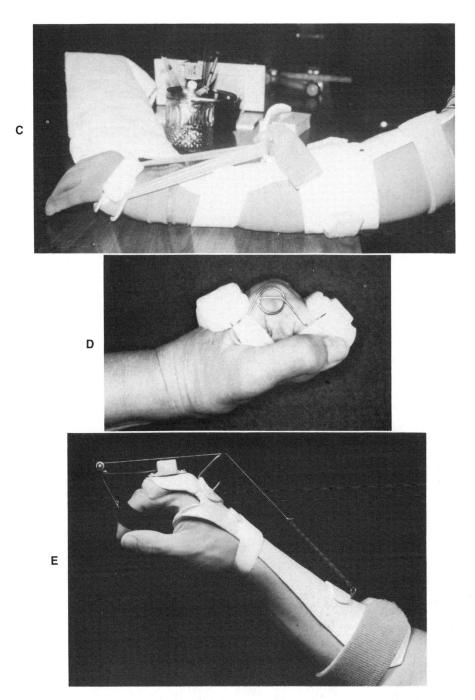

Fig. 6-1, cont'd. Dynamic assists may be fabricated from a wide variety of materials: Theraband **(C)**, spring coil **(D)**, and springs **(E)**. (**C** courtesy Robin Miller Wagman, O.T.R./L., Ft. Lauderdale, FL.) *Continued.*

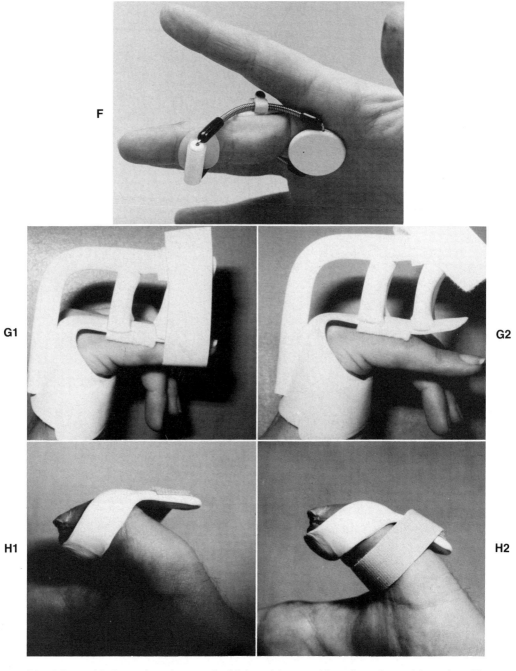

Fig. 6-1, cont'd. Dynamic assists may be fabricated from a wide variety of materials: springs (**F**) and Velcro (**G** and **H**). (**F** courtesy Renske Houck-Romkes, O.T., Rotterdam, Netherlands; **G** courtesy Janet Bailey, O.T.R./L., Columbus, OH; **H** courtesy Susan Glaser-Morales, O.T.R., Virginia Beach, VA.)

The purpose of this chapter is to discuss those principles which govern the use of dynamic assists, including identification of optimal force and torque magnitudes, physical properties of assist materials, correlation to patient requirements and splint design, and concepts from the principles of mechanics and fit.

Identify optimum force magnitude parameters. When discussing dynamic assists and the forces they impart, it is important to understand the fundamental differences between a splint designed to substitute for absent or weak active motion and a splint that corrects passive motion limitations. A substitution splint is applied to a passively supple hand, requiring a force that is just sufficient to pull or push the splinted segment into predetermined alignment. Due to the presence of normal passive motion, determination of the amount of force to use is not imperative. The dynamic assist is simply adjusted until the desired position is achieved (Fig. 6-2). This, however, cannot be done with splints designed to correct fixed articular deformities. Because of the *lack* of normal passive motion, knowledge of the magnitude of the force generated by the dynamic assist is critical when applying a corrective splint. Regardless of the force used, the segment cannot readily be brought into alignment without disrupting tissue continuity. The key, therefore, is to provide enough tension to control collagen alignment and to stimulate tissue growth. Too much force will cause damage, escalating the inflammatory response and scar formation, while too little will not effect joint motion.

Just how much force is required to influence growth and collagen alignment without causing additional tissue damage? Although this question seems elemental, and a few researchers and hand specialists have tried to define the parameters of splinting forces, quantitative statistical data are almost nonexistent in the literature. Some authors have correlated lack of skin blanching or no increase in joint inflammation with appropriate splinting forces, and others have attempted to apply numerical values to better define force magnitude. Delineating the important interrelationship between magnitude and time, Kosiak (1959) found that the amount of pressure causing damage in laboratory animals was related to a combination of force and duration. Based on experience, Malick (1974) used 0.5 pound of force to illustrate her splint manual; in 1978 and again in

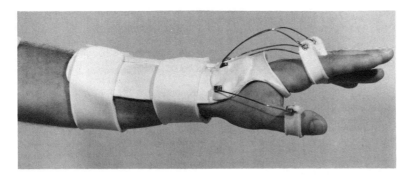

Fig. 6-2. Dynamic assist force measurements are not necessary for substitution splints because normal passive range of motion is present. (Courtesy Christine Heaney, B.Sc., O.T., Ottawa, Ontario.)

1985 Brand recommended splinting forces ranging between 100 and 300 gm. Pearson (1978) noted that joint deformity could be corrected with as little as 3 ounces of rubber band traction, and Fess, Gettle, and Strickland (1981) used 8 ounces of force to describe resolution of forces and the need for a 90-degree angle of approach of traction used in hand splinting. Despite these attempts, most clinicians currently rely on feel to judge the amount of force they apply to the hand.

Therapists' abilities to select rubber band tensions. Recognizing that most splints are fitted without measuring assist force, Fess (1984) assessed the abilities of 47 therapists (36 Registered Occupational Therapists, 3 Registered Physical Therapists, and 8 Occupational Therapy Students) to select rubber band tensions. Clinical experience of the therapists ranged from none to 18 years; hours spent in academic splinting class ranged from none to more than 40 hours; and 24 of the 47 subjects reported that they considered themselves specialists in hands. The average number of splints made per subject ranged from 0 to more than 20 per week; and of total patient loads the percent of hands treated ranged from 0% to 100%. Of those who considered themselves specialists in hands, experienced ranged from none to 17 years in hand rehabilitation.

Using a standard set of instructions, subjects selected rubber band tensions appropriate to two case histories from two tension adjustment frames (Fig. 6-3). The case histories involved two proximal interphalangeal joint flexion deformities of 50°/90° of left index fingers, one acute (6 weeks) and one chronic (6 months). The splints pictured in the two case histories were of identical design (Fig. 6-4). To ascertain the reliability of the therapists' skills, subjects chose their rubber band tensions from two frames, which were identical except for the color of the top surface and the number of rubber band choices. The blue frame allowed nine options of randomly weighted rubber bands in 50 gm increments; the yellow frame had five options of randomly arranged bands in 100 gm increments (Fig. 6-5). Band tensions were obtained by attaching standardized brass weights to high-quality no. 33 rubber bands (Fig. 6-6), which had been checked for consistency of length. Tensions in both frames ranged from 100 to 500 gm.

Subjects were asked to read the first case history, select and record the number of an appropriate tension from the blue frame, and then (without returning to the blue frame) select and record the same tension on the yellow frame. The same format was then used for the second case history. Statistical instruments used to analyze the data included frequency distributions, mean, median, and mode, score range, standard deviation from ungrouped data, standard error of difference between means, and probability.

Results indicated that of the four major groups tested—(1) students, (2) not specialists in hands, (3) specializing in hands but not members of the American Society of Hand Therapists (ASHT), and (4) members of ASHT—no statistical differences were found between the 50 gm increment frame and the 100 gm increment frame for both flexion deformities. Therapists at all levels of experience were capable of identifying a rubber band tension and replicating that tension in a second set of rubber band options ($p < .05$).

For three of the four groups tested it was found that therapists applied less force to the acute flexion deformity than they did to the chronic deformity. This was found to

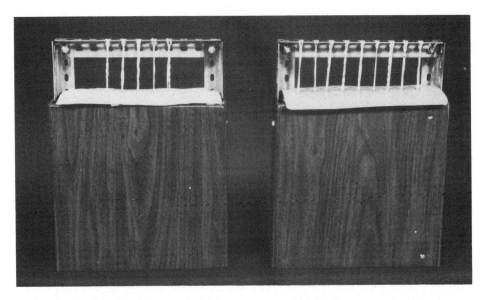

Fig. 6-3. In accord with two case histories, therapists selected rubber band tensions from two tension adjustment frames.

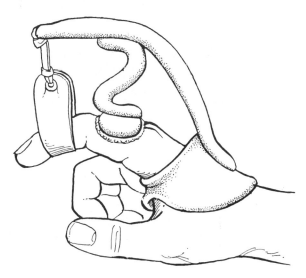

Fig. 6-4. The splints described in the case histories were identical for both the chronic and acute injury.

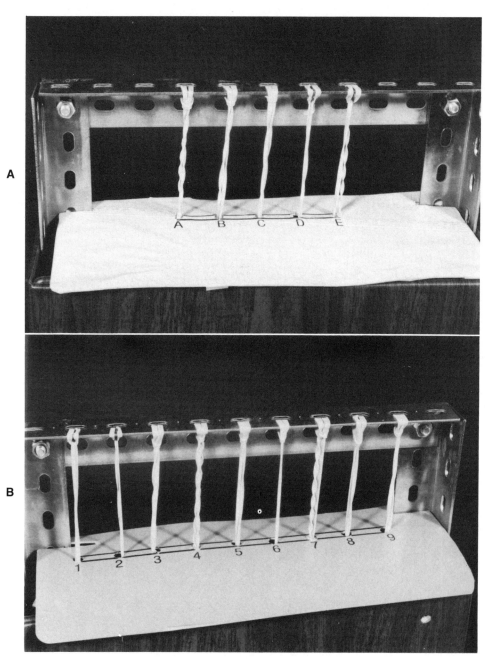

Fig. 6-5. To test selection reliability, rubber bands were randomly arranged in 100 gm (**A**) and 50 gm (**B**) increments.

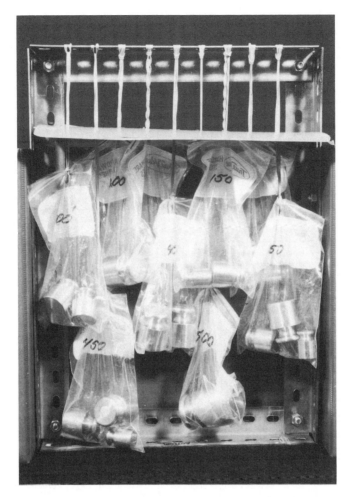

Fig. 6-6. Standard brass weights were attached to no. 33 high-quality rubber bands and suspended from the tension adjustment frames.

be statistically significant in the ASHT group and the "not specialized" group. Students did not alter the forces when treating the acute and chronic cases.

Variables that were found to correlate positively with lighter tension selections (Fig. 6-7) included (1) a 91% to 100% case load of hand patients; (2) six or more hand splints made per week; (3) 6 or more years specializing in hands; and (4) member of ASHT. Of this group mean tension selections ranged from 164.3 to 197.5 gm (5.8 to 7.0 ounces) for the acute proximal interphalangeal flexion deformity, and 265.0 to 293.8 gm (9.4 to 10.4 ounces) for the chronic proximal interphalangeal flexion deformity.

Those variables which did not correlate with lighter tension selections included years of experience other than hands, hours spent in academic splint class, a case load of up to 30% hand problems, not specializing in hands, and students. Interestingly, stu-

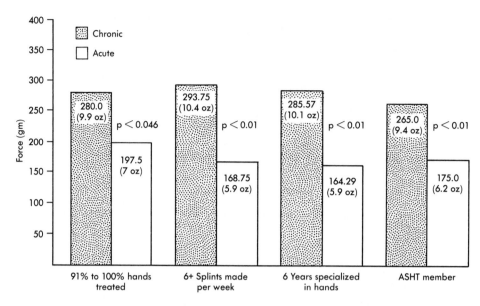

Fig. 6-7. Statistically significant positive correlations were found between four variables and lighter rubber band tension selections.

dents and less experienced therapists almost universally selected greater tensions than did the more experienced hand specialists. In other words, if a mistake was made, it was most often made in the direction of applying too much tension rather than too little.

In conclusion, this investigation indicates that experienced hand specialists alter their rubber band tensions according to diagnosis. These selections are not haphazard, but instead can be replicated at a statistically significant level. And, verifying some of the parameters suggested in the literature, the overall magnitude of tension used ranged from 164 to 294 gm, depending on the acuteness of the injury.

Appropriate boundaries. Although the research just cited needs to be further correlated with clinical studies, a general concept of the ''safe boundaries'' of the force magnitude required to influence tissue growth and collagen alignment, as identified by highly experienced hand specialists, begins to emerge. These parameters may be used as a standard with which any type of dynamic assist component affecting the small joints of the hand may be compared and evaluated, whether possessing elastic, inelastic, or spring wire properties. Further investigation needs to be undertaken to determine whether this tension range is effective for larger joints such as the elbow or for more complicated articulations such as those found in the wrist.

Identify optimum torque magnitude parameters. While knowledge of force magnitude is fundamental to good splint fabrication and fit, it is not the only important factor in understanding the complex mechanical interrelationships involved in mobilizing a joint through prolonged gentle traction. The point on the finger at which the rotational force is applied is also an essential factor. In the previous section, an optimal range of forces was identified, but are these parameters applicable to all splinting situations? In other words, how may the concepts of the above study may be expanded to apply to other splint designs that direct corrective forces to different levels of a finger? The answer is through torque measurements. Torque acts as a common denominator for interpreting the mechanical stresses of rotational force placed on a given joint at different levels of a digit. As described in Chapter 5, torque is defined as the product of the amount of rotational force and the perpendicular distance between the axis of joint rotation and the force line of action, or torque equals force times distance (T = FD). For example, a force of 200 gm placed 2 cm, 4 cm, and 6 cm, away from a joint would result in torque measurements of 400 gm/cm, 800 gm/cm, and 1200 gm/cm, respectively. A splinting force that is appropriate at one level may not be appropriate at another. The "safe boundaries" of force described in the previous section were derived from a study involving deformities at the proximal interphalangeal joint and an application of rotational force to the midportion of the middle phalanx, a distance of approximately 1 cm from the joint axis. What then, are appropriate forces proximal and distal to this point, and what are force parameters for the metacarpophalangeal and distal interphalangeal joints? To date there are no published research studies specifically addressing these issues, but if one assumes that forces similar to those defined for the proximal interphalangeal joint would be applicable to the metacarpophalangeal and distal interphalangeal joints, "safe boundaries" of force may be deduced through torque parameters for each joint of a finger. The previously defined force range of 164 grams-294 grams may be converted into torque measurements by multiplying each by 1 cm, resulting in a torque margin of safety of 164 cm/gm to 294 cm/gm. Utilizing these torque parameters as standards, safe force magnitudes may be equated for various distances from a joint axis by applying the basic torque formula (164 cm/gm = F · D; 294 cm/gm = F · D):

Distance from axis (cm)	"Safe force boundaries" (gm)
1	164-295
2	82-147
3	55-98
4	41-74
5	33-59
6	27-49
7	23-42
8	21-37

These forces may in turn be applied to each of the three joints of a finger (Fig. 6-8). Although these force parameters may not be considered absolute without further research, it is graphically apparent that there is no single force or force range that is appropriate for all splinting needs. Forces for correction of joint deformity are directly related to the distance between the point of force application and the axis of rotation of the joint being mobilized: the greater the distance, the less the force required. Torque also allows comparison of forces imparted by prefabricated splints of differing sizes (Fig. 6-9). Representing the actual amount of stress applied to a joint, the determination

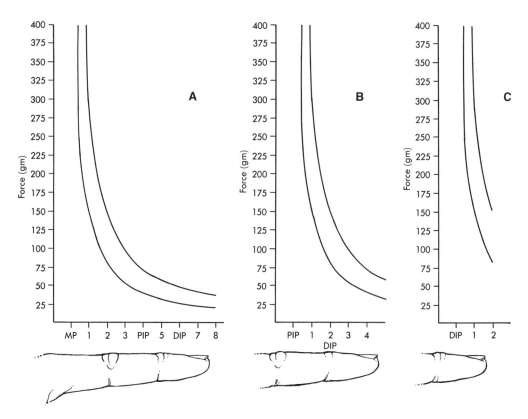

Fig. 6-8. Using torque parameters, "safe boundaries" for different levels of force application may be computed for the metacarpophalangeal (**A**), proximal interphalangeal (**B**), and distal interphalangeal (**C**) joints.

of torque magnitude parameters is essential to understanding and utilizing prolonged gentle traction for mobilization of stiffened digital joints.

Correlate physical properties of the dynamic assist with patient requirements. The physical properties of the material making up a dynamic assist regulates the range of forces it generates. For example, rubber bands of a given size and quality produce a fairly predictable force spectrum, whereas spring coil assists produce another range of forces. Unfortunately, however, not all coil splints create similar tensions, nor do rubber band components. Even among assists made of similar substances, variables such as shelf life and quality may alter the amount of force created. Durability must also be considered. An assist that requires frequent adjustments to keep it within the required force parameters creates more work for the therapist and unnecessary inconvenience and expense for the patient. To increase patients' opportunities to achieve their full rehabilitative potentials, those responsible for fabricating mobilizing splints should be well acquainted with the basic similarities and differences of the many materials currently available to generate forces in the form of dynamic assist components.

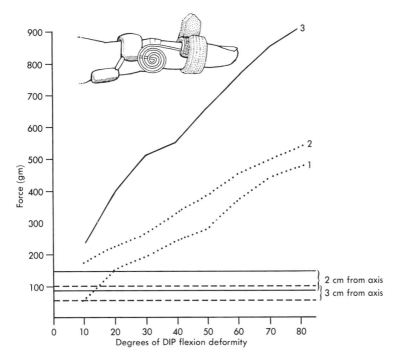

Fig. 6-9. Although not representative of all splints of this design, these commercially available spring coil splints produced excessive force measurements. Splints 1 and 2 apply force 3 cm from the proximal interphalangeal joint axis of rotation; and 3, 2 cm from the axis. Splint 1 meets "safe force" criteria (parallel horizontal solid and dotted lines) for a flexion deformity ranging between 10 and 15 degrees.

As described by Brand (1985) one may identify the conditions at which dynamic assists produce optimal ranges of tension by plotting their reactions to progressive loading on length-tension curves. These graphic representations are invaluable in understanding why, when, and how mobilizing splints work.

Rubber band tensions are directly influenced by length and thickness of the bands. If two rubber bands of the same length but with differing thicknesses are subjected to similar loads, the narrower of the two bands elongates more quickly with less tension but is not as durable in splinting situations (Fig. 6-10). Force ranges are also influenced by the quality of the rubber bands (Fig. 6-11).

The forces produced by spring coil splints are regulated by the thickness and resiliency of the wire, the size of coils, and the distance from the coil to the distal end of the splint. Larger wire diameters, tighter coils, and longer distances generate greater forces. Longer and larger diameter spring wire splints follow a similar pattern.

Like those for rubber bands, length tension curves for springs vary according to the properties of the materials from which the springs are made. Tracking a more linear pattern than rubber bands, some springs may double or triple their resting length with

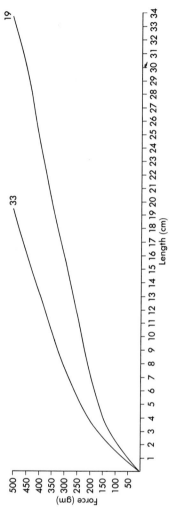

Fig. 6-10. Rubber band thickness influences length tension and durability. Comparison of identical resting length rubber bands indicates that the thinner bands (*19*) elongate more quickly with less force than do the heavier bands (*33*).

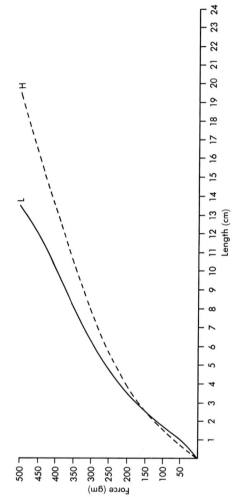

Fig. 6-11. High quality rubber bands (*H*) stretch more with less force than do lower quality bands of the same size (*L*).

minimal to moderate increases in force, while others quickly exceed safe force parameters with very little change in length (Fig. 6-12). Springs are often more durable than rubber bands and shelf life is excellent.

Other materials such as elastic thread, Exer-tubing, orthodontic elastics, Velcro, and cotton webbing exhibit widely differing force tension curves (Fig. 6-13).

Since the physical properties of a dynamic assist influence durability and regulate the amount of tension produced, the choice of material comprising the assist is extremely important and should be carefully coordinated to meet the individual needs of the patient. For example, if a splint is needed to correct a 30-degree flexion contracture of a proximal interphalangeal joint, none of the spring coil splints illustrated in Fig.

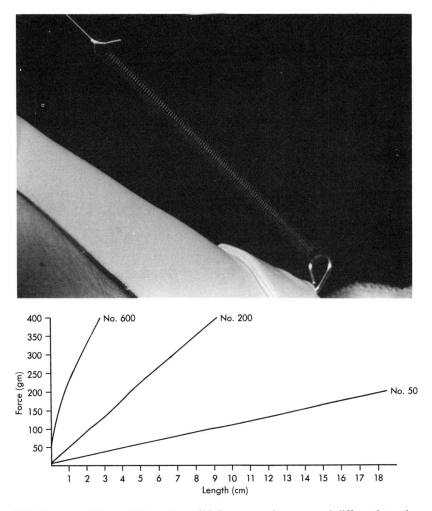

Fig. 6-12. These no. 50, no. 200, and no. 600 Scomac springs respond differently to the application of increasingly greater forces.

6-9 would produce appropriate forces, but elastic traction in the form of rubber bands or Exer-tubing cut to given lengths could be used. Cotton webbing or Velcro could provide inelastic traction when tightened to specific tensions and should also be considered.

Correlate physical properties of the dynamic assist with the design of the splint. Splint design also influences the type of dynamic assist that may be used. Because of their physical properties, some materials may not be compatible with certain splint designs. For example, a dynamic assist that requires length to generate appropriate force parameters would probably have limited effectiveness with a hand-based splint design simply because of the relative shortness of the splint. Because of inherent mechanical bias, some splints and assist components are more effective under specific conditions. For example, a three-point pressure splint, such as the commercially available safety pin splint that utilizes a Velcro or webbing assist to generate force, would not be effective in correcting a 45° flexion deformity. In this instance it is not the material from which the assist is made that is the problem, but rather the design of the splint itself. Mechanically, three-point pressure splints are ineffective when used to correct deformities greater than 35 degrees (see Chapter 5). Velcro, however, could be used as a dynamic assist to correct a 45-degree flexion deformity if it were attached to an outrigger to provide a 90-degree angle of approach.

Outrigger height influences the type of dynamic assist that may be used. If the outrigger is a high profile design or if a low profile outrigger is used on a hand-based splint (Fig. 6-14), the length at which the assist produces an optimal force range is critical. Too much elasticity in the assist requires an excessively tall outrigger to generate an appropriate force range. Conversely, an assist should be long enough to prohibit

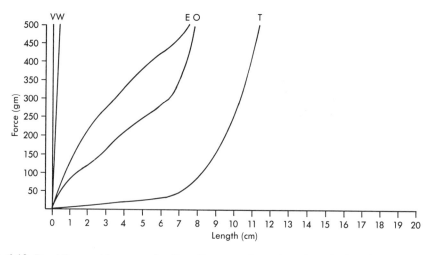

Fig. 6-13. Providing a wide range of options for use as dynamic assists, the length tension curves for velcro *(V)*, cotton webbing *(W)*, Exer-tubing *(E)*, orthodontic rubber band *(O)*, and elastic thread *(T)* differ considerably.

forces from grossly exceeding the upper limits of the acceptable force range when the finger is actively moved in a direction opposite to that of the assist. Since an elastic assist may increase in length by as much as 6 cm as a finger moves away from its pull, it is important also to identify the forces generated by the assist in its elongated position (Fig. 6-15). Although active compression is beneficial to the nutrition of articular surfaces by stimulating synovial fluid infusion, and normally occurring forces, transmitted to joints as objects are grasped, reach considerable magnitudes, care should be taken to avoid excessive resistance to the digits as dynamic assists are stretched through func-

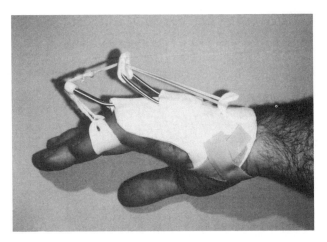

Fig. 6-14. A dynamic assist that requires excessive length to generate the force range necessary for splinting stiff joints would be inappropriate for a relatively short splint such as this. (Courtesy Susan Emerson, M.Ed., O.T.R., Dover, NH.)

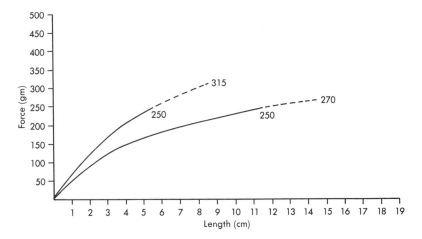

Fig. 6-15. Forces increase as a finger is moved in a direction opposite to the pull of the dynamic assist. When stretched an additional 3 cm, the original 250 gm force is increased by 20 gm for the no. 19 rubber band as compared to a 65 gm increase for the no. 33 band.

tional motion patterns. These concepts are also applicable to forearm based low-profile outrigger designs, but the criteria are often easier to attain because of the additional length of the splints. The acceptable force range does not change, but assists with greater elastic properties may be used, facilitating adjustment.

Consider the principles of mechanics and fit. Dynamic assists should apply a force that is 90 degrees to the longitudinal axis of the segment being mobilized. This eliminates joint compression and distraction and allows the full magnitude of the force to be directed toward correcting the deformity or moving a passively supple joint through an arc of motion. To avoid unequal stress to ligamentous structures surrounding the immediate joint and those more proximal on the ray, the angle of traction should also be perpendicular to the axis of the joint being mobilized. Providing final increments of refinement, guides or pulleys can control the direction of force (Fig. 6-16).

Pressure applied by the finger attachment device should also be carefully monitored. To distribute forces over a larger area and decrease pressure, finger cuffs should be as wide as possible without impeding adjacent joint motion. Generally speaking, cuffs should be constructed of a strong but pliable material, since the combination of a rigid finger cuff and lack of a 90-degree angle of approach may create an unfavorable situation (Fig. 6-17). A low-profile finger cuff designed by Brand (Fig. 6-18) eliminates the potentially dangerous leverage effect produced by conventional cuffs. This type of cuff is especially helpful when dealing with a hand that lacks sensibility. If hooks, suture loops, or Velcro are attached to the fingernails, the amount of traction should not jeopardize the vascular status of the nailbed or surrounding tissue.

Friction between a finger cuff and the underlying cutaneous surface often indicates lack of a 90-degree angle of approach of the traction, allowing the cuff to migrate proximally or distally. By altering the length of the outrigger as joint motion changes, this friction may be controlled. Friction may also occur between the surfaces of the dynamic assist and the outrigger at the fulcrum point in low-profile splint designs. As the portion of the assist that comes in contact with the outrigger moves back and forth, friction is created, eventually undermining the strength of the assist. An interface of nylon line or unwaxed dental floss between the elastic assist and the finger attachment device increases durability (Fig. 6-19), as do pulleys on the outrigger (Fig. 6-20). Another site of friction that may jeopardize the longevity of a dynamic assist component is the junction of the elastic assist and the interface. As stress is applied, the harder interface material (nylon line, dental floss, etc.) cuts into the softer elastic assist. Protective liners or special looping techniques may alleviate this problem.

Control and maintain force magnitude. Once correct tensions are set (Fig. 6-21), corrective splints require careful monitoring and frequent readjusting to maintain their effectiveness (Fig. 6-22). An elastic assist may lose some of its rebound ability, creating excessive length and a concomitant inability to generate forces within the desired range. These types of assists may require adjustment or replacement as often as every 2 or 3 days, depending on physical properties and use. The optimum range of forces for a spring coil splint occurs at very specific joint ranges. These ranges differ from one type of coil splint to another, resulting in splints of limited use if they cannot be readily

Text continued on p. 186.

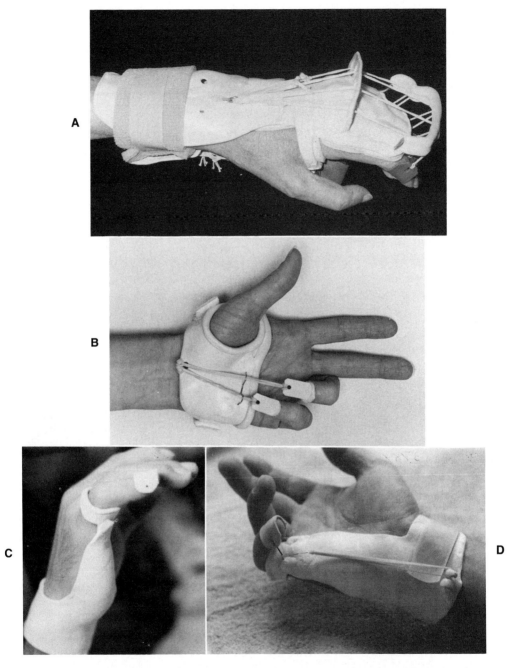

Fig. 6-16. Pulleys and guides refine the direction of pull of dynamic assists. (**A** courtesy Diana Williams, O.T.R., Danville, PA; **B** courtesy Barbara Allen, O.T.R./L., Oklahoma City; **C** and **D** courtesy Carolina deLeeuw, M.A., O.T.R., Tacoma, WA.)

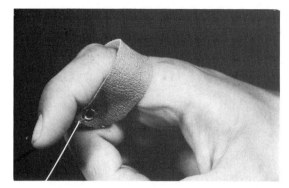

Fig. 6-17. In the absence of a 90-degree angle of pull the area of force application of a rigid-material finger sling decreases and resultant pressure increases.

Fig. 6-18. Designed by Paul Brand, MD, this low-profile finger cuff allows the full width of the cuff to remain in contact with the dorsum of the finger even if a 90-degree angle of pull is not present.

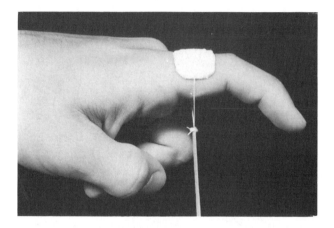

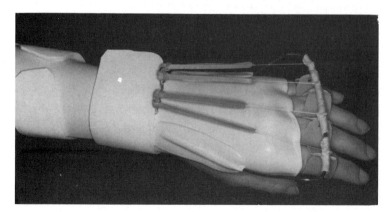

Fig. 6-19. Using an inelastic material as an interface between a dynamic assist and a finger cuff diminishes friction at the outrigger fulcrum. (Courtesy Barbara Raff, O.T.R., Park Ridge, IL.)

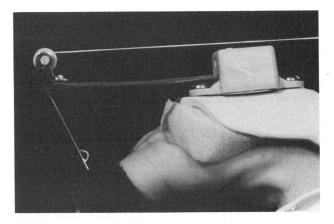

Fig. 6-20. By decreasing friction, outrigger pulleys increase the durability of the assist unit and ease active finger motion.

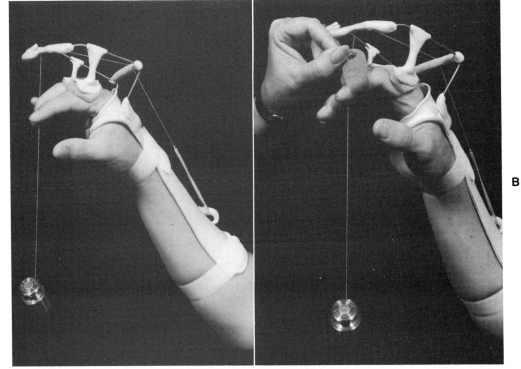

A   B

Fig. 6-21. A simple method of setting tension, an appropriate size standard brass weight is attached to the untrimmed end of the assist unit and is suspended from the outrigger at a 90-degree angle (**A**). The finger is then pulled gently into position and a mark is placed on the fishing line at the point where the cuff will be attached (**B**).

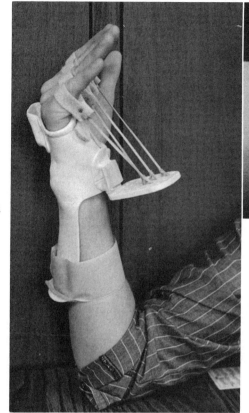

A

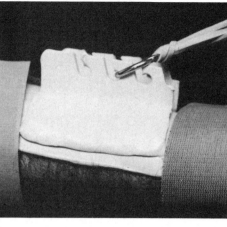

B

Fig. 6-22. Constructed of a solid piece of material in which multiple holes have been drilled, this "slab" outrigger facilitates maintenance of a 90-degree angle of pull (**A**). A series of attachment sites in the form of progressive notches eases tension adjustment (**B**). (**A** courtesy Joyce Roalef, O.T.R./L., Dayton, OH; **B** courtesy Karen Schultz, M.S., O.T.R., C.V.E., Santa Monica, CA.)

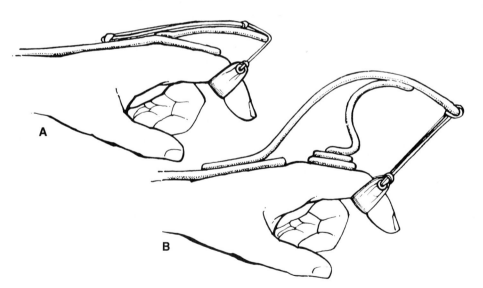

A

B

Fig. 6-23. For legend see opposite page.

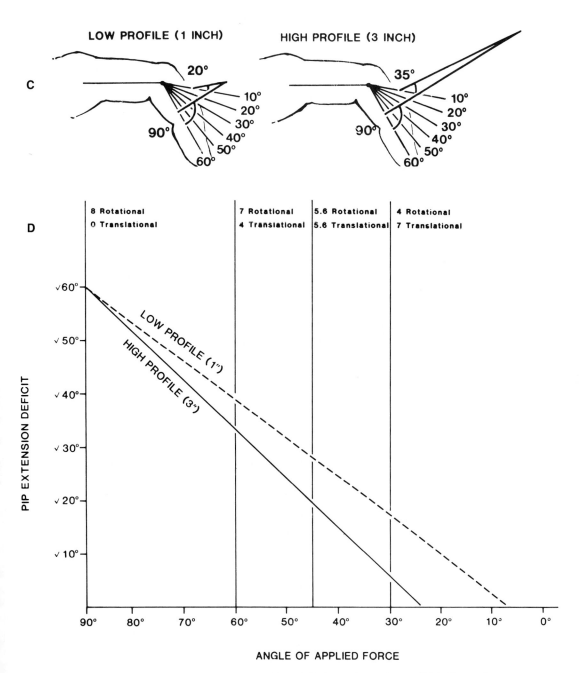

Fig. 6-23. Comparison of low-profile outriggers (**A**) and high-profile outriggers (**B**) indicates that as passive motion improves, the high-profile design maintains a better angle of pull without adjustment than does the low-profile design (**C** and **D**). (From Fess, E.E.: Principles and methods of splinting for mobilization of joints. In Hunter, J., et al., editors: Rehabilitation of the hand, ed. 2, St. Louis, 1985, The C.V. Mosby Co.)

adjusted. Inelastic traction must be adjusted frequently as joint motion changes, as must the length of an outrigger to maintain a constant 90-degree angle of approach of the mobilizing force.

Although outrigger height does not influence force magnitude of dynamic assists, it does influence adjustment schedules. Low-profile outriggers lose the required 90-degree angle of approach more quickly than do their high-profile counterparts (Fig. 6-23). This, however, is a concept applicable only when working with correctional forces. If the purpose of a splint is to substitute for weak or absent active motion, full passive joint motion is a prerequisite, and the need for sequential adjustments to accommodate motion improvements is nonexistent. Low-profile outriggers are appropriate design options for control or substitution splints because they do not need sequential adjustments. Conversely, high-profile outriggers provide longer increments of near 90-degree angle of pull than do the low-profile designs, indicating that for correctional splints the higher design option requires fewer adjustments as improvements in motion are gained. Whether this is an important concept in designing a correctional splint depends entirely on the patient's ability to return to the clinic for adjustments and the time demands of the therapist's case load.

With the creation of a splint comes the responsibility for maintaining its effectiveness. To set only the initial force is not sufficient. Hands and dynamic assists change with time, making previously set tensions ineffective and obsolete. To date, no dynamic assist component exists that maintains optimal force parameters throughout the full arc of joint motion without adjustments. Frequent measurements of joint motion, tension checks, and monitoring of the traction angle of approach identify the need for alterations.

SUMMARY

Providing the power source for mobilizing splints, dynamic assists are constructed from elastic, inelastic, or spring wire materials. They are influenced by the physical properties of the materials from which they are made and therefore generate different ranges of forces. It is the hand specialist's responsibility to determine optimum force and torque parameters, to set the dynamic assist at an appropriate tension, and to maintain its adjustment according to the individual needs of each patient. Angle of approach, pressure, friction, and ligamentous stress also must be carefully monitored so that the patient reaches full rehabilitative potential as quickly as possible. If these factors are not attended to, expensive and disappointing delays may occur.

CHAPTER 7

Design principles

GENERAL PRINCIPLES OF DESIGN

Consider individual patient factors.
Consider the length of time the splint is to be used.
Strive for simplicity and pleasing appearance.
Allow for optimum function of the extremity.
Allow for optimum sensation.
Allow for efficient construction and fit.
Provide for ease of application and removal.
Consider the splint/exercise regimen.

SPECIFIC PRINCIPLES OF DESIGN

Identify key joints.
Review the purpose: to immobilize; to increase passive motion; to substitute
    for active motion.
Determine if the wrist should be incorporated.
Consider kinetic effects.
Identify areas of diminished sensibility.
Decide whether to use static or dynamic forces.
Determine the surface for splint application.
Use mechanical principles advantageously.
Adapt for anatomic variables.
Choose the most appropriate material.
Adapt to general properties of the material.

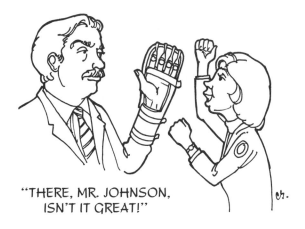

"THERE, MR. JOHNSON,
ISN'T IT GREAT!"

The principles of splint design evolve from the integration of the principles of fit, mechanics, and construction. The most important consideration in splint design is the exact function expected of the splint for a specific patient. A thorough understanding of the particular problem and therapeutic goals for which a splint is required is essential to the design process. Armed with this knowledge, one can determine the ultimate configuration of the splint to be constructed. Nineteen fundamental principles must be considered in the designing of a given splint. These principles range from general to specific and result in a series of decisions that lead to the final splint design.

The principles of design may be divided into two categories. Eight general principles based on individual patient characteristics form a framework for the overall designing process of hand splints. The consideration and incorporation of these broad principles implements the creation of a splint that is practical for both the patient and the therapist. Adherence to the remaining eleven more specific principles concerned with the particular pathologic situation help to ensure the optimum functional benefit and patient tolerance of the splint. It should be emphasized that the principles discussed in this chapter are used only after there has been an appreciation of all factors unique to each patient. Decisions are made based on personal, technical, and medical considerations. The result is often substantially different splint configurations for patients with similar therapeutic needs but different logistic or personal requirements. With experience, these decisions can be made automatically, without the need to review a detailed ''checklist'' of the principles listed here. Consultation with all persons involved in the rehabilitative effort must precede the actual design process, for this information strongly influences decisions as to splint configuration.

All of these principles are integrated and considered by the hand specialist almost simultaneously as assessment of the patient progresses, eventually leading to a splint design that is unique to the situation. Astute observation and careful objective measurement provide the foundation on which critical decisions are made, allowing design creation ''from the inside out'' rather than haphazard application of a preconceived or standard configuration without regard to important individual variables.

GENERAL PRINCIPLES OF DESIGN

The basic considerations for splint design are discussed in the following principles.

Consider individual patient factors. The individual requirements of each patient are the most influential factors in determining the ultimate size and configuration of a given splint. After the functional requirements of the splinting program are established, additional individual factors must be addressed: How much of his pathologic condition and rehabilitation program does the patient understand, and how much of the program can he intelligently accomplish for himself? How accessible is the splinting facility, and how often will he be able to return for splint adjustments or changes? To what extent will his family be able to assist him in splint application and exercises? What are the age and occupational factors?

All these factors come into careful consideration at the onset of a splinting program. Serial splints that must be changed every 3 or 4 days may present a hardship to a patient located many miles from the therapy department, and the use of an elaborately designed

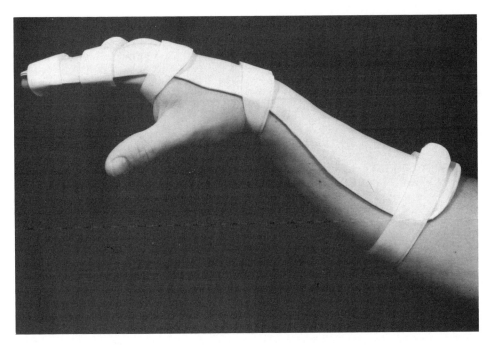

Fig. 7-1. This complex finger immobilization splint used in early passive range-of-motion of flexor tendon repairs would be contraindicated for a young child because of its ease of removal.

splint for a patient with poor motivation or an inadequate understanding of proper splint application will almost certainly result in improper use of the splint. In addition, modifications may be dictated by patient age (Fig. 7-1). Splints designed for use on adults may be poorly tolerated by or inappropriate for a child.

Consideration of specific circumstances such as these allows for the appropriate creation of a design that is more likely to be successful because of its adaptation to the wearer's specific situation.

Consider the length of time the splint is to be used. In general, the shorter the anticipated need of the splint, the simpler its design, material type, and construction should be. An elaborately designed splint that required numerous hours to design, construct, and fit and is expected to be discarded or replaced within a few days can rarely be justified to cost- and efficiency-conscious consumers, hospital administrators, and third-party participants. However, if the same splint were to be employed for 3 or 4 months, its preparation would certainly be more appropriate. Similarly, if the device is expected to be used for several years or more, consultation with an orthotist may be indicated to allow for splint construction with more durable materials such as aluminum, steel, and some of the polyester resins.

Strive for simplicity and pleasing appearance. Attempts should be made to keep the overall design as simple and cosmetically pleasing as possible (Fig. 7-2). At best, a hand splint is a strange-looking device, attracting attention to its wearer and further emphasizing the deformity. A poorly designed splint becomes even more obvious, less-

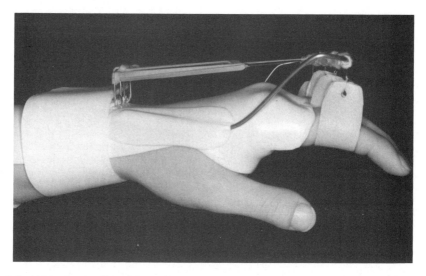

Fig. 7-2. Although complicated in design, this splint presents an excellent appearance because of its neatness and finishing details. (Courtesy Barbara Raff, O.T.R., Arlington Heights, IL.)

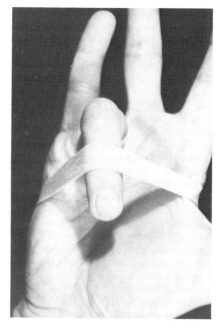

Fig. 7-3. A wide rubber band can be an effective splint for increasing proximal interphalangeal joint flexion.

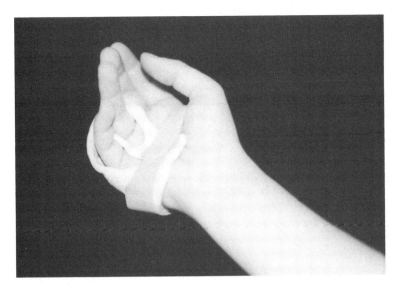

Fig. 7-4. This simple metacarpophalangeal extension block splint for ulnar nerve paralysis allows full flexion of the fourth and fifth digits. (Courtesy Sandra Artzberger, M.S., O.T.R., Milwaukee, and Bonnie Ferhing, L.P.T., Fond du Lac, WI.)

ening patient acceptance, increasing frustration, and possibly decreasing the potential for successful rehabilitation. Sometimes only a large, somewhat cumbersome splint will accomplish the desired objectives, but in many instances a simple adaptation functions equally well (Fig. 7-3). Above all, consideration for the wearer should take precedence over any impulse to design a complicated and elaborate masterpiece that may serve only as a monument to its creator!

   Allow for optimum function of the extremity. The upper extremity has the unique ability to move freely in a wide range of motions, which allows for the successful accomplishment of a tremendous variety of daily tasks. The segments of the arm and hand function as an open kinematic chain, with each segment of the chain dependent on the segments proximal and distal to it. Compensation by normal segments when parts of the chain are limited by injury or disease often provide for the continued functional use of the extremity. Because of this adaptive ability, splinting of the upper extremity should be carefully designed to prevent needless immobility of normal joints (Fig. 7-4). For example, if digital joint limitation is caused by a capsular pathologic condition alone, the wrist might not require incorporation in the splint design. If, however, wrist position, by virtue of its effect on the osseous chain or the extrinsic musculotendinous units, directly influences distal joint motion, immobilization of the wrist may be required to obtain maximum splint efficiency. Although the mechanical purchase on a stiff joint may be enhanced by stabilization of joints proximal (Fig. 7-5) or distal to the joint, care should be taken to apply this concept in appropriate circumstances only. If

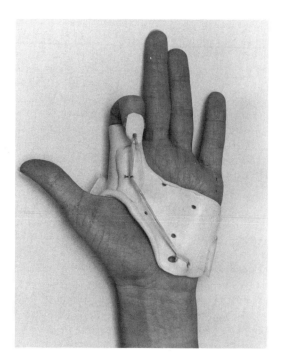

Fig. 7-5. Stabilization of the metacarpophalangeal joint allows the mobilizing force of the rubber band traction to be directed to the interphalangeal joints. (Courtesy Barbara Allen, O.T.R., Oklahoma City.)

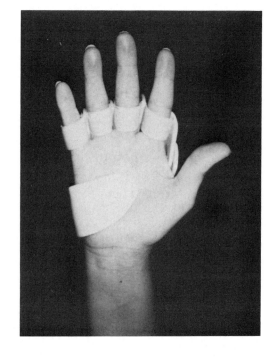

Fig. 7-6. Splints designed to leave large palmar tactile surface areas of the hand free from splint material enhance functional use. (Courtesy Joan Farrell, O.T.R., Miami.)

similar results can be obtained by leaving these adjacent joints free, the kinetic chain will have the advantage of added motion.

Allow for optimum sensation. Without sensation the hand is perceptively blind and functionally limited. Because cutaneous stimuli provide feedback for activity, splint designs should leave as much of the palmar tactile surface areas as free from occlusive material as possible (Fig. 7-6).

Allow for efficient construction and fit. The splint design should also allow for quick, efficient construction. With increasing concern for medical costs, long construction and fit times are for the most part inappropriate. Proper design can expedite construction and fit and decrease expense. Because each part that must be bonded or joined increases the construction time, the incorporation of multiple components into the main body of the splint at the design stage results in improved efficiency. For example, providing contour at the time of designing eliminates the need for separate reinforcing strips that must be cut, formed, and bonded during the splint preparation phase. However, at times the addition of a separate piece such as a dorsal phalangeal bar (lumbrical bar) can facilitate future splint adjustments without the need to modify the entire splint. Anticipation of the fit and construction factors at the design level also eliminates much of the need for time-consuming experimentation and innovation during patient contact stages.

On occasion, a commercially available splint may seem to meet the requirements of a given hand problem (Fig. 7-7). If the splint satisfies all the individual variables, if a good fit is obtained, and if the cost does not exceed that of a similar design custom-made splint, the use of a prefabricated commercial splint may actually be more expedient in regard to overall time and expense.

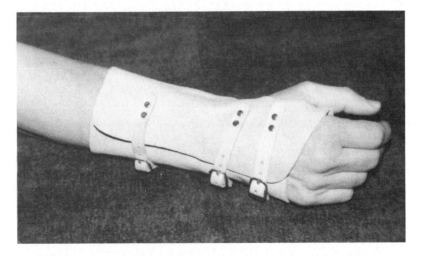

Fig. 7-7. If it meets all the individual criteria and if a good fit can be obtained, a commercially available splint may save time and expense. (Courtesy Elizabeth Spencer, O.T.R., and Lynnlee Fullenwider, O.T.R., Seattle.)

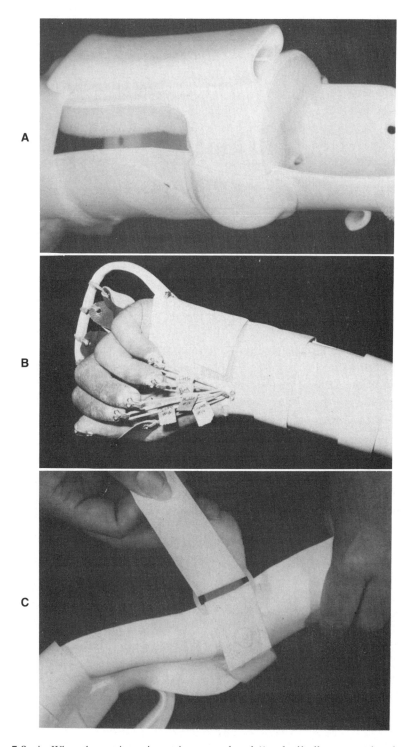

Fig. 7-8. A, When the outrigger is not in use, a dorsal "pocket" allows easy detachment from the splint. **B,** Rubber band "tags" ensure correct application of traction. **C,** Adjustable D-ring straps facilitate application and removal of bilateral long finger and thumb immobilization splints such as resting pans or safe position splints. (**B** courtesy Joan Farrell, O.T.R., Miami.)

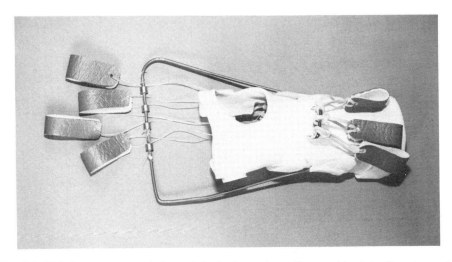

Fig. 7-9. This long metacarpophalangeal flexion/extension splint provides two alternate passive motions in a single splint. (Courtesy K.P. MacBain, O.T.R., Vancouver, BC.)

Provide for ease of application and removal. Whenever possible, patients should be able to apply and remove their splints. Dependence on others for assistance may lead to frustration of both patient and family, resulting in poor wearing habits or discarding of the splint. To allow for ease of wear and removal, the splint should be designed for simple hand and forearm insertion with straps provided that can be tightened or loosened without great difficulty. Individual adaptations in the splint design, fastening devices, or method of splint application may be necessary to further facilitate patient independence (Fig. 7-8).

Consider the splint/exercise regimen. In some instances the designing of several functions into one splint may lessen patient confusion and simplify the wearing and exercise routines. For example, the amalgamation of a finger flexion/extension system into a single splint eliminates the need for a more complicated alternating two-splint routine. Efficient design considerations such as these are more clearly understood by the patient, allowing him to direct his attention more fully to rehabilitation (Fig. 7-9).

SPECIFIC PRINCIPLES OF DESIGN

The individual considerations, including age, intelligence, location, and life-style, of the particular patient are the general principles of design, with primary emphasis directed toward splint function, appearance, economy, and patient acceptance. The remaining eleven specific principles of design stress the accomplishment of predetermined goals as defined by the unique pathologic condition:

1. What is the exact disease, injury, or deformity for which splinting is needed?
2. What are the immediate and long-term goals of the splinting regimen?
3. What is the most efficient and effective means of reaching these goals?
4. What anatomic and material variables must be considered?

These are the questions to which the specific design principles pertain.

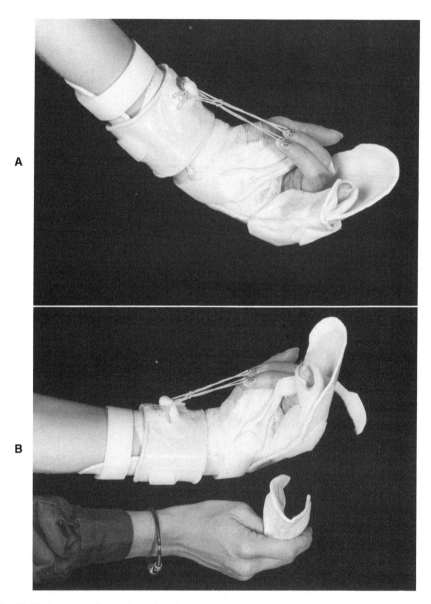

Fig. 7-10. Because of associated injuries to the ring and small fingers, this splint **(A)**, designed to be used for early passive mobilization of index and long flexor tendon repairs, has a removable component **(B)** that immobilizes the fourth and fifth digits in extension. (Courtesy Joanne Kassimir, O.T.R., Plainview, NY; photography by Owen Kassimir.)

Identify key joints. A careful evaluation of the hand with regard to existing and potential joint mobility is perhaps the single most important consideration in determining the ultimate configuration of a hand splint. Specific recorded data obtained from active and passive range-of-motion measurements provide the examiner with an accurate assessment of motion discrepancies and allow for splint design that may effectively improve the problem areas.

After careful identification of the problem joints, decisions are made as to which joints are to be immobilized and which will receive mobilization efforts. Drawing on the ingenuity and creativity of those responsible for creating splints, it is not unusual to have joints that must be immobilized and joints that require mobilization efforts in the same hand (Fig. 7-10). Because of the often highly complicated pathology and physiology involved in treatment and reconstructive procedures of a diseased or injured hand, close communication between the surgeon and the therapist is absolutely imperative. Misunderstood, misdirected, or poorly timed intervention to healing tissue could seriously jeopardize the rehabilitation potential of a hand. The referring physician's evaluation, rehabilitative goals and prognosis, operative notes, x-rays, and arteriograms, are essential information on which splinting and exercise programs are based. Once these data are obtained, splints may be designed to impart controlled forces on various digital joints or to improve the passive motion and provide for a corresponding improvement in active motion.

Immobilization splinting is usually employed to allow rest or healing, to strategically position the part with the expectation of motion loss, or to gain an increased mechanical advantage at an adjacent joint. Simple gutter or close-fitting support splints (Fig. 7-11) are commonly used to promote healing of osseous, capsular, ligamentous, or tendon structures and to provide rest to inflamed joints with the goal of lessening or preventing deformity. Badly damaged joints with no expectation of functional salvage may be splinted to allow stiffening in the most favorable position.

A static splint may also be used on one or more joints to augment the mechanical forces at another joint by allowing an increase or decrease of tension on musculotendinous units. Maximum benefit of a mobilization splint is obtained by immobilizing joints proximal or occasionally distal to the injured or diseased joint. When loss of motion is a problem at only one joint of a given digital ray, dynamic traction to the entire segment results in the dissipation of force on the normal joints with little effect on the problem area. When all joints of the segments are equally impaired, the necessity of immobilizing proximal or distal joints is less important (Fig. 7-12).

When dealing with a particularly difficult situation in which numerous joints are involved, it is sometimes helpful to mark the joints with a water-soluble felt-tip pen, using an easily identifiable code for the joints to be mobilized and those to be immobilized (Fig. 7-13). This method or other graphic techniques that allow clear visualization of the splinting objectives are extremely important to correct splint design.

Review purpose: to immobilize; to increase passive motion; or to substitute for active motion. After identifying key joints, one must review the specific functional objective of a given splint. Is it desirable to increase or to maintain the passive range of motion or to substitute for absent active motion? Are joints to be immobilized to

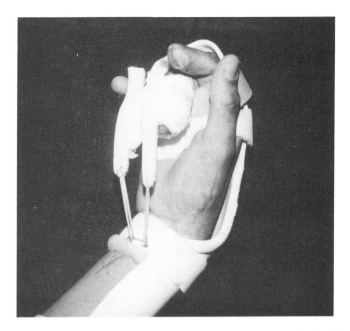

Fig. 7-11. Circumferential casts immobilize the distal joints of the long and ring fingers to allow fracture healing while the metacarpophalangeal and proximal interphalangeal joints are mobilized for early passive mobilization of flexor tendon repairs. (Courtesy Robin Miller Wagman O.T.R./L., Ft. Lauderdale, FL.)

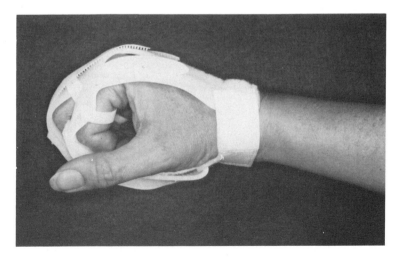

Fig. 7-12. This type of simple finger flexion splint employs inelastic traction to increase passive flexion of the digital joints.

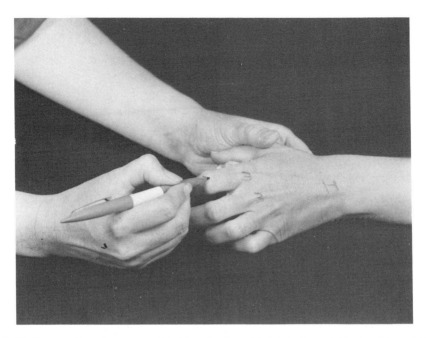

Fig. 7-13. In complicated cases, graphic identification of joints to be mobilized and immobilized may aid the novice in splint design.

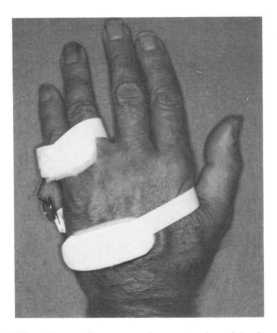

Fig. 7-14. A modified Wynn Parry splint prevents hyperextension of the fourth and fifth metacarpophalangeal joints in ulnar nerve paralysis.

allow healing? Substitution splints frequently provide control of function and may be fabricated of more durable, less adjustable materials because of their expected length of use. An example of a substitution splint is the use of a wrist immobilization splint to provide wrist extension in radial nerve paralysis or a piano wire splint (Fig 7-14) to restore a flexion restraint at the metacarpophalangeal joints in ulnar nerve paralysis. To be effective, a substitution splint requires full passive joint motion. If full joint excursion is not present, a different splint is first required to decrease the existing deformity. Splints designed to increase passive range of motion are often temporary and should be easily adaptable because configurative alterations must be made as the arc of motion changes. Immobilization splints are also worn for relatively short periods. The more pliable plastic materials should be employed for these splints.

It is imperative that the designer of the proposed splint clearly understand the reason for the application of the splint and adapt the design accordingly.

Determine if the wrist should be incorporated. Deciding whether a splint should be hand based or forearm based is a major step in the design process. An incorrect choice may needlessly immobilize the wrist or result in a splint that is ineffective in increasing range of motion or providing protection to healing structures. The key question concerns wrist position and whether it alters or affects the motion or stability of more distal structures. If wrist posture does influence articular motion or changes the tension on vulnerable structures, the wrist should be incorporated in the splint. If, however, wrist motion does not influence articular motion or inappropriately stresses tissue, a hand-based splint design may be considered.

The option of including the wrist in a splint influences fabrication and fit time, splint cost, splint effectiveness, and patient comfort and acceptance. Although the longer forearm-based splints require more preparation time, are less acceptable to patients, and are more expensive, the function they provide in controlling the effects of extrinsic musculotendinous units on digital joint motion cannot be attained with a smaller hand-based splint. Conversely, if a small wrist-free splint will suffice, economy of cost and time are achieved and the potential for patient acceptance is enhanced.

Consider kinetic effects. Because the upper extremity functions as an open kinematic chain, the inclusion of a joint in a splint can alter external and internal forces to proximal or distal joints. Recognition of the potential problems and understanding how to positively control and use these altered forces are important weapons in the astute hand specialist's armamentarium. For example, if a thumb metacarpophalangeal joint is immobilized, the stresses of normal use of the first ray are increased at both the carpometacarpal and interphalangeal joints. A splinted wrist may create a greater demand for shoulder and elbow motion to substitute for the impeded wrist movement. Increased force on unsplinted joints becomes a significant factor in designing splints when adjacent joints cannot tolerate the extra stress, necessitating the creation of splints that produce minimal compensatory effects to proximal or distal structures.

Kinetic concepts may also be used advantageously to enhance motion or to prevent deformity. By immobilizing the wrist and interphalangeal joints of the fingers, the specialist may harness the full power of the extrinsic digital flexors and extensors to produce metacarpophalangeal joint motion in a postoperative replacement arthroplasty pa-

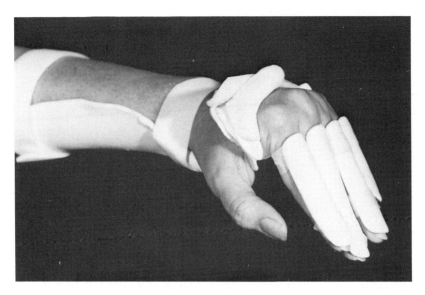

Fig. 7-15. Simple interphalangeal immobilization splints, such as these dorsal gutters, concentrate active extrinsic motion on the metacarpophalangeal joints.

tient (Fig. 7-15). A flexed wrist enhances finger extension and abduction, and an extended wrist requires greater proximal excursion of the extrinsic extensors to produce full simultaneous digital extension. Flexed metacarpophalangeal joints in an intrinsic minus hand facilitate interphalangeal extension via the intact extrinsic extensors. A thorough understanding of upper extremity anatomy and kinesiology are prerequisites to identifying and using kinetic concepts to their full potential in splint designs.

Identify areas of diminished sensibility. It is important to identify areas of decreased or absent sensibility before finalizing a splint design. Because of the increased possibility for pressure necrosis, special care should be taken to create splints that prevent or minimize forces over those areas where sensibility is impaired. Widening of narrow components, contiguous fit, and the judicious use of padding are effective methods of decreasing splint forces on insensitive portions of the extremity.

Decide whether to employ static or dynamic forces. Concomitant with the recognition of splint purposes and the identification of key joints is the decision regarding whether the proposed splint should function statically or dynamically. Static splints may be used to immobilize or to mobilize joints and generally are more simple in concept and design than are dynamic splints. These splints affect primarily the joints that they cross, and their success depends on the use of favorable mechanical advantage and the recognition of kinematic and anatomic variables. Static splints may also be used serially to enhance passive range of motion of a joint (Fig. 7-16), providing a form of "inelastic traction."

Dynamic splints are often more complicated in design and necessitate the use of specific mechanical principles to achieve optimal functional results. The choice between elastic and inelastic traction for mobilizing joints frequently depends on the joint to be

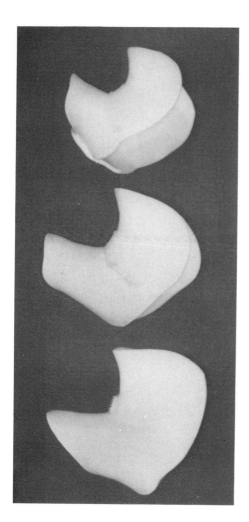

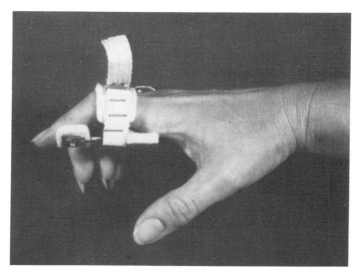

Fig. 7-16. Static thumb ''web spacers'' may be used serially to increase carpometacarpal joint passive motion.

Fig. 7-17. Inelastic traction is often more efficient than elastic traction in decreasing interphalangeal flexion stiffness of 30 degrees or less.

mobilized and its specific range of motion. For example, inelastic traction in the form of serial web spacers often produces better results in increasing motion at the thumb carpometacarpal joint than will conventional dynamic splints using elastic traction. This has also proved true for increasing extension of a proximal interphalangeal joint whose extension deficit is 30 degrees or less (Fig. 7-17). Decisions at this level in the design result in major changes in the final configuration of the splint.

Determine the surface for splint application. The decision as to what surface or surfaces of the hand or forearm the splint is to be applied is the next step in the progression through the hierarchy of design principles. This decision is influenced by the interrelationships of anatomic and mechanical factors. Although pressure is usually better tolerated on the palmar surface of the extremity, one must be aware that this side makes the greatest contribution to function and sensation. A dynamic extension splint is mechanically more efficient when based dorsally, and a palmar splint provides a stable base for dynamic flexion forces. Ulnar deviation of the wrist may be statically controlled from either the ulnar or radial surface, but if passive ulnar deviation is to be increased through elastic traction, the splint should be based on the ulnar aspect of the forearm. In summary, for the greatest mechanical advantage in a dynamic traction splint, the direction of pull and the base of the splint should be on the same side of the hand.

Use mechanical principles advantageously. The employment of mechanical principles adds detail and dimension to the development of the hand splint. These principles determine the length and width of the splint, regulate splint position, define the angles of attachment of the traction devices, and may help identify additional splint components. Failure to consider and adapt to these principles may result in an ineffective or uncomfortable splint that may have otherwise been designed appropriately.

Adapt for anatomic variables. Individual anatomic variables, abnormal structures, defects, or limited allowable motion (Fig. 7-18) may also influence the design of the splint and are important in the choice of surface on which the proposed splint will be based. A skin graft over the dorsum of the forearm may preclude dorsal construction, as would the presence of significant dorsal synovial swelling over the carpus. A prominent radial styloid process is a frequent problem in palmarly applied splints that incorporate the wrist.

Choose the most appropriate materials. The wide variety of splinting materials currently available allows the hand specialist to selectively match materials to meet the specific requirements of individual patients. Each material has idiosyncratic properties that are more or less beneficial to given situations. Some are stronger or more durable (Fig. 7-19), while others mold so closely and evenly that fine skin creases are duplicated on the internal surface of the splint. The property of becoming translucent during the malleable stage may help with hard-to-fit anatomic variables, and the ability to form a rapid and strong bond economizes construction time. Some materials are soft (Fig. 7-20), some are less expensive, and others withstand the high temperatures required for certain types of sterilization techniques.

The more knowledgeable hand specialists are regarding the multitude of available materials, the more options they have for making the best selections to meet the special

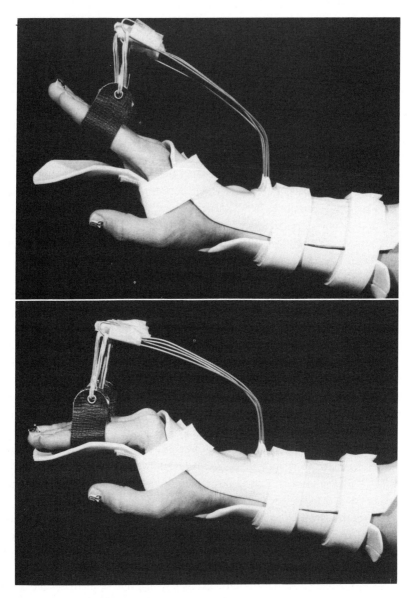

Fig. 7-18. Designed to permit early passive mobilization to extensor tendon repairs in Zone V, this splint allows active flexion and passive extension of the metacarpophalangeal joints within a predetermined limited arc of motion. (Courtesy Roslyn Evans, O.T.R., Vero Beach, FL.)

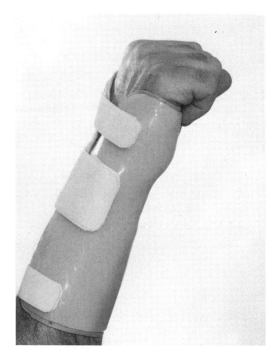

Fig. 7-19. Bonding polyethylene to Plastazote produces a comfortable and extremely durable wrist immobilization splint that may be used with early return to work patients. (Courtesy Theresa Bielawski, O.T.[C], and Jane Bear-Lehman, M.S., O.T.R., Toronto, Ont.)

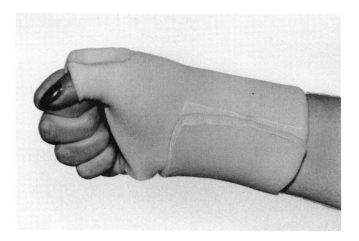

Fig. 7-20. This polyurethane foam splint permits protected motion of the wrist and thumb carpometacarpal and metacarpophalangeal joints. (Courtesy Rivka Ben-Porath, O.T., Jerusalem, Israel.)

needs of their patients. The day of the "universal" splint material ended more than a decade ago. Contemporary specialists understand the implications of the differing material properties as they apply to treatment situations and use them to their advantage.

Adapt to general properties of the selected splint material. Adaptation of design to incorporate the properties of available materials is also an important consideration in the fabrication of hand splints. Many of the low-temperature materials require splint designs that provide strength and support through increased contour of the material to the hand. A bar type of splint constructed from these materials would be an inappropriate design choice because of the inherent weakness of the material. Technical difficulties in splint fabrication must also be considered to avoid poor results when working with a particular material. If the material has a high cohesive or bonding factor, a circumferential design may increase fit problems when overlapping ends bond together unexpectedly, and the choice of a rigid material for a design whose success depends on a close fit may predispose frustration and failure.

●   ●   ●

The general principles of design provide the basic framework on which the fabrication of any hand splint must be based, whereas the specific principles, altered by individual patient variables and functional requirements, influence the final configuration of the splint. The experienced hand specialist does not employ these principles one by one in checklist fashion but considers them simultaneously, adding, eliminating, and supplementing them with innovation and creativity. The challenge is to create a splint that not only meets the functional objectives but is acceptable and well tolerated by the patient.

CHAPTER 8

Construction principles

Strive for good cosmetic effect.
Use equipment appropriate to the material.
Use type of heat and temperature appropriate to the material.
Use safety precautions.
Round corners.
Smooth edges.
Analyze mechanical principles.
Stabilize joined surfaces.
Finish rivets.
Provide ventilation as necessary.
Secure padding.
Secure straps.

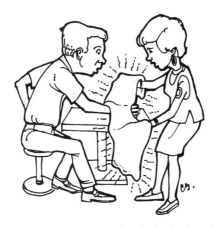

"MY, THIS NEW MATERIAL CERTAINLY
IS STRETCHY."

Once a splint has been designed and a pattern prepared, construction is technically not as difficult as are the preceding stages and those to follow. The principles of construction represent concepts that are directly related to the durability, cosmesis, and comfort of the finished product. Adherence to the 12 principles listed at the beginning of this chapter should produce a splint that will be well tolerated, durable, and visually acceptable.

The construction of a splint may be divided into five phases: (1) transfer of the pattern to the material, (2) heating of the material, (3) cutting of the material, (4) joining of separate parts, and (5) finishing details of the splint. Because fitting of unassembled parts of the splint usually occurs after the cutting phase, there is an obligatory time separation between the initial construction phases and the final phases of joining and finishing. Many of the principles of construction are applicable to more than one phase and should be considered as overall guidelines rather than as techniques specific to a single phase.

Strive for good cosmetic effect. Since a splint is an unusual looking, extraneous piece of equipment, it has little inherent cosmetic value however well designed, constructed, or fitted it may be. It is therefore important that all efforts be directed toward making the external appearance of the splint as pleasing as is possible. Splints that resemble an aberrant assortment of discarded junk have no place in the today's therapeutic armamentarium. Material or fabrication expense should not significantly influence splint cosmesis. Inexpensive materials can be neatly assembled into a functional splint, and, conversely, more costly materials can be poorly constructed and assembled with resultant splint discoloration, fatigue, and irregular surfaces. Good splint appearance is achieved through careful attention to detail during the various phases of construction.

Materials should not be overworked. Bubbles and burn spots from overheating are unacceptable, as are rough edges, sharp corners, pen marks, fingerprints, and dirty smudges. When possible, the number of different materials used in a splint should be kept to a minimum, and, when joining pieces of a material whose opposing surfaces differ in texture, take care to align the surfaces so that the external surface textures match (Fig. 8-1).

Use equipment appropriate to material. The availability of a wide variety of splinting materials helps meet the unique splinting needs of patients. It is vital that the hand specialist be thoroughly versed in the idiosyncrasies of the physical properties and the specific equipment requirements of these materials; the use of dissimilar substances mandates that construction methods be carefully adapted to meet specific criteria of the materials. This is especially important when switching between low and high temperature–forming substances. For example, an indelible marking device should be used when transferring a pattern to a material that requires wet heat for cutting and forming, whereas the use of a water-soluble pen with a dry heat material is advantageous, since the pen marks can be washed off when no longer needed. Although metal files or an electric sander can be used to smooth edges on high temperature–material splints, these devices cause friction gumming and exaggerate roughness on low temperature–material edges. Power saws produce burrs on the edges of cold, low temperature–forming ma-

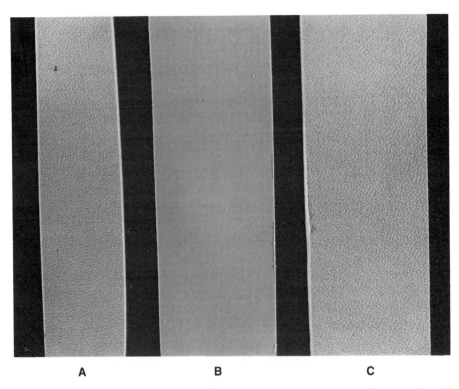

A   B   C

Fig. 8-1. Matching textured surfaces improves splint cosmesis. *Correct combination,* **A** and **C;** *incorrect,* **A** and **B** or **B** and **C.**

terials, whereas cutting the same material with scissors after it is warmed produces a continuous, smooth-finished splint edge.

When working with wire, it is important to understand the purpose of the component being constructed and the stresses to which it will be subjected, for the type of wire selected will dictate the tools required for shaping. Ordinary coat hanger wire may be molded with the aid of pliers, but a bending bar is often necessary to shape more resilient wire, such as the steel welding rod frequently used in outriggers (Fig. 8-2, *A*). To produce smoothly contoured, tightly coiled springs from heavy-gauge piano wire, other specialized bending jigs are required (Fig. 8-2, *B*).

Use type of heat and temperature appropriate to material. The reaction of splinting materials to heat varies with the type of material, but temperature extremes in either direction (too much heat or not enough) directly influence construction techniques. Overheating causes blistering, stretching, and surface irregularities; underheating may produce rough-cut edges and uneven pliability. Bonding of low-temperature materials is also not as reliable when the temperature is not at optimum level.

Splint construction is not only influenced by temperature; it is also affected by the type of heat used. Some materials, such as Orthoplast, bond more readily to themselves when dry heat is employed, eliminating both the possible surface contamination caused

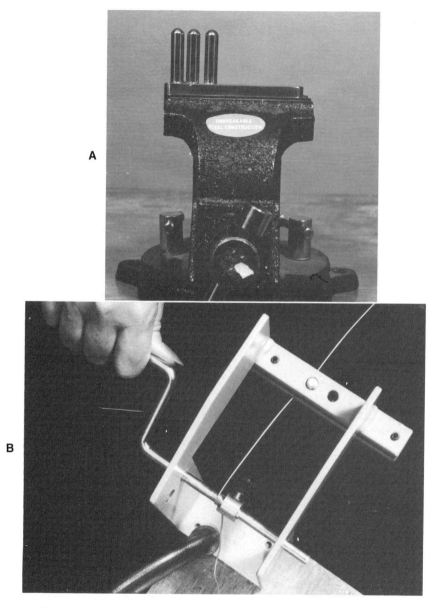

Fig. 8-2. Special equipment is necessary when shaping heavy-gauge wire. **A,** Bending bar. **B,** RESCAP jig. **C,** Adapted Wynn Parry jig.

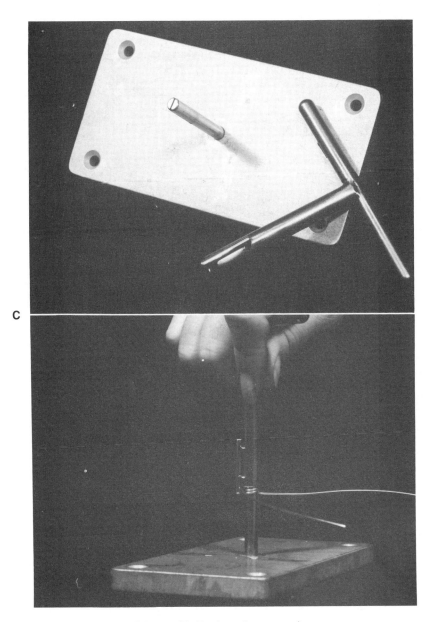

Fig. 8-2, cont'd. For legend see opposite page.

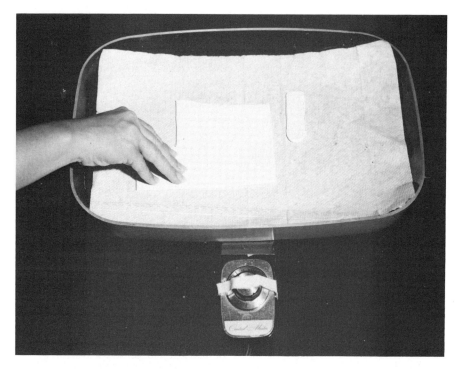

Fig. 8-3. Large pieces of Orthoplast may be heated in a dry skillet lined with a paper towel to prevent sticking and surface impregnation. Use of a dry skillet allows the material temperature to be consistently maintained over many hours, providing malleable plastic whenever it is needed throughout the treatment day.

by wet heat and the need for additional cleaning with chemical solvents (Fig. 8-3). The type of heat may also influence the speed at which the material becomes malleable. Most low-temperature materials respond more quickly and uniformly to wet heat, especially if they have been contoured previously. However, if only a small section of a splint needs heating (Fig. 8-4), the use of dry heat from a heat gun allows adjacent structures to remain unaltered.

Use safety precautions. Exposure to a large volume of hand trauma patients results in an awareness of the potential dangers of working with both manual and power tools and an appreciation of the need for high safety standards. Eyes should be protected, rings removed, and loose hair and clothing secured (Fig. 8-5) before any piece of power equipment is turned on. Since studies have shown that dull or poorly maintained tools cause accidents, both hand and power tools should be inspected and repaired routinely. Careful attention should be directed to the wiring of wet-heat electrical appliances.

Protection of the patient and the therapist from potential harm by sharp or hot materials during splint formation and construction stages is of utmost importance. Gloves and stockinette provide a heat barrier when working with high-temperature substances, and sharp edges of metal and wire should be taped to prevent inadvertent injury. Ma-

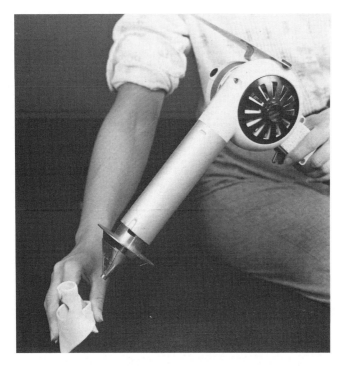

Fig. 8-4. A heat gun and a spot heater direct dry heat to small areas.

terials warmed with wet heat should be dried thoroughly before handling and application.

Round corners. Both inside and outside corners of a splint should be rounded for
increased strength, durability, cosmesis, and comfort. Uniformity of the curves may be
attained by drawing around a coin at each corner during the transfer phase of splint
construction (Fig. 8-6). To enhance the overall cosmetic effect and to prevent pointed
edges from causing damage to clothing or injury to the patient, corners should also be
rounded on straps and accessory splint parts such as outriggers and finger cuffs (Fig.
8-7).

Smooth edges. Splint edges should be smoothed and slightly rounded (Fig. 8-8).
Nicks and points lessen the comfort and cosmetic appearance of the splint and decrease
its strength.

When cutting low-temperature materials, to help eliminate edge imperfections care
should be taken to use smooth, easy cutting strokes, avoiding complete closure of the
scissor blades (Fig. 8-9). A finished edge on a separate splint part that has been tubed
or doubled for strength may be attained by first bonding the appropriate surfaces together and then cutting around the bonded edges with scissors (Fig 8-10). Minor edge
defects may be repaired by heating the edge and gently rubbing a fingertip over the
defect, compressing the material into a more desirable configuration.

Text continued on p. 218.

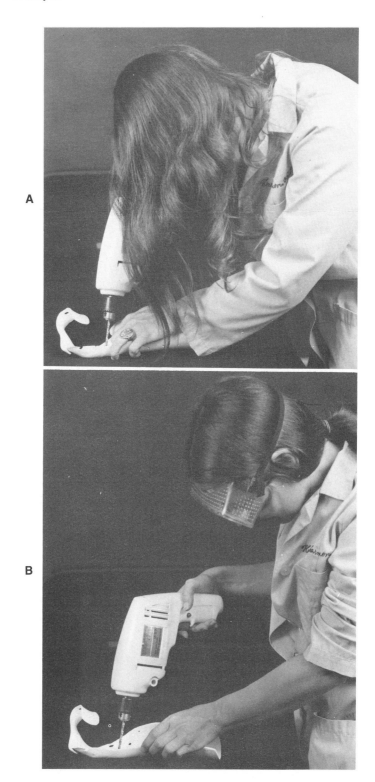

Fig. 8-5. Safety precautions should be carefully observed when working with hand tools or power equipment. **A,** Incorrect. **B,** Correct.

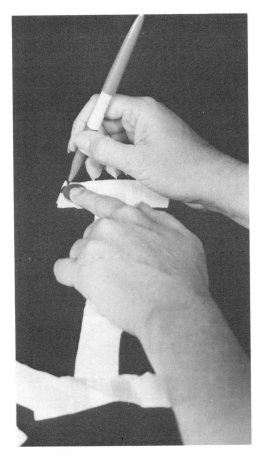

Fig. 8-6. Splint cosmesis is improved if corners are uniformly rounded. This may be accomplished during the transfer stage by drawing a coin on both external and internal corners.

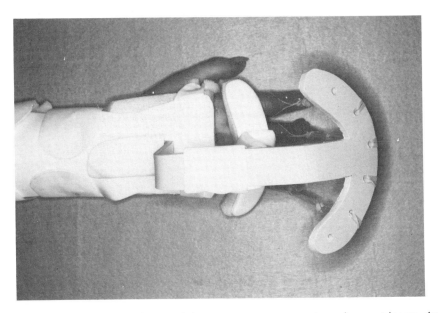

Fig. 8-7. Corners should also be rounded on accessory components such as outriggers, dorsal phalangeal bars, finger cuffs, and straps.

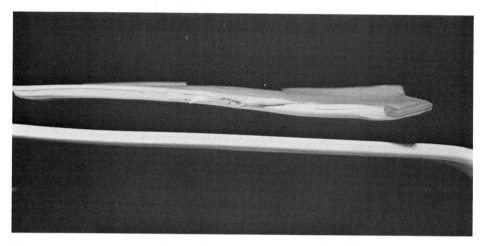

Fig. 8-8. Edge nicks and points should be smoothed into even and slightly rounded surfaces. *Top,* Poor finishing techniques; *bottom,* correctly finished edge.

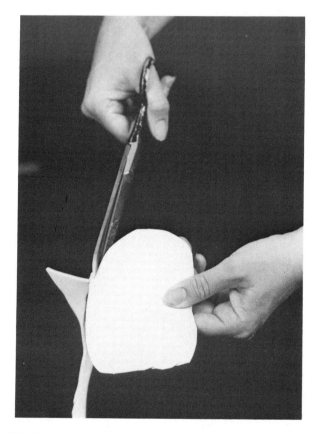

Fig. 8-9. Improper use of scissors results in rough, uneven splint edges.

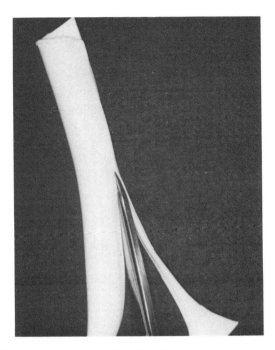

Fig. 8-10. Simultaneous cutting of bonded pieces creates a smooth single edge.

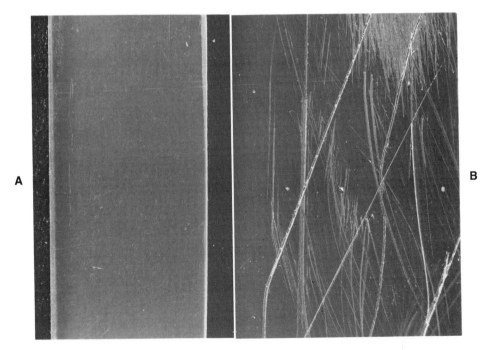

Fig. 8-11. Overextension of sanding or filing onto the flat surfaces of the material lessens the cosmetic appearance. **A**, Correct. **B**, Incorrect.

High-temperature materials, wire, and metals require the use of files, sandpaper, emery cloth, or steel wool for finishing edges and ends. A novice using these materials may spend a prolonged period of time finishing edges, but with experience most splints can be finished in a maximum of 3 to 5 minutes of filing and sanding. When smoothing edges, care should be taken to avoid marring the wider, adjacent surfaces of the material (Fig. 8-11).

Analyze mechanical principles. Mechanical principles may be applied to enhance strength and durability to splints through adaptation of leverage systems and careful consideration of the area of force application during splint construction. Rounding inside corners increases the area of force application, diminishing the chances of material fatigue and fracture at more vulnerable corner sites. The placement of a small drill hole at the end of inside cuts also disperses pressure by widening the area of force application (Fig. 8-12).

Leverage concepts may also facilitate the fabrication process itself. For example, with wire, the application of the bending force at a point 12 or 15 cm away from the actual site of the bend creates a long lever arm and decreases the force required, thus making the shaping process easier (Fig. 8-13).

When joining splint parts, the use of one rivet allows axial rotation, whereas two or more rivets afford a solid and stable splint joint. Providing longer sites of attachment for outriggers (Fig. 8-14) increases the durability of the bonded or riveted interface by increasing the ratio between the lengths of the resistance arm and the force arm of the outrigger.

A careful analysis of a broken splint or splint part is an important step in determining why a splint has failed. The resulting evaluation of the force systems involved in the splint should facilitate repair and aid future splint preparation through technique improvement.

Stabilize joined surfaces. With the many self-bonding splinting materials on the market today, the need for riveting splint components together has diminished consid-

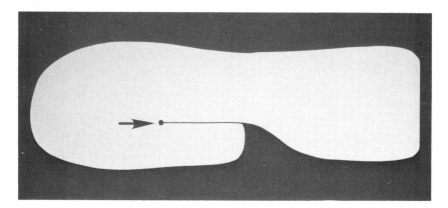

Fig. 8-12. A small hole *(arrow)* at the terminal end of an inside cut will disseminate cracking forces and increase splint durability.

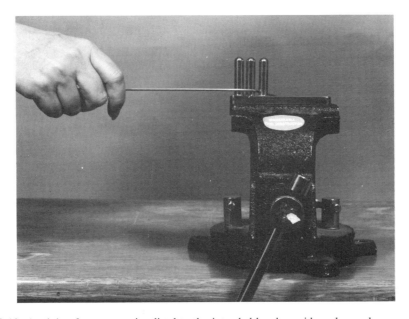

Fig. 8-13. Applying force at a point distal to the intended bend provides a longer lever arm with which to shape wire.

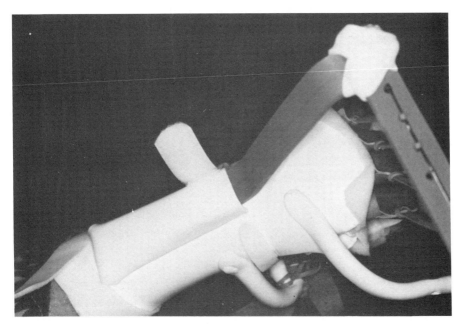

Fig. 8-14. The increased mechanical advantage (MA) afforded by a long attachment site allows for a stronger bond at the proximal end of the outrigger.

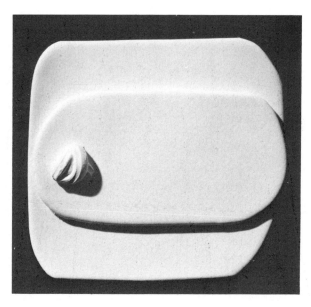

Fig. 8-15. Plastic rivets of a homologous low-temperature material provide a stable bond but may fracture with constant stress.

erably. However, occasions arise when the extra strength afforded by a rivet is useful, if not mandatory. When a separate part must be joined to a splint, consideration of the function of the part and its requirements with regard to joint immobilization or mobilization is important. An understanding of mechanical principles and the use of equipment appropriate to the material selected will ensure a more favorable result. It is important to reemphasize that, although one rivet allows motion between the joined surfaces, two or more rivets, surface bonding, or gluing results in a secure coupling of splint components. The choice of rivet type depends on the specific parts to be joined and the characteristics of the materials used (Fig. 8-15). If motion is desired in a splint, a metal rivet is more durable, and the placement of a paper spacer between the two surfaces to be joined allows smoother rotation of the joint after the setting of the rivet and removal of the paper. Surface bonding and gluing require adherence to the techniques specific to individual materials. This frequently depends on proper cleaning and heating of the contiguous surface areas for optimum results.

When adding a wire component to a splint, it is important to provide a durable and solid union. The combination of the smoothness and narrow diameter of wire, plus the torque created from the distally applied forces of dynamic assists, makes it difficult to stabilize a wire component such as an outrigger to the supporting body of the splint. A secure union of plastic and wire parts is accomplished by forming a zig-zag or open loop on the proximal end(s) of the wire component at the point(s) of attachment (Fig. 8-16, *A*). The adapted end(s) prevents dislodging once thermoplastic reinforcement strips are bonded over the wire, onto the body of the splint (Fig. 8-16, *B*).

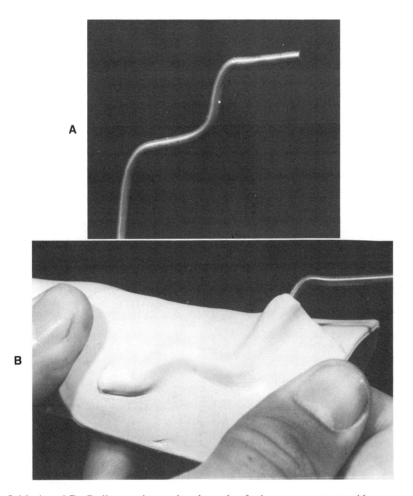

Fig. 8-16. A and **B,** Curling or zig-zagging the ends of wire components provides a more stable attachment site.

Finish rivets. For comfort and a more pleasing appearance, rivets should be flush with the material surface, particularly when they will contact the patient's skin. This is accomplished by countersinking high-temperature materials or, in the case of the softer, low-temperature materials, by heating and molding of the rivet or the surrounding surface area. Tape or moleskin placed over an "internal" metal rivet prevents deterioration and rusting of the rivet caused by perspiration. External rivet parts should be smooth and nonobtrusive, providing good appearance, comfort, and function.

Provide ventilation as necessary. The ventilation of a splint should be done judiciously and prudently, depending on the patient, the patient's life-style, splint configuration, the materials employed, and the environment. Splints with large skin contact areas more frequently require adaptation to improve air circulation. Ventilation holes

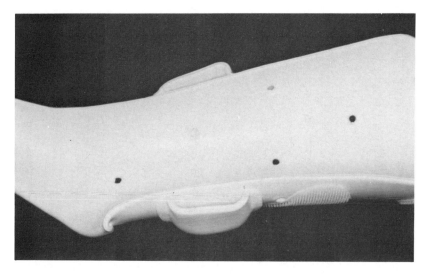

Fig. 8-17. Ventilation holes should not be placed over bony prominences, near edges, across narrow components, or in areas of high stress forces.

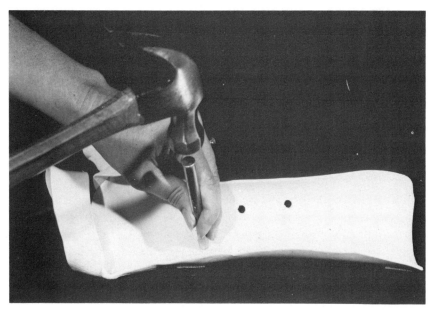

Fig. 8-18. Ventilation holes should be made from the inside of the splint to ensure a comfortable inner surface.

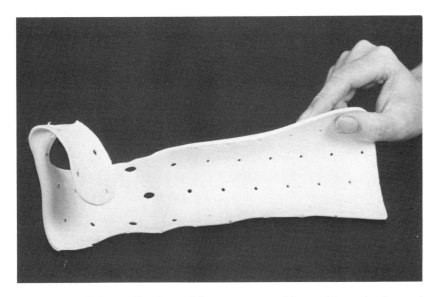

Fig. 8-19. Commercially ventilated materials may create problems with rough edges and over-stretched holes.

should be small enough to prevent tissue protrusion and should be randomly positioned away from splint edges to eliminate weakening of the material (Fig. 8-17). Holes should not be situated over areas such as bony prominences that require close material contact to decrease pressure.

Low-temperature materials may be ventilated with a hand tool such as a drive punch or rotary punch (Fig. 8-18). The use of an electric drill, although suitable for high-temperature materials, is inadvisable with softer materials because it causes friction melting around the holes, resulting in rough everted edges. Perforations should be made from the inside out to give a smoother inner splint surface, and all external hole edges should be smoothed by heating or sanding, according to material type.

Commercially available perforated materials may produce poor finished products because of the preset hole pattern and the inevitable enlargement that occurs with heating and stretching during fit. Multiple, large stretched openings, rough edges, and structural weakness are often the result of poor planning and fitting (Fig. 8-19).

If perforated material is used, extra attention to detail must be taken during the pattern transfer and molding stages of splint construction. Careful placement of the pattern on the material diminishes the chance of cutting through perforations, and avoidance of overheating lessens the potential for overstretching and enlargement of the preset holes. If the perforation pattern is such that it is impossible to eliminate edge imperfections, it is important to ensure that the edges of the splint are finished in a manner that prevents injury to the patient and destruction of clothing (Fig. 8-20).

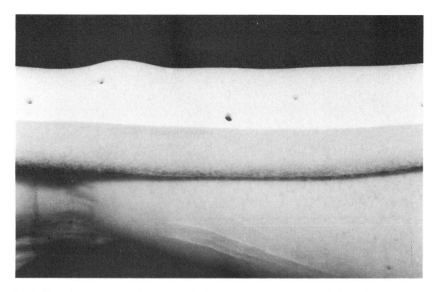

Fig. 8-20. To achieve a smooth protected edge on splints constructed from heavily perforated materials, a narrow band of self-adhesive Moleskin may be adhered to splint edges.

Secure padding. Padding should be used appropriately and should be anchored securely to the splint, allowing ease of splint application and removal. Increased comfort is provided when the padding material is cut slightly larger than the part to which it is to be adhered, allowing it to curl around splint edges (Fig. 8-21).

Secure straps. Straps should be strategically placed to provide splint stability on the extremity and should facilitate independent splint application and removal. Generally, straps should be placed at the far distal and proximal limits of the splint: this allows the full mechanical advantage of the design to be used. They should be securely attached to the splint by riveting or gluing. The fastening and unfastening procedure should be easily accomplished by the patient. Strap ends should be treated to prevent fraying, corners should be rounded for a more pleasing appearance and increased durability (Fig. 8-22), and overlapping soft materials should lie flat and be joined securely (Fig. 8-23), as should fastening devices such as Velcro, buckles, and snaps.

With pressure-sensitive interlocking materials such as Velcro, the hook portion should be used sparingly because of its abrasiveness to skin and clothing. It should not comprise the length of straps themselves, but will prove durable as a fastening device when used in single lengths rather than multiple, smaller buttons (Fig. 8-24). Velcro loop straps should be long enough to provide complete coverage of the portion of hook that has been adhered to the splint, to prevent snagging and tearing of clothing, and to provide tabs that are easier to grasp (Fig. 8-25).

Straps may be adapted to facilitate use through the addition of loops or tabs (Fig. 8-26) and may be converted to adjustable straps by increasing the length and pulling through a D ring.

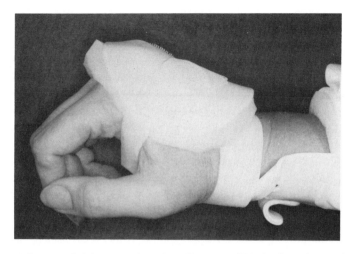

Fig. 8-21. Padding cut slightly larger than the splint part will help disseminate edge pressure.

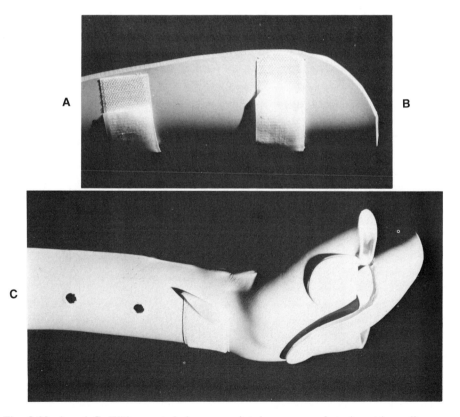

Fig. 8-22. A and **C,** With repeated closures, pointed corners on fastening strips pull away and curl, eventually resulting in detachment of the entire strip. **B,** Rounding the ends of Velcro straps and fastening strips improves appearance and increases durability.

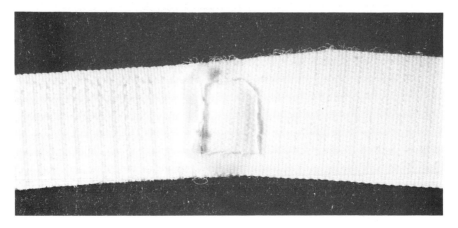

Fig. 8-23. Stitch or glue overlapping soft materials to provide a smooth durable union.

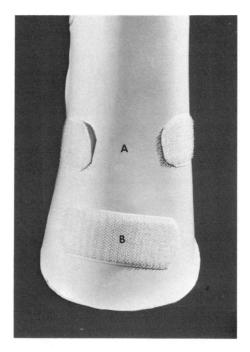

Fig. 8-24. Small button-fastening strips (**A**) that are self-adhesive or glued in place are not as durable as is a single fastening strip (**B**) that directs the unlocking forces to the center of the strip rather than to the structurally weaker edge.

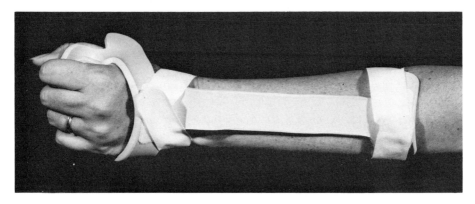

Fig. 8-25. A slight overlap of strap ends eases opening and closing and provides complete protection from hook snagging.

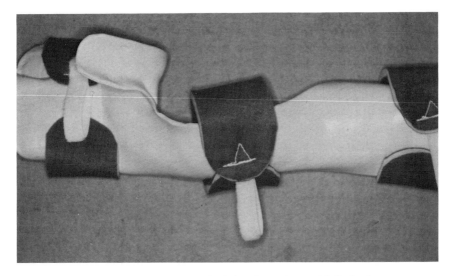

Fig. 8-26. Loops ease strap manipulation for patients with limited grasp.

SUMMARY

The principles of splint construction provide the strategic guidelines for the actual fabrication of a given splint after the design and pattern-making stages have been completed. When combined with the important principles of splint fit, the creation of a comfortably fitting, durable, and cosmetically satisfactory splint should be ensured. Failure to adhere to these principles as they pertain to the sometimes trivial details of splint manufacture may result in splint disuse because of patient discomfort, splint breakage, or, more important, failure of the splint to correct the problem for which it was originally designed. To this end meticulous attention to detail is the overriding consideration; attempts to ''short-cut'' these construction principles to speed splint preparation inevitably result in failure.

CHAPTER 9

Fit principles

MECHANICAL CONSIDERATIONS

Use principles of mechanics.
 Reduce pressure.
 Use optimum rotational force.
 Eliminate friction.
 Use optimum leverage.

ANATOMIC CONSIDERATIONS

Accommodate bony prominences.
Incorporate dual obliquity concepts.
Consider ligamentous stress.
Maintain arches.
Align splint axis with anatomic axis.
Use skin creases as boundaries.

KINESIOLOGIC CONSIDERATIONS

Allow for kinematic changes.
Employ kinetic concepts.

TECHNICAL CONSIDERATIONS

Develop patient rapport.
Work efficiently.
Change method according to properties of materials used.

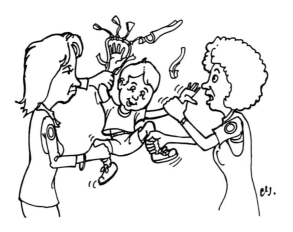

"NOW YOU TELL ME HE'S HYPERACTIVE."

The accurate fitting of hand splints to accommodate the individual anatomic variations of patients with a wide variety of clinical diagnoses is a necessary and demanding process. Prefabricated splints designed for universal wear or poorly contoured splints created without a thorough knowledge of the principles of proper splinting are uncomfortable and result in pressure problems or noncompliance, often with substantial functional loss to the patient.

With the availability of a wide spectrum of fabrication materials that may be individually adapted to each patient's needs, no excuse may be given for the use of splints that do not fit comfortably and are poorly tolerated. The basic principles of splint fitting should be thoroughly understood by anyone engaged in the management of hand problems.

Following the design and construction phases, the principles of fitting comprise the next major step in the production of a well-functioning splint. These principles encompass mechanical, anatomic, kinesiologic, and technical factors. Fit concepts relating to anatomic structures include consideration of bones, joints, ligaments, arches, and mechanical principles that are directly applied to the shaping of hand splints. Kinesiologic concepts deal with the hand in motion and with the forces that implement this motion; and technical principles incorporate techniques based on practical application and efficiency. The mechanical principles described in Chapter 5 and dynamic assist principles in Chapter 6 must be applied to the fitting of a hand splint in order to attain ultimate design effectiveness.

MECHANICAL CONSIDERATIONS

Use principles of mechanics. Employment of the principles of mechanics during the fitting of a hand splint is paramount, since the use of improper forces can damage cutaneous, ligamentous, or articular surfaces. To increase motion of a joint, the mobilizing force should always be directed perpendicular to both the segment being moved and to the rotational axis of the joint. When traction is applied simultaneously to several joints of the same digital ray, a perpendicular pull must be attained at each rotational axis. Other mechanical principles that must be considered in splint fitting include leverage as applied to the placement of straps, finger cuffs, and fingernail hooks, dissemination of the applied force to reduce pressure, and elimination of friction. Care should be taken periodically to reevaluate the dynamic forces employed in each splint, and it is imperative that alterations be incorporated as the condition of the hand changes; otherwise the effectiveness of the splint may be compromised considerably.

ANATOMIC CONSIDERATIONS
Bone

Accommodate bony prominences. The bony prominences of the extremity must always be considered when fitting a splint. Subcutaneous soft tissue is at a minimum over these areas, rendering them more vulnerable to externally applied pressure. Improper contouring of the splint material may cause pressure ischemia, which often results in tissue necrosis.

In the upper extremity the most common problematic bony prominences include the ulnar styloid process, the pisiform, the radial styloid process, the heads of the metacarpals, and the base of the first metacarpal (Fig. 9-1). Additionally, the dorsal surface of the hand is particularly vulnerable in comparison to the palmar surface because of its relative lack of pressure-disseminating subcutaneous tissue. Caution must be employed when fitting parts of splints that come into contact with or are adjacent to these bony prominences, such as forearm bars or troughs, opponens bars, wrist bars, dorsal phalangeal bars, and dorsal metacarpal bars. Care should be taken to either avoid these protuberances or to decrease the pressure over them by widening the area of application through increased material contact or the use of selective padding (Fig. 9-2).

Incorporate dual obliquity concepts. Dual obliquity is a second important consideration in splint fitting that is determined by the skeletal configuration of the hand. This principle has two anatomic ramifications: the progressive decrease of length of the metacarpals from the radial to the ulnar aspect of the hand and the immobility of the second and third metacarpals as compared to the mobile first, fourth, and fifth metacarpals. Due to this unique structural formation, two oblique lines may be drawn that particularly relate to splint design and fit. The first, from a dorsal aspect, is created by the progressive metacarpal shortening (Fig. 9-3); the second, from a distal transverse view, is the result of the progressive metacarpal descent from the radial to the ulnar side of the normal hand in a resting posture (Fig. 9-4).

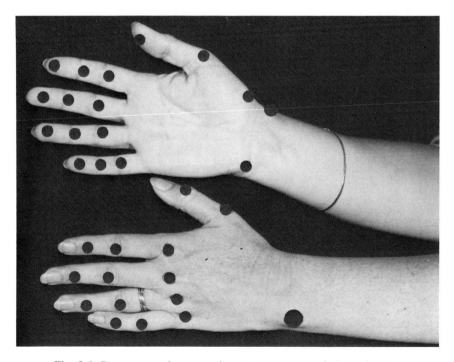

Fig. 9-1. Pressure over bony prominences may cause soft tissue damage.

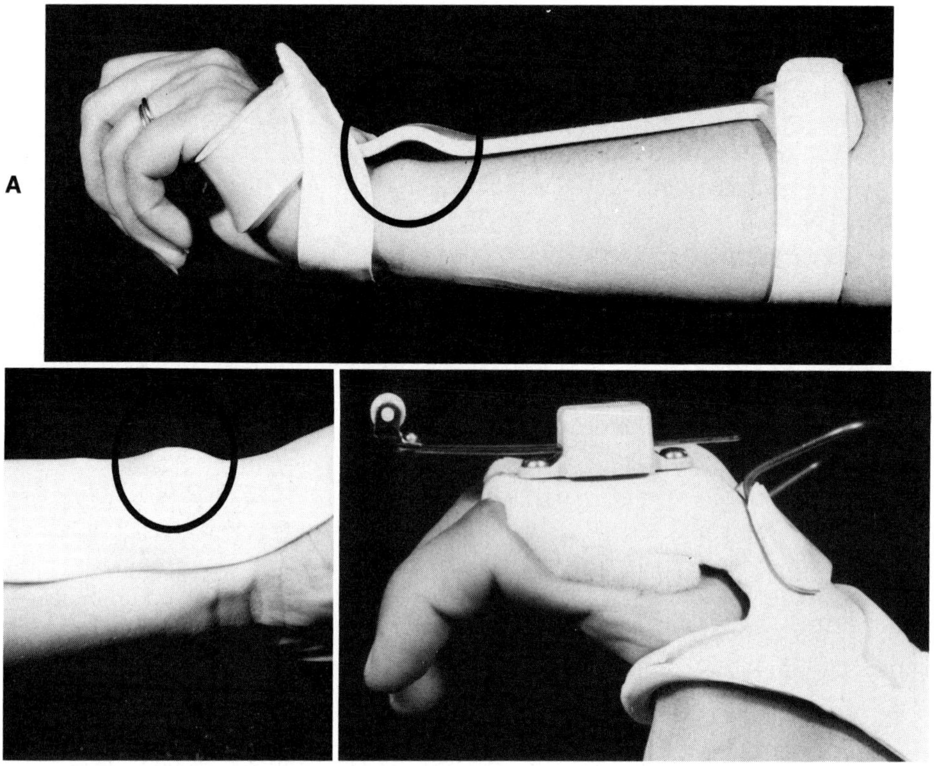

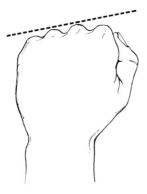

Fig. 9-2. Pressure over bony prominences may be decreased by avoidance **(A)**, wider area of contact **(B)**, or contoured padding **(C)**.

Fig. 9-3. Dorsally, the consecutive metacarpal heads create an oblique angle to the longitudinal axis of the forearm.

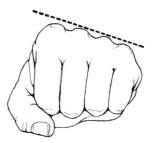

Fig. 9-4. Distally, the fisted hand exhibits an ulnar metacarpal descent that creates an oblique angle in the transverse plane of the forearm.

Functionally, this anatomic arrangement means that, with the forearm fully supinated and resting on a table, a straight object gripped comfortably in the hand will not be parallel to the table but will be slightly higher on the radial side. When the wrist is held in a nondeviated posture, the object will also not be held perpendicular to the longitudinal axis of the forearm but will form an oblique angle with the more proximal portion of the angle occurring on the ulnar side of the hand and the distal portion on the radial aspect.

This principle of dual obliquity must then be translated to any splint part that supports or incorporates the second through fifth metacarpal bones. That is, a splint should be longer and higher on the radial side (Fig. 9-5) and at no time should end or bend perpendicular to the longitudinal axis of the forearm when the wrist is not deviated to either side (Fig. 9-6).

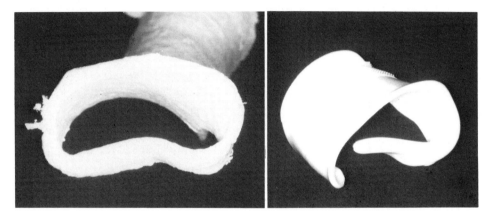

Fig. 9-5. Providing support for the transverse arch, the metacarpal bars should be slightly higher on the radial side when viewed distally.

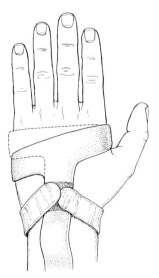

Fig. 9-6. The metacarpal bars should follow the oblique configuration of the metacarpal heads. *Solid lines,* Correct; *broken lines,* incorrect.

Ligaments

Consider ligamentous stress. The preservation of ligamentous structures in correct position and tension is another fundamental anatomic principle of proper fitting of hand splints. Since ligaments normally provide for joint stability and direction, it is important that their functions be considered when attempting to augment hand function with splinting devices. The application of incorrect forces via an improperly fitted splint may cause further damage to an injured or diseased hand by erroneously stressing periarticular structures, resulting in inflammation, attenuation, and occasionally disruption of ligamentous tissue.

From a simplistic point of view, each metacarpophalangeal and interphalangeal joint has three similar ligaments whose presence directly influences the construction of hand splints: two collateral ligaments and a palmar plate ligament. In hinged joints, such as the interphalangeal joints, the collateral ligaments prevent joint mobility in the coronal plane, that is, ulnar and radial deviation. Because of this anatomic arrangement, splints designed to mobilize these joints must be constructed so that their line of pull or application of force is perpendicular to the joint axis (Fig. 9-7). It is also important to monitor splints carefully as passive joint motion improves so that ligamentous structures are not overstretched. Immobilization splints should also be designed to protect this ligamentous support system to prevent instability. It is believed that after digital injury,

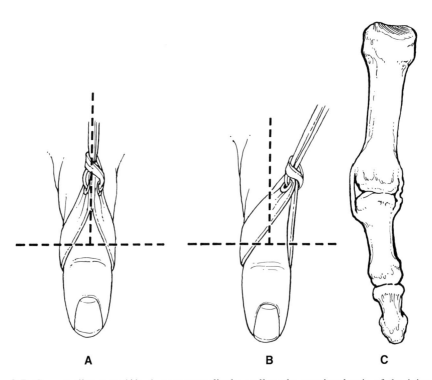

A   **B**   **C**

Fig. 9-7. Correct alignment (**A**). A nonperpendicular pull to the rotational axis of the joint (**B**) will produce unequal stress on the collateral ligaments (**C**).

which requires proximal interphalangeal joint immobilization, a splint that maintains the joint in near-full extension will best preserve collateral ligament length and prevent flexion contracture.

Because of the camlike structure of the heads of the metacarpals, the collateral ligaments of the metacarpophalangeal joints are not taut until the proximal phalanx is brought into near-full flexion, allowing finger abduction-adduction in extension and limited lateral motion when the fingers are flexed. This is an important concept to recognize when fitting splints that act on the metacarpophalangeal joints. If the full length of the collateral ligaments of the metacarpophalangeal joints is not maintained, a loss of flexion may occur, and the ensuing fixed contracture may be impossible to improve by conservative means. So-called safe position splints, such as the Michigan burn splint (Fig. 9-8), embody this concept by positioning the metacarpophalangeal joints in flexion to maintain collateral ligament length. More difficult to envision, but equally important, is the action of a dorsal phalangeal bar (lumbrical bar) that determines the degree of extension allowed to the metacarpophalangeal joints. If the potential for metacarpophalangeal joint stiffness is present, the dorsal phalangeal bar should be adjusted to hold the proximal phalanges in near-full flexion (Fig. 9-9).

A concept that is frequently misunderstood is the function of the metacarpophalangeal collateral ligaments (2-5) and the carpometacarpal ligaments of the fourth and fifth digits during simultaneous finger flexion. Bunnell (1944) correctly noted that in the normal hand each finger points toward the scaphoid when flexed. However, over the years this observation has created some confusion when it was too literally applied to the fitting of hand splints designed to increase passive finger flexion. It is essential to understand the kinematic differences between digital alignment in single finger flexion and simultaneous multiple finger flexion. When the fingers are individually flexed, the tips of the digits touch the palm in a small area near the thenar crease. The distal transverse arch maintains a concave configuration, and the longitudinal axis of each digit aligns toward the scaphoid as Bunnell described. However, when the fingers are flexed simultaneously, the distal transverse arch flattens and digital palmar contact occurs from the middle of the first metacarpal to the hypothenar eminence (Fig. 9-10). The dorsal rotation of the fourth and fifth metacarpals changes the alignment of the longitudinal axis of the ring and small fingers away from the direction of the scaphoid toward a more ulnar orientation. Functionally this allows the hand to grasp objects without the fingers overlapping each other. It also permits optimal palmar surface contact of the hand on larger objects during palmar grip.

The lengths of the metacarpophalangeal joint collateral ligaments and the ligaments of the fourth and fifth carpometacarpal joints are critical to this digital spreading and mobility of the distal transverse arch. In splinting it is essential that the lengths of these ligaments be preserved. When flexion traction to more than one digit is required, the proximal ends of the traction devices at the wrist level should not be anchored at a single point, but should individually originate, allowing maintenance of the lengths of the metacarpophalangeal and carpometacarpal joint ligaments and permitting digital separation (Fig. 9-11). If, however, the traction anchor point is placed at a midforearm position, then a single attachment may be appropriate because the distally widening fan

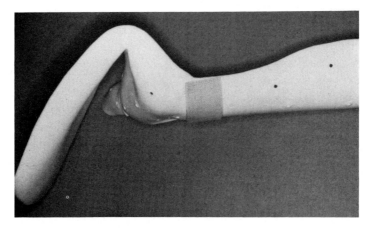

Fig. 9-8. To preserve periarticular tissue length, this safe position splint maintains the metacarpophalangeal joints in flexion and the interphalangeal joints in extension.

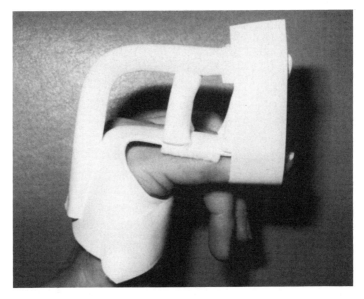

Fig. 9-9. A dorsal phalangeal bar is used to position the metacarpophalangeal joints in near-full flexion to maintain the length of the collateral ligaments. (Courtesy Janet Bailey, O.T.R./L., Columbus, OH.)

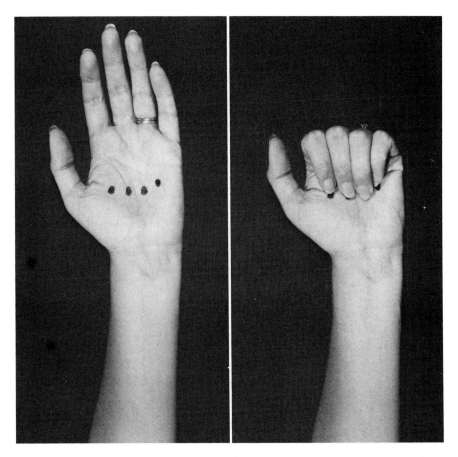

Fig. 9-10. Digital palmar contact occurs from the middle of the first metacarpal to the hypothenar eminence when the fingers are flexed simultaneously.

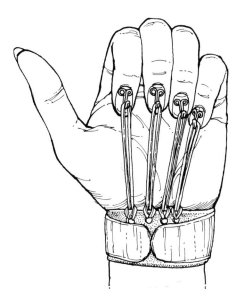

Fig. 9-11. To maintain the necessary ligament length at the 4-5 carpometacarpal and (2-5) metacarpophalangeal joints to allow simultaneous finger flexion, dynamic flexion assists should not overlap at the level of the wrist.

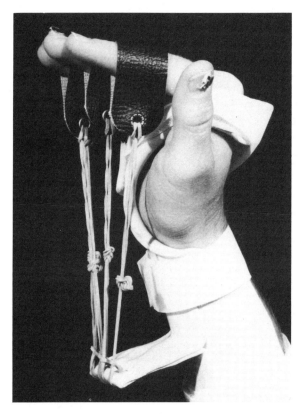

Fig. 9-12. Midforearm attachment of the dynamic assists allows a separation of forces at the wrist level when simultaneously mobilizing multiple digits into flexion. (Courtesy Roslyn Evans, O.T.R., Vero Beach, FL.)

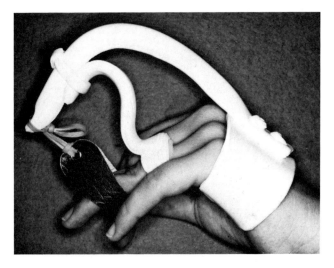

Fig. 9-13. Attenuation of the palmar plate with resultant hyperextension of the joint may occur with prolonged unsupervised extension traction.

configuration of the dynamic assists results in separation of the traction forces at the wrist level (Fig. 9-12). Because the rotation afforded by the ulnar two metacarpals varies from patient to patient, it is important that the angle of approach of the mobilizing force be evaluated carefully for each digit incorporated in the splint.

Palmar plate ligaments prevent hyperextension of the metacarpophalangeal and interphalangeal joints of the hand. When employing mobilizing splints to increase passive joint extension, such as outriggers, serial cylinder casts, or three-point pressure splints, caution should be taken to prevent attenuation of these structures. This may be done by tension adjustment and by careful monitoring of the progress of the joint as it is brought to the neutral position (Fig. 9-13).

The thumb carpometacarpal joint is a saddle articulation that allows motion of the first metacarpal through all planes. There are five primary thumb carpometacarpal ligaments; when fitting thumb splints, one should give careful thought to the position in which the thumb is placed and the ultimate functional ramifications of this position. Maintenance of the first web space must be emphasized, and for most supportive or positioning splints the thumb should be held in wide abduction. If a splint is required to increase passive range of motion of the thumb carpometacarpal joint, it must be fitted so that the mobilizing force is directed to the first metacarpal. Force applied incorrectly to the proximal phalanx creates undue stress on the ulnar collateral ligament of the metacarpophalangeal joint, potentially causing further damage by attenuating the ligament and creating an unstable joint (see Chapter 12).

Arches

Maintain arches. The three skeletal arches of the hand (proximal transverse, distal transverse, and longitudinal) must also be taken into consideration in attaining congruous splint fit. The distal transverse or metacarpal arch consists of an immobile center post, the second and third metacarpal heads, around which the mobile first, fourth, and fifth metacarpals rotate (Fig. 9-14). The longitudinal arch (Fig. 9-15) on a sagittal plane embodies the carpals, metacarpals, and phalanges and allows approximately 280 degrees of total active motion in each finger. The carpal or proximal transverse arch, although existent anatomically, is of secondary importance in splinting because the flexor tendons and palmar neurovascular structures that traverse through the arch obliterate its concavity exteriorly. These arches, which combine stability and flexibility, allow the normal hand to grasp an almost endless array of items of various sizes and shapes with a maximum or minimum of surface contact.

To maintain the maximum potential mobility of the hand, the distal transverse and longitudinal arches must be preserved throughout the duration of treatment. The distal transverse arch should be apparent in any splint that incorporates the metacarpals (Fig. 9-16), provided significant dorsal and palmar swelling is not present. If this type of edema exists, care should be taken to adjust the parts of the splint that are responsible for supporting the arch as the edema subsides. Care should also be taken to continue the transverse arch configuration in splint parts that extend distal to the metacarpophalangeal joints, such as dorsal phalangeal bars or finger pans (Fig. 9-17).

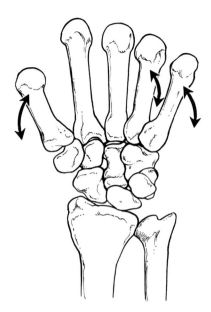

Fig. 9-14. The mobile first, fourth, and fifth metacarpals allow the hand to assume an anteriorly concave configuration, which is fundamental to coordinate grasp.

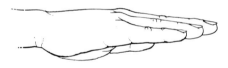

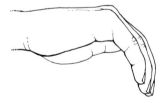

Fig. 9-15. In the sagittal plane the motion potential of the segments comprising the longitudinal arch is approximately 280 degrees.

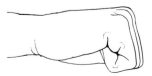

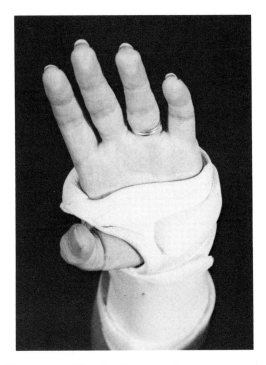

Fig. 9-16. The metacarpal bar should support the transverse metacarpal arch.

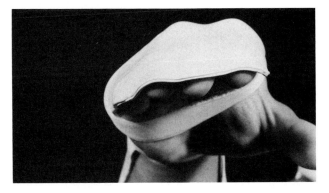

Fig. 9-17. The transverse metacarpal arch should be continued to splint parts that affect the fingers.

Because of the mobility afforded by the longitudinal arch, splints that affect it are varied. Basically, any splint that incorporates the phalanges, either statically or dynamically influences the state of this arch. The use of a finger pan, either in a resting pan splint or a safe position splint, statically provides support for the entire length of the longitudinal arch. Extension or flexion outriggers, metacarpophalangeal flexion cuffs, and elastic traction applied through the use of fingernail clips are examples of splint parts that are used to augment the passive range of motion of the longitudinal arch. When fitting splints that support only certain segments of the longitudinal arch, care must be taken not to block the motion of the remaining adjacent components of the arch, either distally or proximally. This may be done through careful attention to the dorsal and palmar skin creases and their relationships to each end of the splint (Fig. 9-18). Whenever support of any part of the longitudinal arch is to be achieved, the desired position of the involved metacarpophalangeal and interphalangeal joints must be predetermined before fitting may commence. This determination of joint posture depends on the specific purpose of the splint and the individual hand condition with which one is dealing.

Joints

Two principles prevail when fitting splints that are designed to mobilize joints: (1) achievement of the correct alignment of the splint axis with the anatomic joint axis and (2) use of a 90-degree angle that is also perpendicular to the rotational axis of the joint.

Align splint axis with anatomic axis. Articulated splints (Fig. 9-19) must provide correct splint and joint alignment to allow achievement of full motion of the joint being splinted. If this is not accomplished, the splint may not only prove ineffective in increasing motion, but may actually limit joint range and cause friction burns as splint components move independent of the joint. The approximate location of a specific anatomic joint axis may be found through observation of the joint as it moves in the plane in which it is to be splinted.

Use optimum rotational force. When dynamic traction is used to increase the passive range of motion of a joint, the splint should be fitted to eliminate all translational forces and permit only rotational force in the desired plane. This is accomplished by positioning the distal end of the dorsal or palmar outrigger at a point that allows the dynamic assist, such as a rubber band, to pull at a 90-degree angle on the bone to be mobilized. This pull should also be perpendicular to the rotational axis of the joint so that the supporting ligamentous structures are equally stressed. If a 90-degree angle of pull is not employed, and if the force is applied in the direction of the joint, significant pressure may be imparted to the cartilaginous surfaces of the joint as a result of compression of the two bones. If the force is directed away from the joint to be mobilized, the joint surfaces may be distracted, and the patient will have difficulty keeping the traction cuffs on the fingers. As the joint range of motion improves, the length of the outrigger must be changed to accommodate a continuous 90-degree angle of pull (Fig. 9-20).

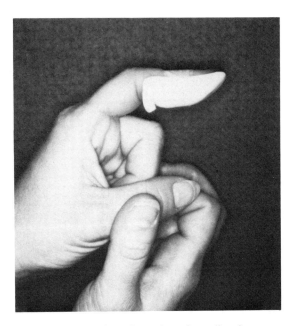

Fig. 9-18. Care should be taken not to impede motion of unsplinted segments of the longitudinal arch.

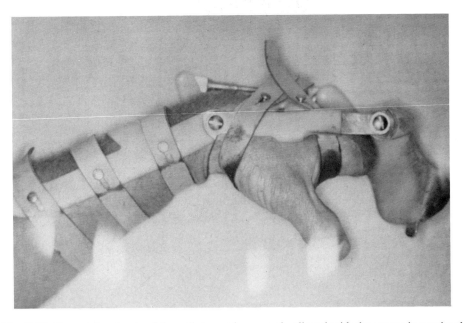

Fig. 9-19. The rotational axis of the splint must be correctly aligned with the anatomic rotational axis of the joint to allow unhampered simultaneous movement of both joints. This partial hand prosthesis exhibits good alignment at the wrist joint. (Splint by Lawrence Czap, O.T.R., orthotist, Columbus, OH.)

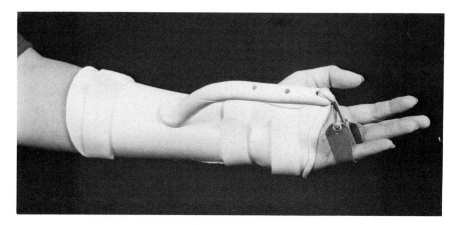

Fig. 9-20. As the finger position changes, the length of the outrigger must be altered to accommodate a 90-degree angle of the traction assist to the segment being mobilized. This palmar outrigger is designed to allow the patient to adjust the traction assist.

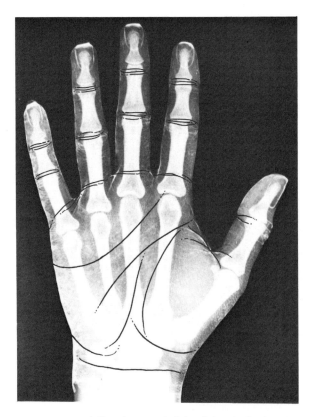

Fig. 9-21. Skin creases correspond directly to underlying joints indicating the boundaries of motion for each segment. (NOTE: Although this is a palmar view, the dye outlines the fingernails and shows through from the dorsum.)

Skin

Concepts of fitting splints with regard to the cutaneous surfaces of the hand include the consideration of skin creases and mechanical principles regarding the dissemination of pressure, elimination of friction, and use of optimum leverage.

Use skin creases as boundaries. Since the dorsal and palmar skin creases correspond directly to the underlying joints (Fig. 9-21), their presence graphically indicates the areas at which motion takes place in the hand and provides tangible boundaries for splint preparation. If the metacarpophalangeal joints are to be unencumbered by a splint, the distal aspect of the splint must not be applied beyond the distal palmar flexion crease; if the thumb is to retain full mobility, the splint material should not lie radial to the thenar crease; and full mobility of a proximal interphalangeal joint may be achieved by terminating the splint slightly proximal to the middle flexion crease of the digit.

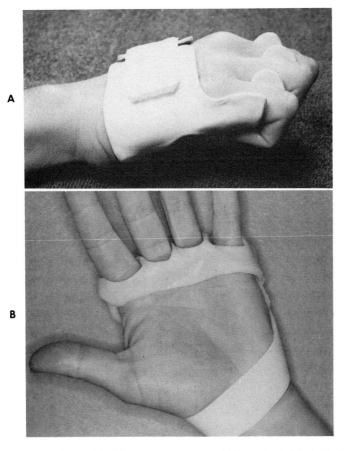

Fig. 9-22. Immobilization or blocking components should be extended to include at least two-thirds the length of the proximal and distal segments that the splint incorporates. **A,** Flexion of the metacarpophalangeal joints is blocked because the palmar phalangeal bar is of sufficient length. **B,** This palmar phalangeal bar was not fitted far enough distally and thus allows metacarpophalangeal flexion. (**A** courtesy K.P. MacBain, O.T.R., Vancouver, BC.)

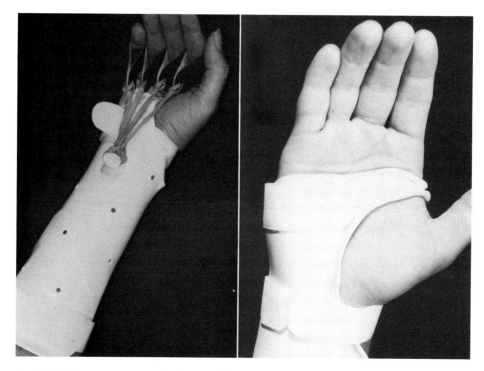

Fig. 9-23. Edge pressure may be decreased by rolling the proximal and distal ends of the splint.

Conversely, if a joint is to be immobilized, the splint should be extended as close as possible to the next segmental crease, both proximally and distally, to provide maximum mechanical purchase (Fig. 9-22).

Use principles of mechanics

Reduce pressure. The dissemination of pressure is another important concept in the design and fitting of hand splints. Excessive pressure, regardless of good splint design and construction, may render the splint intolerable and unwearable. Pressure may be decreased by increasing the area of application. This should be considered in the original design of the splint and may be augmented at the time of fitting by rolling the proximal and distal ends of the splint (Fig. 9-23) and contouring the material nearly to the full length of the segment being fitted.

Padding may be used appropriately to decrease the influence of splint parts that cannot be widened because of their specific functions or place of application. It may also be used to disseminate pressure over especially problematic areas where contouring of the splint material and achievement of a contiguous fit are insufficient to prevent underlying soft tissue damage. When using padding within a contoured space, it is important to achieve a fit that will accommodate the addition of the padding without effectively diminishing the area of the concavity and compromising the fit of the splint (Fig. 9-24). However, one should beware of the overuse of padding because, in addition to its eventual contamination by moisture and dirt, it is frequently indicative of a poorly fitted splint.

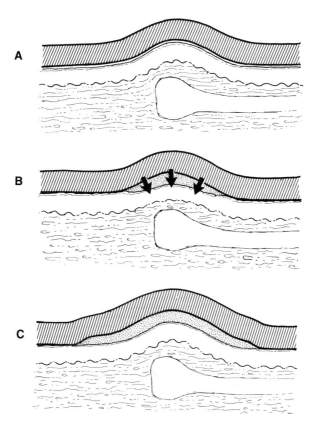

Fig. 9-24. The addition of padding must not compromise splint fit by diminishing contoured space (**A**). **B,** Incorrect. **C,** Correct.

Cutting holes in splints to alleviate pressure is a common mistake that may result in greater pressure around the circumferential border of the cutout with potential tissue injury. It is important to follow the contours of the extremity as closely as possible; if full wound coverage is not present, the splint may be applied over an appropriate dressing. In some instances, application of a splint may be detrimental to specific local tissue viability. The splint should then be designed to avoid this area and any adjacent tissue that may be of questionable viability. The splint border encroaching on this defect should be contoured outward to increase the area of application and decrease the edge pressure (Fig. 9-25).

Eliminate friction. The elimination of friction is the third principle associated with skin. Friction of the splint material against the skin or friction caused by skin against skin, as with adjacent fingers, often is the result of an improperly designed or poorly fitted splint. The splint may be too large, the angle of pull incorrect, or the splint axis may not correspond to the anatomic joint axis. A careful observation of the area of friction and a reevaluation of the various principles of fitting hand splints will probably uncover the problem. Placement of an appropriate material between two cutaneous surfaces may also alleviate troublesome contact areas (Fig. 9-26). Initially, patients should be instructed to remove their splints every 1 to 2 hours to check for areas of skin embarrassment.

Optimum leverage. Fingernail attachment devices such as dress hooks or Velcro buttons should be applied to the proximal and center aspect of the nail. Distal attachment results in considerable discomfort because of the leverage effect of the nail away from the proximal nail bed (Fig. 9-27). This excess leverage could also cause damage to the nail itself.

Proximal and distal straps should be attached as closely as possible to the respective ends of the splint; for optimum mechanical advantage a strap that functions as the middle reciprocal force should be positioned over the joint on which it acts, provided it will not jeopardize tissue viability.

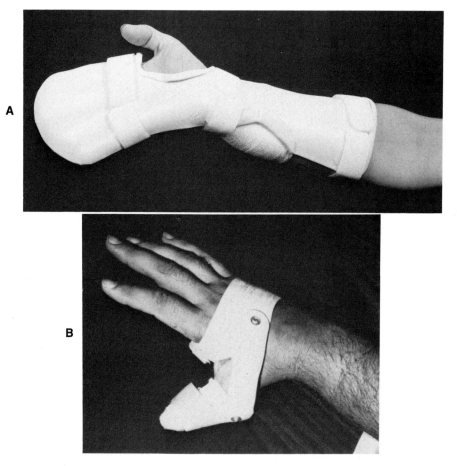

Fig. 9-25. Splint edges that must be adjacent to areas of soft tissue of questionable viability should be contoured outward to decrease pressure. (**B** courtesy Joan Farrell, O.T.R., Miami.)

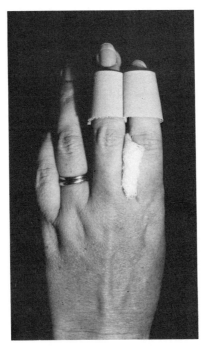

Fig. 9-26. Placement of gauze between two adjacent cutaneous surfaces will decrease friction.

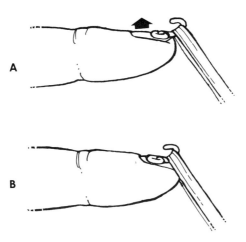

Fig. 9-27. Care should be taken to minimize the leverage effect of a fingernail attachment device on a fingernail bed by avoiding distal attachment. **A,** Incorrect. **B,** Correct.

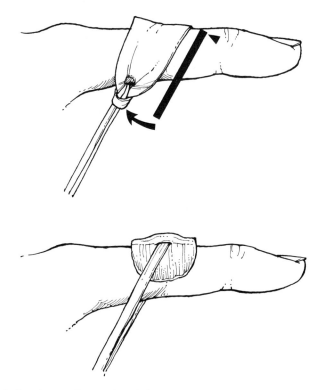

Fig. 9-28. By placing the attachment site of the dynamic assist closer to the finger, the leverage effect of the finger cuff is diminished and pressure is decreased.

Leverage effects on finger cuffs may be diminished by placing the attachment site of the traction device closer to the surface of the digit as advocated by Brand (1985) (Fig. 9-28). This is especially helpful when dealing with the insensitive hand.

KINESIOLOGIC CONSIDERATIONS

Kinesiologic considerations encompass two additional concepts pertaining to the actual shaping of a hand splint: kinematic principles and kinetic principles. Kinematic principles deal with the differences between the hand at rest and the hand in motion, and kinetic principles concern the dynamic force relationship between the hand and the splint. Both the design and form of a hand splint should reflect an understanding of these two major concepts.

Allow for kinematic changes. As the fingers and thumb move through an arc of motion from a fully extended position to an attitude of full flexion, basic external anatomic configurations change their relationships. In flexion, palmar skin creases approximate, arches deepen, dorsal bony prominences become more apparent, the dorsal surface area elongates, and the palmar length lessens. As the thenar and hypothenar masses

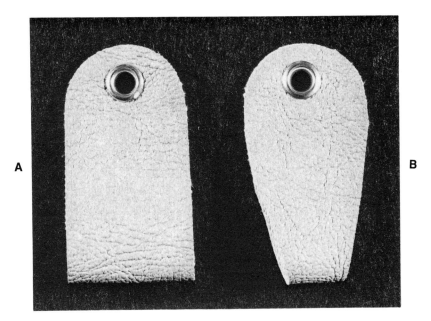

Fig. 9-29. Depending on hand size, extension finger cuffs (**B**) should be cut to allow finger flexion. Flexion cuffs may be used without alteration (**A**).

move palmarly in opposition, the breadth of the hand changes to become convex dorsally and concave palmarly, resulting in the increase of dorsometacarpal surface area. A splint designed to allow motion must be fitted to accommodate anticipated changes in the arches and bony prominences. For example, finger extension cuffs must be cut to permit full proximal and distal phalangeal flexion (Fig. 9-29), whereas the entire width of flexion cuffs may be preserved to decrease pressure. Hypothenar bars should not inhibit motion of the first metacarpal, and phalangeal bars should allow unencumbered motion of the segments they do not support. If these types of adaptations are not executed, motion of the hand may be inhibited, pressure and friction injury of the skin may occur, and the splint may be rendered ineffective.

Employ kinetic concepts. The actual positioning of specific splint parts will augment or retard muscle action. An extension finger cuff placed on the proximal phalanx assists the long extensor tendons, while interossei and lumbrical forces are reinforced when the cuff is positioned at the middle phalanx. The fitting of a dorsal phalangeal bar to prevent metacarpal hyperextension augments extension of the fingers by maximizing the extrinsic extensor action at the interphalangeal joints (Fig. 9-30). Because of the relative lengths of the extrinsic digital flexors and extensors, a wrist bar fitted for extension enhances finger flexion, and conversely a flexed wrist bar favors finger extension. A knowledge of kinetic principles as they pertain to the hand is important in achieving the full potential of splints to increase hand function.

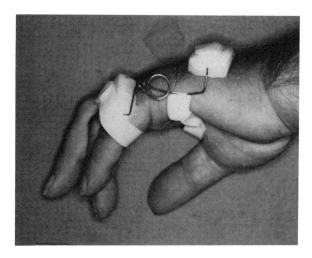

Fig. 9-30. This dorsal phalangeal bar prevents metacarpophalangeal joint hyperextension and allows the excursion of extrinsic extensors to be focused on the interphalangeal joints.

TECHNICAL CONSIDERATIONS

Numerous techniques of fitting hand splints are based on practical everyday experiences. These additional clinical considerations increase efficiency and make the fitting process run more smoothly.

Develop patient rapport. An explanation about the proposed splint—its functions, material, and method of forming—implement the development of patient rapport and trust. A rehearsal of the desired position in which the hand is to be splinted before the actual application of the splint material also expedites the fitting process. If thermal materials are used, the patient should be warned that the material will feel warm. Allowing a child to play with scraps of the material before fitting commences is ultimately well worth the extra time and effort!

Work efficiently. The use of devices or methods that increase the efficiency of the molding time may also be of considerable benefit. Lightly wrapping a warmed, low-temperature, thermal material splint to the patient's hand and forearm with an Ace bandage allows for full attention to be directed to the positioning of the hand. Strategically applied tape holds splint parts in position as they cool (Fig. 9-31), and, in working with more slowly setting materials such as plaster, a hand rest or positioning device (Fig. 9-32) lessens muscle fatigue during the cooling phase.

Allowing gravitational forces to augment splint fabrication is another efficiency consideration of fit. If the splint is to be worn palmarly, molding is facilitated by placing the forearm and hand in supination; a dorsal splint is best fitted in pronation.

Change method according to properties of materials used. Different materials require the use of diverse approaches to the forming procedure (Fig. 9-33). For example, if a protective stockinette is used during the shaping of a splint constructed of high-

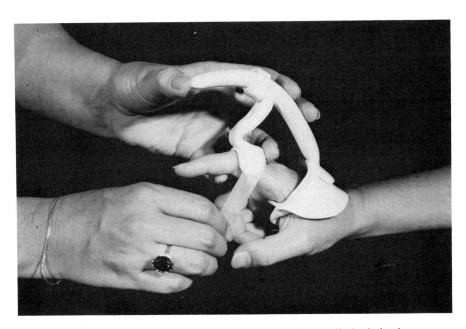

Fig. 9-31. Tape may be used to maintain splint position until plastic hardens.

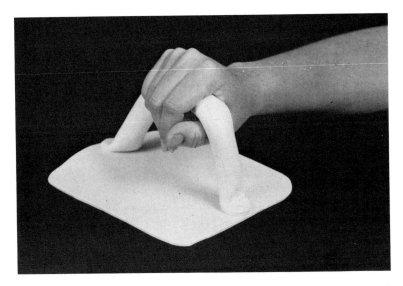

Fig. 9-32. A positioning device may be of assistance when the curing phase is prolonged.

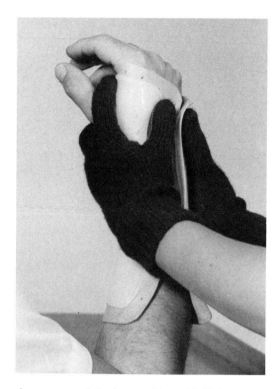

Fig. 9-33. Protective gloves are needed when working with high-temperature materials such as polyethelene. (Courtesy Theresa Bielawski, O.T.[C], and Jane Bear-Lehman, M.S., O.T.R., Toronto, Ont.)

temperature material, the resulting splint will be somewhat large for the unprotected hand, requiring further adjustment. Moisture should be eliminated from the surfaces of a material requiring wet heat before application to the patient, and the use of a separating substance such as petroleum jelly augments the removal of newly applied cylindrical plaster splints.

SUMMARY

Those involved in the splinting process must arm themselves with a knowledge of the anatomic, mechanical, kinesiologic, and technical principles that are an absolute prerequisite for proper fit. Failure to adhere to these principles often results in embarrassing pressure areas, splint disuse, and patient distrust, with the probable attendant decrease of hand function.

The decision to use a splint on the hand of a particular patient is a serious consideration involving the physician and the therapist; a close communication between the two must exist so that the exact function expected from each splint may be realized. If the proper fit techniques are employed, the opportunity for maximum hand function and patient satisfaction is provided.

PART THREE

Anatomic site

CHAPTER 10

Splints acting on the wrist and forearm

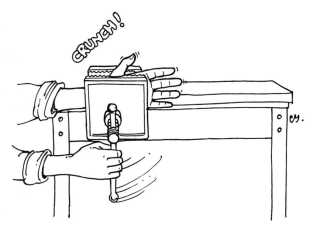

"MR. BROWN, THAT'S NOT GOING TO HELP!"

Two osseous structures, the ulna and the radius, which are connected by a fibrous interosseous membrane, form two articulations—the proximal radioulnar joint and the distal radioulnar joint. These integrated forearm components provide critical rotational movement to the entire distal portion of the upper extremity open kinematic chain. With an axis of motion that travels proximally through the head of the radius and distally through the head of the ulna, the radius rotates in relation to the ulna. The two bones are positioned parallel to each other in supination, and the radius crosses over the ulna in pronation. Following the arc of the radius, the hand may be rotated approximately 180 degrees. Combined, the radioulnar joints allow a single arc of transverse rotational motion—pronation-supination—and form a uniaxial joint with 1 degree of freedom of movement. The coalescence of forearm and wrist motion results in hand positioning in the sagittal, coronal, and transverse planes.

The osseous anatomy of the wrist consists of the distal radius and ulna and eight carpal bones. The wrist is classified as a condylar diarthrosis with a wide range of motion resulting from its many small internal joints and intrinsic stability provided by a complex ligamentous arrangement. As the most proximal segment in the intercalated chain of hand joints, the wrist is the key to function at the more distal joint levels. The wrist is vulnerable to a wide assortment of injuries and diseases, thus making it subject to acute or secondary patterns of deformity, instability, or collapse, that may significantly interfere with hand performance.

The collective carpal bones form the anteriorly concave proximal transverse arch, whose functional position directly influences the kinetic interaction of structures composing the longitudinal arch. It appears that the traditional concept of the wrist carpus as two transverse four-bone rows is a substantial oversimplification of its complex dynamic motion patterns. Taleisnik (1978), in refining the work of Navarro, defines the carpal scaphoid as the lateral or mobile column of the wrist, with the triquetrum serving as the medial or rotation column and the remaining six bones comprising the central or flexion-extension column. Taleisnik points out that the anatomic positioning of the wrist ligaments, particularly on the palmar side, permits these intricate columnar movements and provides the best rationale for understanding the dynamic anatomy of the wrist, its function, and its behavior during injury.

Direct or adjacent trauma, particularly when accompanied by crushing or prolonged edema, may result in fibrotic changes in the tightly articulated wrist joints, resulting in limited range of motion. The obligatory immobilization of fracture, tendon, or ligament injuries in this area increases the possibility of motion loss. Conversely, ligamentous rupture or attenuation secondary to inflammatory disease processes may result in wrist instability and collapse patterns that can compromise digital performance to an even greater extent than that produced by wrist stiffening.

The wrist serves as the key joint to distal hand function and influences both digital strength and dexterity. It is therefore important to give very careful consideration to proper joint positioning and protection, as well as the restoration and preservation of a satisfactory range of motion. A program that integrates splinting and exercise often provides the essential elements to maintain wrist function.

It is also important that the effect of wrist position be thoroughly considered in the preparation of any hand splint. Wrist dorsiflexion tightens extrinsic flexor tendons and permits the synergistic wrist extension–strong finger flexion function employed in power grasp. Wrist palmar flexion tightens the long extrinsic extensor tendons, allowing the hand to open automatically, while greatly reducing digit flexion efficiency. Splints designed either to relax or protect extensor tendons or to promote active digital flexion should support the wrist in an appropriate degree of dorsiflexion. This is often determined by the individual problem. Conversely, active digital extension or flexor tendon healing is enhanced by splinting the wrist in a flexed attitude. One must take care, however, to avoid positioning the wrist in either excessive palmar flexion or dorsiflexion, which could lead to attenuation of delicate soft tissue structures or cause pressure on the median nerve as it passes through the carpal canal. Understanding and careful application of these kinetic mechanisms will aid healing and motion programs in the hand.

The purpose of this chapter is to discuss splinting of the wrist and forearm with regard to anatomic, kinesiologic, and mechanical factors. There are six basic reasons for splinting the wrist and forearm:

1. To protect injured or repaired structures.
2. To prevent deformity.
3. To decrease pain.
4. To enhance digital function.
5. To correct deformity.
6. To increase the purchase on more distal joints.

It is much more common to use wrist and forearm splints for immobilization purposes. With the limited exception of splints designed to correct deformation, the majority of splints in the preceding list require immobilization techniques.

SIMPLE WRIST SPLINTS

When used to control articular motion, simple wrist splints affect motion of the multiple carpal joints in a similar manner. They may be used to mobilize or to immobilize.

Immobilization

Simple wrist immobilization splints allow healing of injured structures of the distal forearm and wrist. Depending on the purpose of application, these splints may be fitted to affect motion in either or both the sagittal and coronal planes.

The most commonly used simple wrist immobilization splint is the dorsiflexion or cock-up splint, which, except in special circumstances, positions the wrist in approximately 10 to 30 degrees of extension to allow maximum composite hand function (Fig. 10-1). Radial and ulnar deviation bars are frequently employed to prevent coronal movement of the hand. For optimum mechanical advantage, the forearm trough should be two thirds the length of the forearm and half its thickness. The metacarpal bar should allow full metacarpophalangeal flexion and extension, and, if possible, straps should be placed at the far distal and proximal ends of the splint and directly over the wrist axis of rotation. Care should be taken to diminish pressure over bony prominences such as the ulnar styloid process and the head of the radius.

Mobilization

Mobilizing the stiffened wrist by splinting is a most difficult assignment. Certainly no externally applied splinting device may selectively differentiate its force application to the radiocarpal or midcarpal joints. When columnar wrist motion patterns are considered, the problem of mobilizing pathologically fibrosed wrist joints becomes even more difficult. Nonetheless, carefully prepared dynamic splints that attempt to gently mobilize immobile carpal articulations without damaging uninjured ligamentous structures may on some occasions prove beneficial.

Simple wrist mobilization splints may be fitted to produce wrist flexion, extension, or deviation and are usually constructed as a single unit or as two pieces connected by

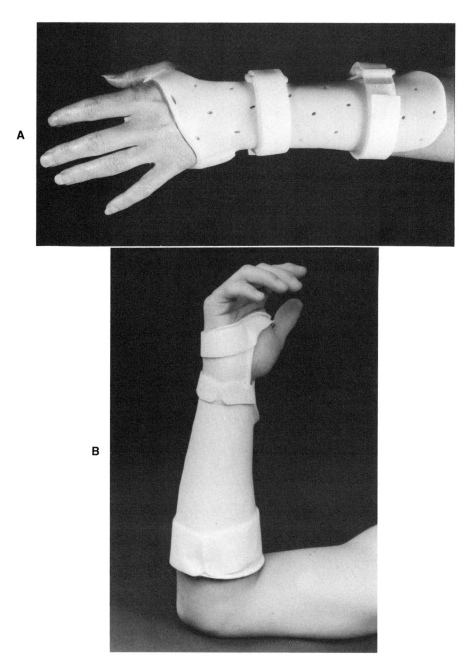

Fig. 10-1. Simple wrist immobilization splints may be fitted dorsally (**A**) or palmarly (**B**). (**A** courtesy Sharon Flinn-Wagner, M.Ed.,O.T.R./L., Cleveland.)

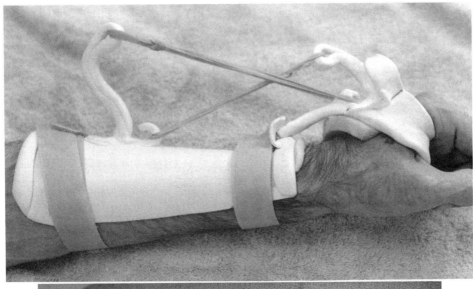

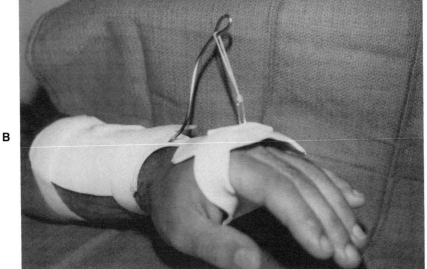

Fig. 10-2. A simple wrist mobilization splint may be designed as a single unit or as two pieces. Depending on the position and mobility of the wrist, use of an outrigger to provide a 90-degree angle of pull to the metacarpals enhances the mechanical function of the splint. (**A** courtesy Carolina deLeeuw, M.A., O.T.R., Tacoma, WA; **B** courtesy Cynthia Philips, M.A., O.T.R., Boston.)

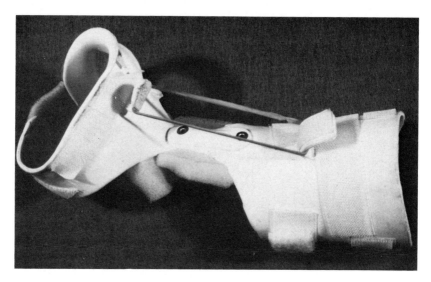

Fig. 10-3. When the wrist is passively supple and the splint is applied to substitute for absent active motion, extended outriggers and a 90-degree angle of pull are not required.

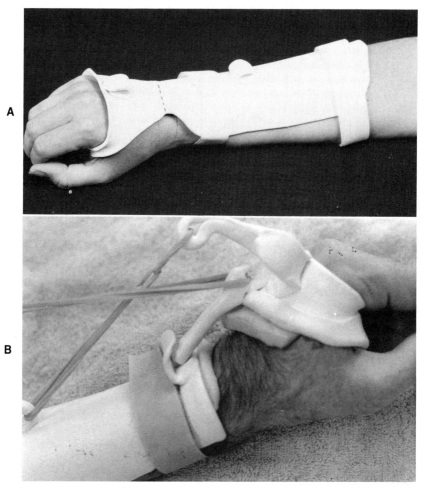

Fig. 10-4. Whether one or two pieces, a hinged wrist bar must be aligned (**A,** *broken line*) with corresponding wrist creases to permit uninhibited motion. (**B** courtesy Carolina deLeeuw, M.A., O.T.R., Tacoma, WA.)

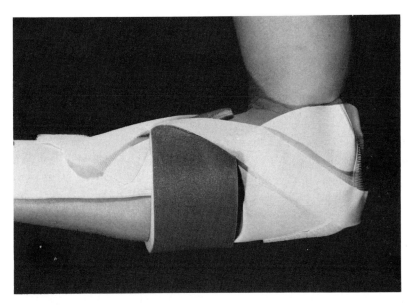

Fig. 10-5. An elbow cuff may assist in maintaining correct position of the splint on the extremity. (This patient was unable to tolerate a triceps cuff.)

a traction device or joints (Fig. 10-2). Both types should allow continuous 90-degree angle of pull to be employed through the use of appropriate length outriggers. If the wrist is passively mobile, an outrigger may not be required (Fig. 10-3). The wrist bar may be absent or hinged (Fig. 10-4). To reduce pressure, the longitudinal length of the metacarpal bar should be as long as possible without inhibiting wrist motion proximally and metacarpophalangeal motion distally. It should also maintain the distal transverse metacarpal arch. Thumb motion should be preserved, and as with the wrist immobilization splints, the forearm trough should be two thirds the length of the forearm and, if using low-temperature plastic, half its thickness. An elbow cuff or triceps cuff may be necessary to prevent distal migration of the forearm trough (Fig. 10-5). Because of the magnitude of the forces involved in mobilizing a wrist, careful attention should be directed to underlying cutaneous surfaces. The splint should be removed for skin inspection a minimum of every hour during the initial wearing phase. Padding is usually necessary at the distal end of the forearm trough and along the length of the metacarpal bar. It is not unusual for a wrist mobilization splint to produce transient median nerve compression with paresthesias in the distribution of the nerve. If a patient complains of numbness in the fingers from wearing the splint, it should be removed and adjusted. If the numbness returns when the adjusted splint is reapplied, the splint should be discontinued.

Some wrist mobilization splints allow motion in one plane but inhibit motion in another, usually through the use of jointed hand and forearm pieces (Fig. 10-6). When fitting this type of splint, it is imperative to match the rotational axis of the splint with the anatomic joint axis. Improper alignment of the two joints produces incorrect forces across the wrist joint, which could lead to further damage, including inhibition of motion and friction abrasions to underlying skin.

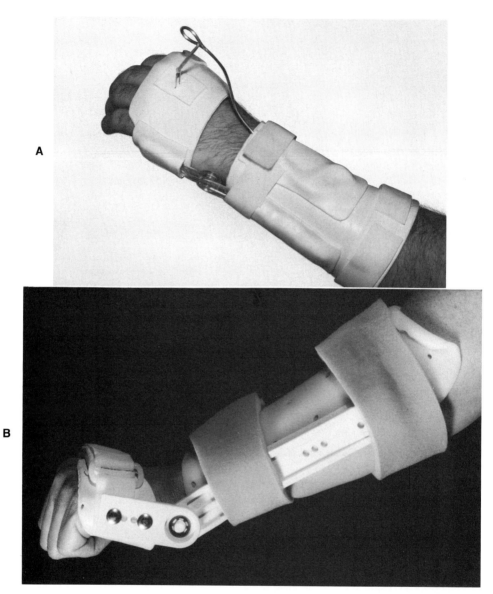

Fig. 10-6. A jointed wrist splint is often used in the postoperative care of a patient who has undergone a wrist arthroplasty procedure. (A courtesy Cynthia Philips, M.A., O.T.R., Boston; **B** courtesy Sharon Flinn-Wagner, M. Ed., O.T.R./L., Cleveland.)

COMPLEX WRIST MOBILIZATION SPLINTS

Despite passively supple joints, tendon adhesions may inhibit simultaneous passive flexion or extension of both the wrist and digital joints secondary to a tenodesis phenomenon. To increase tendon excursion and convert the tenodesis effect, a splint must be designed to either immobilize the wrist and mobilize the fingers or mobilize the wrist and immobilize the fingers. Either method enhances the mechanical focus of the dynamic traction. Although both types of splints would be categorized as long, the mechanical emphasis of each is different, as are their descriptive classifications: long finger mobilization splint and long wrist mobilization splint, respectively.

In a long wrist mobilization splint the posture of the wrist and the direction of the traction are dictated by whether flexor or extensor tendon excursion is limited. When flexor tendon adhesions are present, a finger pan may be used to immobilize the fingers in extension, while dynamic extension traction is applied to the wrist (Fig. 10-7). If extrinsic extensor adhesions limit simultaneous wrist and finger flexion, the fingers may be immobilized in a flexed attitude and gentle flexion traction applied to the wrist. To provide optimum rotational effect, the traction assist for either splint should pull at a 90-degree angle to the metacarpals and should also be perpendicular to the center of the sagittal axis of rotation of the wrist. The metacarpal bar should support the distal transverse metacarpal arch and, in the case of the long wrist flexion splint, should allow full metacarpophalangeal flexion. The forearm trough should be of sufficient length and width to provide good mechanical advantage and strength.

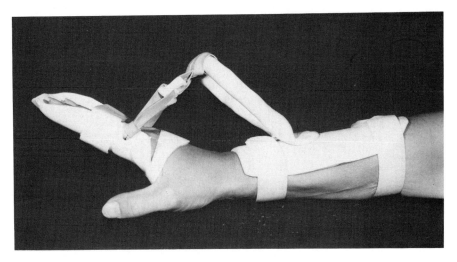

Fig. 10-7. This long wrist extension splint may be used to decrease the tenodesing effect of extrinsic flexor tendon adhesions.

As previously mentioned, efforts to mobilize digital joints may be compromised by the position the wrist is allowed to assume. The tenodesis effect of wrist extensors on digital flexors is an important consideration in the design of long finger splints with wrist immobilization components. Although the wrist is included as an adjunctive measure, the primary purpose of these long finger mobilization or immobilization splints is directed toward influencing digital status. For this reason further discussion of these types of splints is included in the chapter dealing with splints acting on the fingers.

RADIOULNAR MOBILIZATION SPLINTS

Because of the orientation of the rotational axis of the forearm and the problems presented in obtaining a secure mechanical hold from which to base mobilization forces, designing and fitting splints to increase supination or pronation range of motion may be a very difficult task. Understanding that the combined rotational axis of the radioulnar joints almost parallels the lengths of the ulna and radius (Fig. 10-8) is essential in dealing successfully with motion limitations of the forearm. To be effective, mobilizing forces must have a 90-degree angle of approach to the axis of joint rotation. Therefore, dynamic traction that is intended to increase supination or pronation should be applied at an angle perpendicular to the length of the forearm.

Requiring considerable ingenuity (Fig. 10-9), radioulnar mobilization splint designs assume unusual configurations. To obtain maximal purchase on the extremity, the wrist is immobilized and the length of the forearm trough should be at least two thirds the length of the forearm. Outriggers may run perpendicular (Fig. 10-10) or parallel (Fig. 10-11) to the axis of rotation.

A congruous fit is very important in radioulnar mobilization splints. If this is not obtained, friction injury to the underlying cutaneous surface can occur. As with wrist mobilization splints, if the patient complains of numbness or tingling in the digits, the splint should be removed immediately.

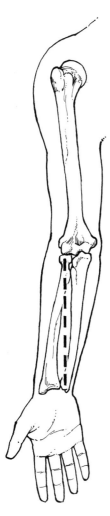

Fig. 10-8. Rotational axis of the forearm runs almost parallel to the lengths of the ulna and radius.

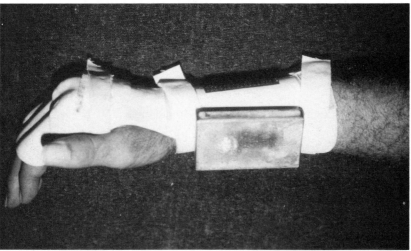

Fig. 10-9. This weighted splint is designed to assist pronation and to block full extension of the metacarpophalangeal joints. (Courtesy Robin Miller Wagman, O.T.R., Ft. Lauderdale, FL.)

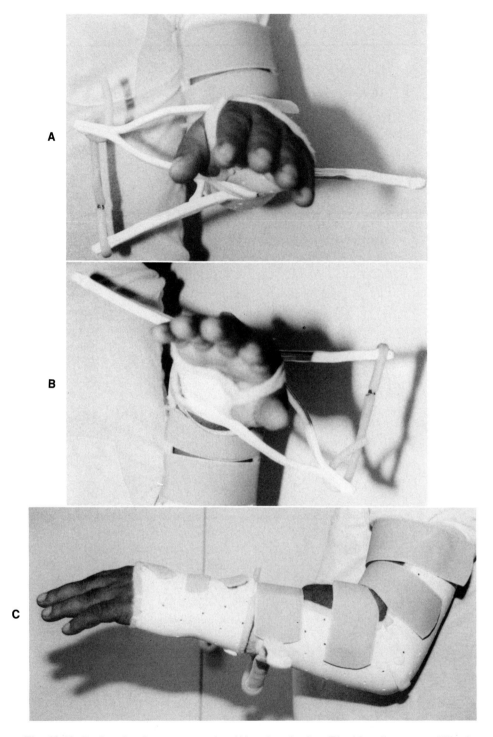

Fig. 10-10. Designed to improve pronation (**A**) and supination (**B**), this splint uses mobilization forces perpendicular to the axis of rotation of the combined radioulnar joints. **C,** Lateral view of (**A**). (Courtesy Janet M. Kinnunen, O.T.R., San Antonio, TX.)

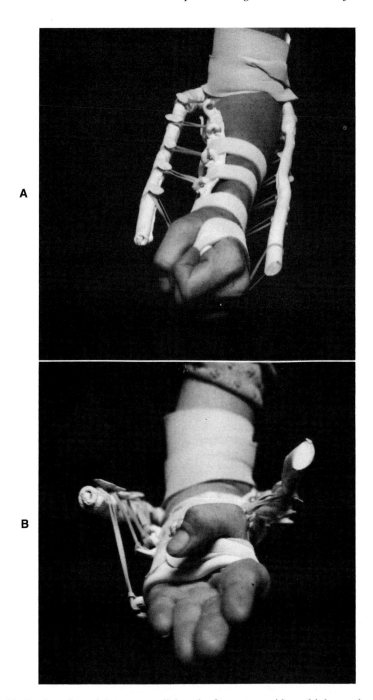

Fig. 10-11. Dual outriggers that run parallel to the forearm provide multiple attachment sites for mobilization forces (rubber bands) that pull perpendicular to the rotational axis of the forearm, enhancing pronation **(A)** and supination **(B)**. (Courtesy Kay Colello, O.T.R., Orange, CA.)

SUMMARY

The integrity of the wrist joint with its complex anatomic and motion arrangements has been established as the "key" to hand function. It is uniquely vulnerable to a variety of injury and disease processes that may result in pain, stiffness, or instability, which may interfere with normal hand function at all levels. The management of these wrist maladies may be substantially enhanced by proper splinting with objectives ranging from pain relief and protection to prevention and correction of deformity. In addition, wrist splinting may be used to negate or augment long extrinsic tenodesis functions in the management of digital pathologic conditions. It is therefore imperative that careful consideration be directed toward the anatomic, kinesiologic, and functional effects of any splint created to traverse this important joint.

The radioulnar joints provide the distal extremity with the very important increment of transverse rotation, allowing the hand to be positioned in a multitude of functional attitudes. In addition to a thorough knowledge of forearm anatomy, the key to splinting these joints lies in understanding their cooperative kinesiologic role.

CHAPTER 11

Splints acting on the fingers

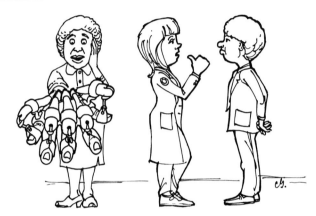

"IT MAY HAVE BEEN BETTER TO INCORPORATE ALL THE FINGERS INTO ONE SPLINT, MR. SIMS."

The purpose of this chapter is to examine the concepts of splinting the fingers. Governed by anatomic, kinesiologic, and mechanical variables, these splints must also adhere to the principles of design, fit, construction, and mobilization. The most common reasons for applying finger splints are the correction or prevention of deformity, the protection of injured or repaired structures and the allowance of controlled active motion to specific joints. Finger splinting may also be used to decrease pain, enhance grasp and release patterns, and provide stability to lax joints.

The functional capacity of the fingers depends on the integrated motion of its four proximally unified, distally independent articulated rays. These triarticular units function as diverging open kinematic chains whose four segments provide a progressive summation of motion in the sagittal and coronal planes. The mobility afforded by the fourth and fifth carpometacarpal joints also provides an element of motion in the transverse plane to the ring and small fingers, allowing palmar and radial approximation of the ulnar border of the hand. The condylar metacarpal joints allow some rotation in addition to flexion, extension, abduction, and adduction of the fingers. Longitudinally each successive joint adds an increment of sagittal mobility until at its maximal limit the cumulative palmar flexion possible per digit is approximately 280 degrees.

The effect of a single joint restriction or the loss of a distal segment on composite hand function is lessened when the rest of the hand has normal motion. However, as the number of stiffened joints or lost segments increases, the compensatory ability of the hand becomes progressively compromised.

In addition to supple joints, it is necessary to have muscles of adequate strength with adhesion-free tendon excursion to produce the highly integrated digital motion required for optimum hand function. In their normal state the fingers represent an equilibrium of intrinsic and extrinsic forces that, in conjunction with the thumb, are capable of functional patterns ranging from delicate prehension to powerful grasp.

Because digital effectiveness depends on mobility, it is important to achieve and maintain adequate motion early in the rehabilitation process. Splinting and exercise programs should be designed to prevent the development of articular and musculotendinous limitations. In the presence of established deformity, emphasis should be placed on restoring lost motion. Programs should acknowledge the structural peculiarities at each joint level and be designed accordingly. The metacarpophalangeal joints of the fingers have a propensity for becoming stiff in extension; the proximal interphalangeal joints more often become stiff in flexion.

Sensibility also plays an important role in finger use. Impaired digital sensibility diminishes the ability of the hand to distinguish texture and pressure variables. This inability to adequately receive, relay, or interpret sensory impulses from the hand severely limits composite hand function. Splints whose designs are meant to encourage hand use should not encumber the palmar surfaces of the fingers, particularly at distal, more tactilely sensitive areas.

IMMOBILIZATION OR BLOCKING SPLINTS

Finger immobilization or blocking splints may be used to promote healing, control early postoperative motion, or enhance functional use. These splints may involve one or more joints and, depending on the specific requirements, may be fitted dorsally, palmarly, laterally, or circumferentially. Care should be taken to maintain correct ligamentous stress at each joint incorporated in the splint and to permit full motion of the uninvolved joints. Maximum three-point mechanical advantage may be ensured by straps placed over key joints and each end of the splint. If, however, the splint is designed to block or partially limit a given motion, the numbers of straps and their placement will be governed by the specific criteria for fitting the splint and the need to obtain a firm purchase on the finger while allowing controlled motion of adjacent key joints (Fig. 11-1). Because of their long narrow configurations, finger immobilization splints should be contoured to half the phalangeal segmental thickness to augment material strength, and splint length should be extended as far distally and proximally as possible without inhibiting motion of uninvolved adjacent joints.

Finger immobilization splints may be categorized as simple or long, depending on whether the wrist is incorporated in the splint. Whereas simple splints prevent articular

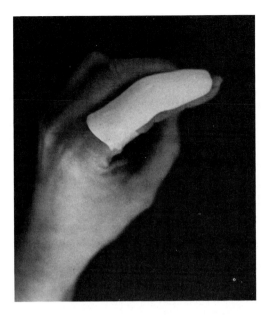

Fig. 11-1. Tape is often used to secure an immobilization or blocking splint to the finger. This splint allows full active flexion of the finger but prevents full extension of the proximal interphalangeal joint.

motion (Fig. 11-2), long finger immobilization splints influence extrinsic musculotendinous units (Fig. 11-3) by means of adjunctive wrist positioning. Wrist position may be used to increase or decrease the amount of tension on these musculotendinous units through alteration of the tenodesis effect. The forearm trough of a long immobilization splint should be half the thickness of the forearm and two thirds its length, for best comfort, strength, and mechanical advantage.

It should be stressed that, for immobilization of finger joints which have not undergone surgical repair, the preferred or "safe" position for the metacarpophalangeal joints is usually considered to be 70 to 90 degrees of flexion, and a 0- to 10-degree flexion posture is best for the interphalangeal joints (Fig. 11-4). These attitudes considerably decrease the potential for ligamentous contractures and the consequent limitation of articular motion.

MOBILIZATION SPLINTS

Although mobilization splints assume a variety of configurations, all must meet certain criteria to be effective. To mobilize stiffened joints, understanding anatomy, kinesiology, surgical procedures, rehabilitation goals, mechanical concepts, properties of dynamic assists, and the physiologic ramifications of applying a splint are equally important. A well-designed splint is rendered ineffective if not worn long enough to produce tissue growth; failure to combine splint and exercise regimens may result in good

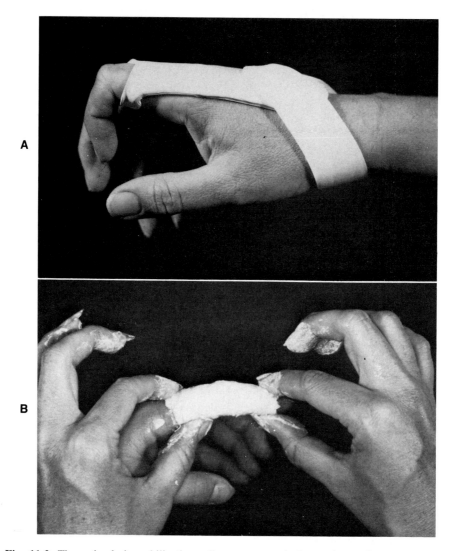

Fig. 11-2. These simple immobilization splints prevent articular motion at the metacarpophalan-geal joint (**A**), at the proximal interphalangeal joint (**B**), and at the distal interphalangeal joint (**C**), as well as of the entire ray (**D**).

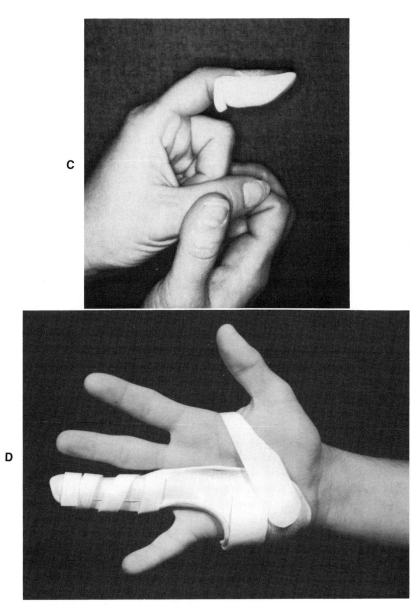

Fig. 11-2, cont'd. For legend see opposite page.

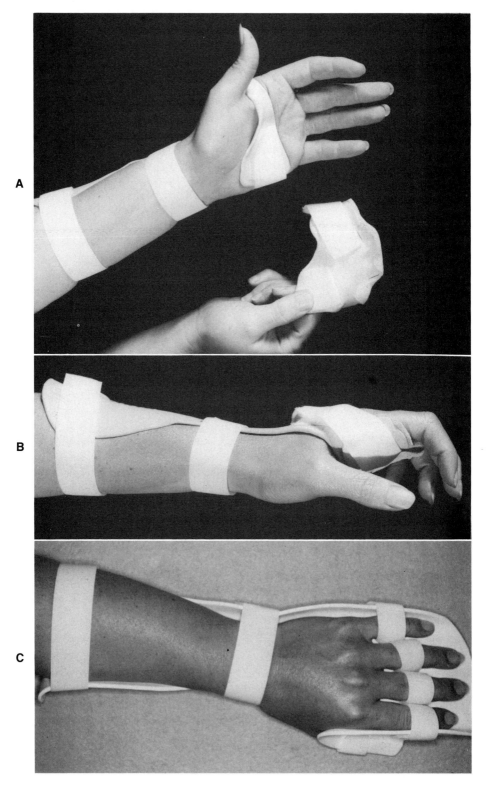

Fig. 11-3. Long finger immobilization splints may partially inhibit motion of the longitudinal rays, as with this adjustable two-piece splint (**A** and **B**), or completely immobilize the fingers (**C**). (**A** and **B** courtesy Sharon Flinn-Wagner, M.Ed., O.T.R./L., Cleveland.)

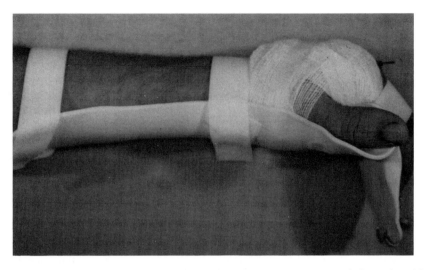

Fig. 11-4. The safe position splint maintains optimum stress on metacarpophalangeal and interphalangeal collateral ligaments.

passive motion but poor active range; application of incorrect forces may actually cause further damage; and a beautifully executed surgical procedure may be jeopardized because of insufficient communication between the physician and the therapist during the postoperative phase. The patient's cooperation is also essential to achieving maximum rehabilitation potential. Too often the fitting of a splint is seen as an isolated experience. Nothing could be further from the truth! A splint that is appropriately used is but one of many tools an astute hand specialist employs in close conjunction with other important aspects of therapy.

Mobilization splints may use elastic or inelastic traction to direct correlative forces. The angle of application of the mobilizing force directly influences the efficacy of the splint, in terms of efficiency in correcting deformity while providing optimum comfort. Elastic traction splints frequently require an outrigger component to serve as a base of attachment or as a fulcrum for dynamic assists. Aside from the obvious difference in mass, the height of an outrigger influences only the number of times it must be adjusted as range of motion of joints changes. As has been shown, high-profile outriggers maintain an angle of pull that is closer to 90 degrees for a longer time and require fewer adjustments as change occurs than do low-profile configurations. Inelastic traction splints usually involve consecutive serial applications or depend on the patient to adjust the amount of force applied as joint motion improves. Selecting type of traction and the configuration of specialized components depends on many factors. Each design option has distinct advantages and disadvantages. There are no universal answers. The more familiar hand specialists become with the many choices available, the better prepared they will be to best meet the needs of their individual patients.

To decrease potential error, careful deductive assessment of the extremity is imperative before final design decisions are reached. It is not unusual for perplexing symptoms to be exhibited by a diseased or injured hand. An inaccurate assumption regarding etiology could lead an unwary person or novice to create a splint that may not only be ineffective but may actually cause further damage. For example, a rotational deformity at the metacarpal level may be misinterpreted as pathology at the more distal metacarpophalangeal or proximal interphalangeal joints. Lack of active motion at a joint may be the result of any number of problems, including shortening of periarticular structures, articular adhesions, intraarticular fracture, tendon rupture, tendon adhesions, and nerve disruption. A splint that is appropriate for one problem may actually be contraindicated for others. It is therefore critical that a complete and accurate concept of the pathology be determined before embarking on the design and fabrication of any mobilization splint.

Metacarpophalangeal level

The metacarpophalangeal joints of the index, long, ring, and small fingers are of the condyloid type in which the rounded metacarpal head fits into a small concavity at the base of the proximal phalanx. The ligamentous arrangement at each joint consists of two collateral ligaments and one palmar ligament that allow anteroposterior and mediolateral motion in addition to a slight amount of phalangeal rotation. Since the ligaments must extend around the cam-shaped palmar portion of the joint, the collateral ligaments are slack when the joint is in extension and taut when the joint is flexed. Pathologic conditions involving the metacarpophalangeal joints of the fingers frequently result in periarticular stiffness and eventually contracture in a position of extension or hyperextension. This type of deformity in a protracted state is extremely difficult to correct through conservative means. It is important to anticipate this problem and make appropriate efforts to maintain adequate length of the metacarpophalangeal collateral ligaments through preventive flexion splinting and exercise programs that emphasize full metacarpophalangeal joint flexion.

Splinting for mobilization of a metacarpophalangeal joint should incorporate a 90-degree rotational force on the distal aspect of the proximal phalanx, which is also perpendicular to the axis of rotation in the desired plane of the involved joint. If a perpendicular pull is not achieved, unequal force will be applied to the periarticular ligaments, which may cause attenuation and result in ulnar or radial deviation of the digit. To allow full flexion, the palmar metacarpal bar of a metacarpophalangeal flexion splint should not extend beyond the distal palmar flexion crease. If distal migration of the splint limits metacarpophalangeal motion, an elbow cuff, triceps cuff, or diagonal splint straps may be added to further stabilize the splint on the extremity. The choice between a simple (Fig. 11-5) or long (Fig. 11-6) splint design depends on the presence or absence of extrinsic adhesions producing a tenodesis effect or poor habitual posturing of the wrist.

Proximal interphalangeal level

The interphalangeal joints of the fingers are true hinge, or ginglymoid, joints and allow motion in only the sagittal plane. The ligamentous structure of these joints is similar to that of the metacarpophalangeal joints in that there are two collateral ligaments and one palmar plate ligament per joint. However, the interphalangeal joints differ from the metacarpophalangeal joints in that the articular surfaces of the interphalangeal joints travel in the same arc throughout their full range and produce an almost

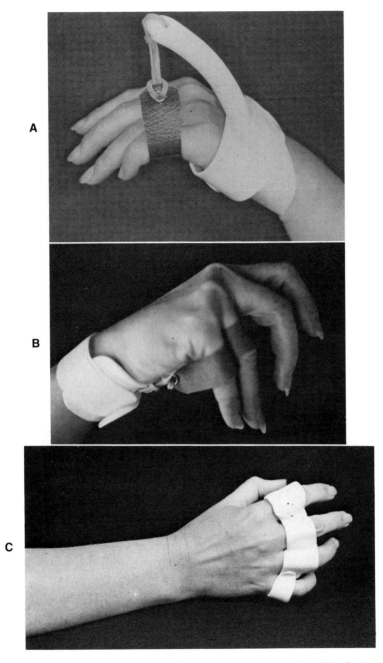

Fig. 11-5. Simple metacarpophalangeal splints may augment extension (**A**), flexion (**B**), or abduction (**C**). *Continued.*

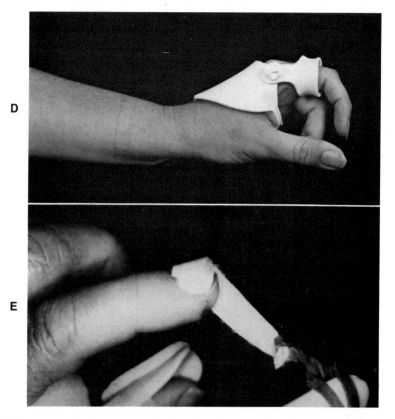

Fig. 11-5, cont'd. Simple metacarpophalangeal splints may augment adduction (**D**) or rotation (**E**).

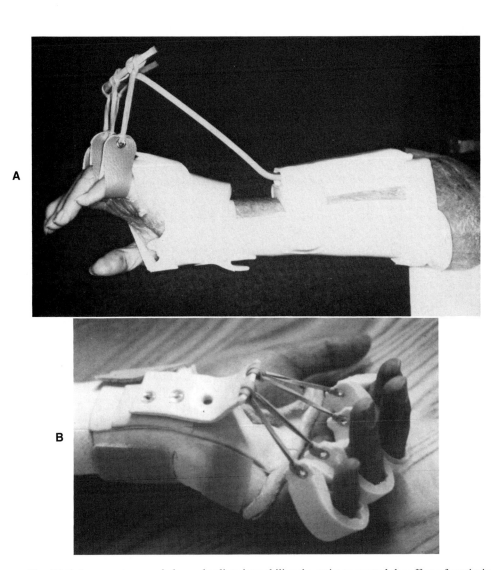

Fig. 11-6. Long metacarpophalangeal splints immobilize the wrist to control the effect of extrinsic musculotendinous adhesions or myostatic contracture on more distal digital joints. (**B** courtesy Karen Schultz, M.S., O.T.R., Santa Monica, CA.)

constant tension on the collateral ligaments regardless of joint position. The changes that do occur vary in the dorsal and palmar halves of the ligaments. When the proximal interphalangeal joint is in extension, the dorsal portion is slack and the palmar portion is taut. When the joint is flexed, the reverse is true. The interphalangeal joints, unlike the metacarpophalangeal joints, have a tendency to develop flexion contractures, although they may become contracted in extension as well.

Splinting for interphalangeal joint mobilization requires that the angle of approach of the rotational force be 90 degrees to the middle phalanx. This force should also be perpendicular to the axis of joint rotation to create equal stress on the collateral ligaments (Fig. 11-7). Because the proximal interphalangeal joint is the intermediate joint of the three digital articulations, splints that influence it often must affect the joints proximal and distal to it. If all the joints within the ray possess similar degrees of mobility, and if wrist position does not affect digital motion, a simple splint design is appropriate (Fig. 11-8). However, if discrepancies exist in the relative mobility of the successive joints within the digital ray, measures should be taken to control the more mobile joint and allow traction to be concentrated on the stiffer joint. Compound splint designs may provide concomitant stabilization of a segment and mobilization of another within the same longitudinal ray (Fig. 11-9). When wrist patterns are poor, or when decreased extrinsic musculotendinous amplitude creates a tenodesing of finger joints, wrist immobilization controls the extrinsic influence at the digital level (Fig. 11-10). A forearm trough and wrist bar may be added to a simple or compound splint design to create an appropriate long splint. When multiple joints of a ray are incorporated within a splint, there is little room for error because the multiple lever arms involved tend to accentuate deformity. Care should be taken to ensure that the mobilizing force influences each joint correctly. *Text continued on p. 287.*

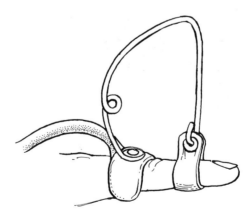

Fig. 11-7. For maximum benefit of traction, the angle of approach should be 90 degrees to the proximal phalanx and perpendicular to the axis of rotation.

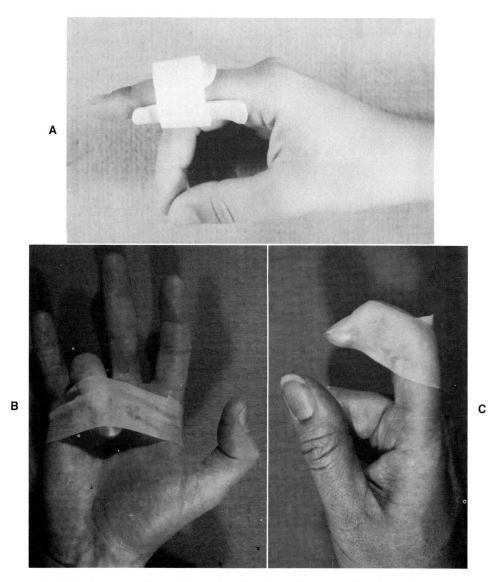

Fig. 11-8. Simple proximal interphalangeal mobilization splints may affect the proximal interphalangeal joint alone **(A)** or influence other joints within the ray in a similar manner **(B and C)**. **(A** courtesy Jill White, M.A., O.T.R., New York.)

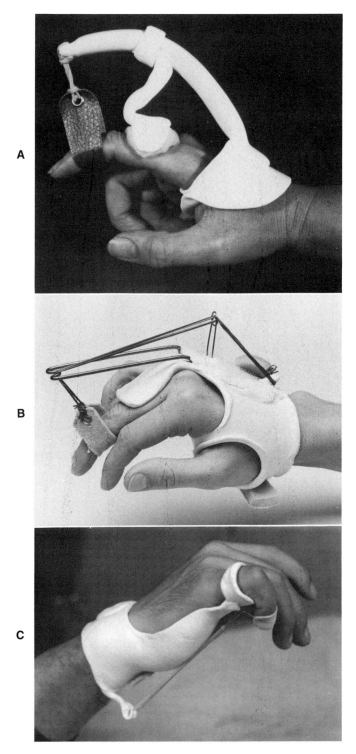

Fig. 11-9. These compound proximal interphalangeal mobilization splints stabilize the proximal phalanx and focus the extension (**A** and **B**) or flexion (**C** to **E**) traction force on the interphalangeal joints. (**B** courtesy Barbara Allen, O.T.R., Oklahoma City; **C** courtesy Carolina deLeeuw, M.A., O.T.R., Tacoma, WA; **D** courtesy Linda Shuttleton, O.T.R., Long Beach, CA; **E** courtesy Donna Reist, O.T.R./L., Akron, OH.)

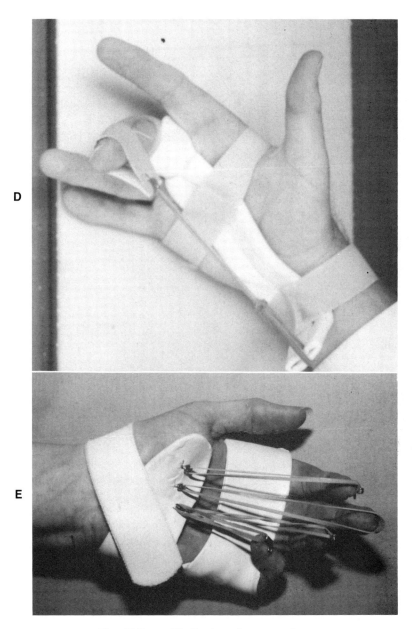

Fig. 11-9, cont'd. For legend see opposite page.

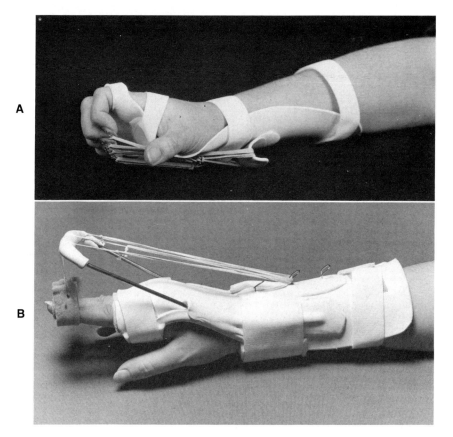

Fig. 11-10. Long proximal interphalangeal mobilization splints resemble their simple and compound counterparts distally but immobilize the wrist proximally. (**B** courtesy Lisa Dennys, B.Sc., O.T., London, Ont.)

Complete immobilization of a metacarpophalangeal joint with a concomitant mobilization force to the proximal interphalangeal joint may be one of the most difficult tasks in splint fabrication. Since the primary intent of the splint is to produce a flexion force, one's initial impulse is to design a palmar-based splint. This, however, often results in frustration and mechanical failure when the distal mobilizing flexion force overpowers the more proximal immobilizing extension force. Upon reassessment, it becomes apparent that the proximal extension force must be equal to or greater than the distal flexion torque to produce complete immobilization of the metacarpophalangeal joint. Therefore a dorsally based splint generates better mechanical advantage for immobilizing the metacarpophalangeal joint against a distal flexion force (Fig. 11-11).

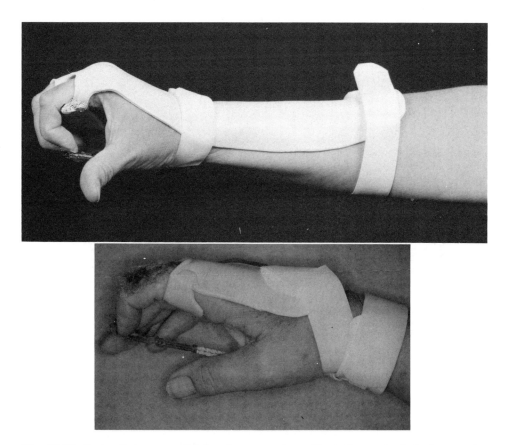

Fig. 11-11. Design that uses a solid dorsal component provides better mechanical advantage for completely immobilizing the metacarpophalangeal joint in compound interphalangeal flexion splints.

Experience and analysis of mechanical factors have shown that three-point pressure inelastic traction splints (Fig. 11-12), including the safety pin or joint jack, are more effective in correcting flexion deformities that measure approximately 35 degrees or less. A joint whose fixed flexion is greater than 35 degrees responds more readily to a compound proximal interphalangeal extension splint or to serial cylinder casts. Experience has also shown that consecutive serial casting of extremely stiff joints results in better passive motion than was achieved with elastic traction on the same joints.

Distal interphalangeal level

Because the distal interphalangeal joints are also hinge articulations, mechanical principles similar to those of the proximal interphalangeal joints are applicable (Fig. 11-13). From a practical point of view, however, the small area of purchase provided by

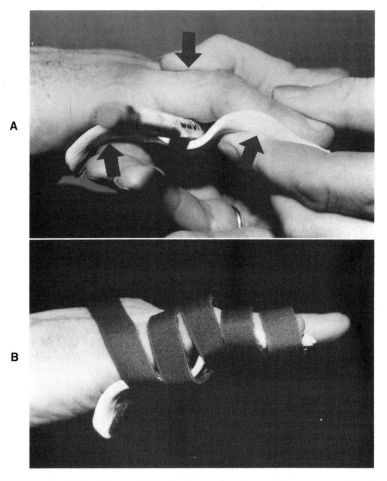

Fig. 11-12. Mechanical advantage for inelastic traction three-point pressure splints is greater for improving proximal interphalangeal joint contractures of 35 degrees or less. During fit stage a gap is created (**A**) to provide three-point purchase *(arrows)* of the inelastic traction on the joint (**B**). (Courtesy Elaine Lacroix, M.H.S.M., O.T.R., Boston, MA.)

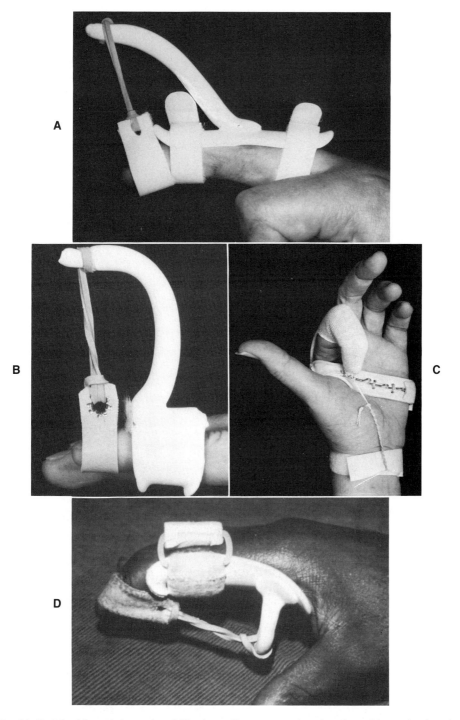

Fig. 11-13. Distal interphalangeal mobilization splints may produce less favorable results than do their proximal interphalangeal joint counterparts. **A,** Compound distal interphalangeal extension splint. **B,** Simple distal interphalangeal extension splint. **C,** Simple distal interphalangeal flexion splint. **D,** Compound distal interphalangeal flexion splint. (**B** courtesy Norma Arras, M.A., O.T.R., Springfield, IL; **C** from Hollis, L.I.: Innovative splinting ideas. In Hunter, J.M., et al., editors: Rehabilitation of the hand, St. Louis, 1978, The C.V. Mosby Co.; **D** courtesy Kathryn Schultz, O.T.R., Altamonte Springs, FL.)

the distal phalanx may make elaborate dynamic traction techniques less successful in correcting stiffness at this joint. Three-point pressure splints that utilize inelastic traction, such as static gutters or cylinder casts, sometimes prove more effective in correcting flexion deformities, and simple straps or rubber bands may best overcome extension stiffness.

MULTIPURPOSE SPLINTS

As experienced hand rehabilitation specialists know, hand problems seldom seem to present themselves in simple textbook formats. Requiring considerable creativity and ingenuity, splints often must be designed to meet multiple rehabilitative goals. For example, the integration of several splints into one eases the changing process from flexion splinting to extension splinting (Fig. 11-14); extension forces to alternate fingers with simultaneous flexion force to the middle adjacent finger help attain final increments of extrinsic tendon excursion (Fig. 11-15); and the commercial availability of articulated splint components considerably simplifies crucial alterations in wrist position on a splint whose primary focus is enhancing digital motion (Fig. 11-16). The concept that each splint must be created ''from the inside out'' to meet individual needs cannot be over-

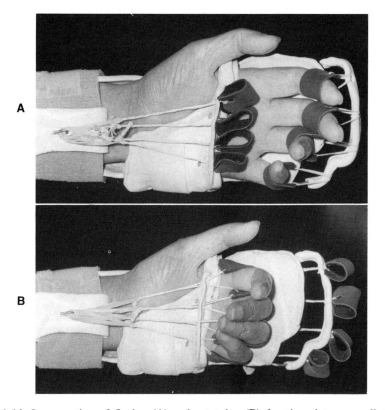

Fig. 11-14. Incorporation of flexion (**A**) and extension (**B**) functions into one splint increases efficiency and patient acceptance by eliminating the need to change from one splint to another. (Courtesy Diana Williams, O.T.R., Danville, PA.)

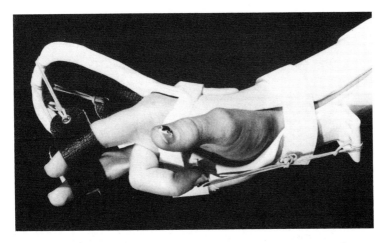

Fig. 11-15. By controlling wrist position and applying a triad of alternate forces to adjacent fingers, final increments of tendon excursion are obtained. (Courtesy Roslyn Evans, O.T.R., Vero Beach, FL.)

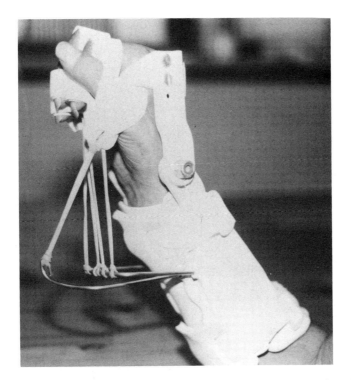

Fig. 11-16. Adjustable wrist unit facilitates tension changes to extrinsic musculotendinous units. (Courtesy Kathryn Schultz, O.T.R., Altamonte Springs, FL.)

emphasized. Attempts at rigid, predetermined assignation or matching of given splint configurations to specific diagnoses might be not only ineffective, but also may be harmful to patients.

SUMMARY

Pericapsular fibrosis resulting in stiffening of the metacarpophalangeal or interphalangeal joints of the fingers represents the most common disabling problem following hand injury, disease, or surgery. The use of preventive splints that immobilize joints in positions least likely to cause stiffness or mobilizing splints designed to overcome existing contracture are important tools to those involved in the hand rehabilitative process. A sound knowledge of normal anatomy and those factors contributing to the pathologic condition at a given joint is required to make decisions about the design of a finger splint. As in any treatment method, the purpose and expected goals of a splint must be well planned and carefully explained to the patient. Once the splint has been applied, it is important to closely monitor progress and to make appropriate alterations in the splint, the wearing schedule, or the exercise routine as changes occur throughout the rehabilitation period.

CHAPTER 12

Splints acting on the thumb

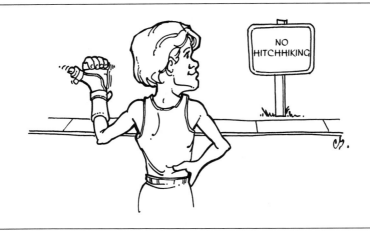

The importance of the thumb in almost all aspects of hand function cannot be overstated. The presence of an opposable thumb gives the human species a manual dexterity that is unparalleled in lower animal forms. Insurance companies assess a 40% functional loss to a hand that is missing the thumb, and the real loss may be substantially greater. Because of the tremendous disability resulting from thumb loss, hand surgeons have long strived to develop techniques to salvage or restore thumb function. Loss may result from congenital absence, traumatic amputation, disease, or injury.

The functional requirements of the thumb differ substantially from those of the other four digits. Thumb stability, for example, is much more important than mobility, and a thumb unit with basilar joint motion alone permits adequate function despite fused distal joints. Even a completely immobile first metacarpal may serve as a stable post for prehension with the mobile adjacent digits if it is in the correct position. In addition to stability, it is important that the thumb unit retain sufficient length for pinch and grasp functions and sensibility of at least a protective grade without pain and hypersensitivity. The maintenance of proper thumb position, therefore, is extremely important. Splints that correct thumb deformities, establish and maintain an adequate first web space, and help mobilize stiffened thumb joints are among the most important discussed in this book.

Consisting of three joints, the thumb ray is a multiarticular, open kinematic chain that moves through three planes and combinations thereof. The distal segment of the chain is allowed a high degree of freedom of movement as the result of the summation of the participating joints. This arrangement helps minimize the disabling effect of the restriction or loss of motion at any of the individual joints as the result of trauma or disease. The circumduction and opposition motions allowed by the CMC joint are critical to positioning the thumb for pinch and grasp tasks. The flexion, extension, and slight rotation of the metacarpophalangeal joint facilitate grasp and release of a wide range of objects of differing sizes. Adding the final increment of refinement, the thumb interphalangeal joint plays an important role in very fine, precision activities.

Splinting may immobilize the thumb or thenar segments to allow healing, control early postoperative motion, or enhance functional use. Inflammatory conditions and soft tissue injuries of thenar structures often require splint immobilization. Postoperative immobilization between exercise periods effectively limits use while allowing early motion, and static positioning of a paralyzed or partially paralyzed thumb aids in the prevention of deformity while permitting continued functional use.

Since optimal effectiveness of the thumb depends on combined mobility and stability, preservation or restoration of motion of the three joints is an important part of the rehabilitation process. Splinting and active range-of-motion exercises, combined with purposeful activity, are the cornerstones of this process. Maximum passive range of motion of the involved joints must be acquired and maintained before a corresponding active range of motion may be achieved or before surgical procedures may be attempted. Splinting is generally accepted as the most effective non-surgical means for achieving an improved passive range of thumb motion.

Regardless of the intent of splint application, the basic principles of mechanics, design, construction, mobilization and fit must be implemented to create a splint that meets the requirements of the specific situation. The purpose of this chapter is to discuss splinting techniques as they relate to the thumb.

IMMOBILIZATION SPLINTS

Simple thumb immobilization splints involve one or more joints and are fitted dorsally, palmarly, or circumferentially (Fig. 12-1). Care should be taken to maintain correct ligamentous stress at each joint traversed, as well as full motion of the unsplinted joints. Straps placed at the level of the axis of joint rotation provide maximum mechanical purchase. Because many thumb immobilization splints have narrow configurations, contouring the material to half the segmental thickness provides splint strength (Fig. 12-2). Circumferential thumb splints eliminate the need for counterforce straps at joints by providing opposing forces along the entire length of the segment (Fig. 12-3).

To control extrinsic thumb musculotendinous units, long thumb immobilization splints statically position the wrist as an adjunctive measure to thumb immobilization.

Wrist position may increase or decrease the amount of tension on these units through alteration of the tenodesis effect (Fig. 12-4). For optimum mechanical design the forearm trough should be at least two thirds the length of the forearm, and the C bar or thumb post should be of sufficient length to fully immobilize the intended segment while allowing unimpeded motion at the more distal unsplinted joints.

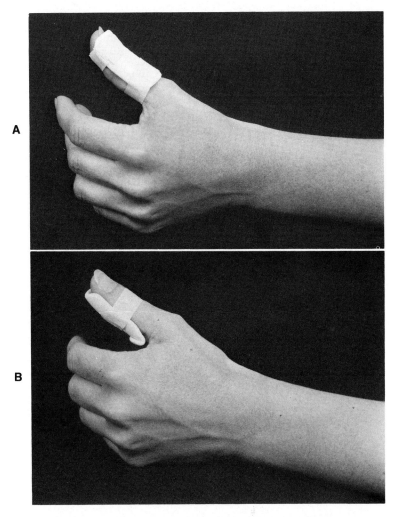

Fig. 12-1. Although the placement of straps differes between dorsal (**A**) and palmar (**B**) simple thumb immobilization splints, the mechanical function of both splints is identical. Proximal and distal pressure is applied palmarly and the opposing middle force is applied dorsally.

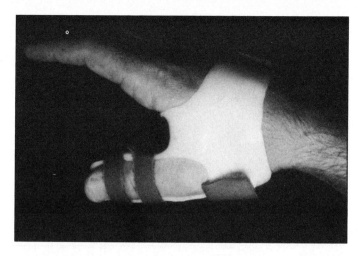

Fig. 12-2. To increase material strength, narrow components such as this thumb post should be contoured to half the thickness of the segment being immobilized. (Coutesy Elaine Lacroix, M.H.S.M., O.T.R., Boston, MA.)

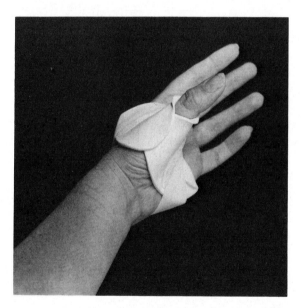

Fig. 12-3. Three-point pressure forces are disbursed along the length of the splinted segment in this circumferential thumb–carpometacarpal-metacarpophalangeal immobilization splint.

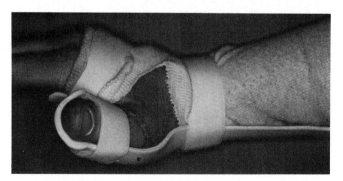

Fig. 12-4. This long thumb immobilization splint limits carpometacarpal, metacarpophalangeal, and interphalangeal joint motion in addition to adjunctively immobilizing the wrist.

MAINTENANCE AND MOBILIZATION SPLINTS

Severe hand injuries, particularly if a component of crush is involved, often produce an insidious contracture of the first web space, which, if permitted to persist, rapidly develops into a rigid adduction deformity that will markedly limit thumb function.

Carpometacarpal level

Pathologic conditions at the carpometacarpal level will often result in limited motion of the first metacarpal with concomitant narrowing of the first web space. Any splint designed to maintain or increase the passive range of carpometacarpal motion must have its site of force application on the first metacarpal. Practically speaking, however, this is difficult because of the intervening soft tissue of the first web space. Many ill-conceived splints fitted with the intent of increasing carpometacarpal motion actually apply most of the rotatory force to the proximal phalanx, resulting in attenuation of the ulnar collateral ligament of the metacarpophalangeal joint, radial deviation of the proximal phalanx, pressure over the radiometacarpal condyle, and instability of the thumb. Care must be taken to ensure that as much of the distal aspect of the first metacarpal is included in the splint as possible and that the primary site of the rotational force is directed toward the metacarpal (Figs. 12-5 and 12-6). To decrease the amount of pressure on the first metacarpal, the area of force application may be widened to include the proximal phalanx. This addition, however, must not jeopardize the stability of the metacarpophalangeal joint by exerting a stretching force on the ulnar collateral ligament. In most instances the splint need not be extended distally beyond the interphalangeal flexion crease, thus allowing full motion of the distal phalanx. The splint should also be fitted proximal to the distal palmar flexion crease, permitting full metacarpophalangeal flexion of the adjacent digits. A thumb carpometacarpal maintenance splint (web spacer) may be used to maintain the width of the first web space and ensure the most useful plane of motion of the thumb carpometacarpal joint. This splint is constructed from either solid (Fig. 12-7) or pliable materials (Fig. 12-8), depending on individual patient requirements.

Since the carpometacarpal joint of the thumb is a triaxial saddle articulation and possesses multiple planes of motion, the splinted position of the first metacarpal should be alternated from full extension to full abduction to minimize the possibility of shortening of the five carpometacarpal articular ligaments as described by Haines (1944) and Napier (1955). This is accomplished through the construction of two splints, one in full extension and the second in abduction and through a carefully supervised exercise routine.

If a full passive range of motion is not present at the carpometacarpal joint, slow, progressive, inelastic traction may be applied through the use of serial carpometacarpal mobilization splints (Fig. 12-9), which are changed and widened every 2 or 3 days. Progressive wedging of the thumb is continued until the passive measurements of abduction and extension duplicate those of the normal thumb or until the passive motion remains unchanged for three or four consecutive splint changes. In most instances, inelastic serial carpometacarpal mobilization splints are more effective than elastic traction splinting for increasing the passive range of motion of the thumb carpometacarpal joint. This of course depends on the patient's ability to return for frequent splint changes.

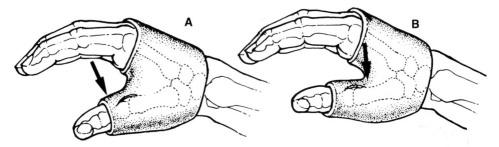

Fig. 12-5. To avoid damage to the metacarpophalangeal ulnar collateral ligament when mobilizing a thumb carpometacarpal joint, force should be directed toward the head of the first metacarpal instead of the proximal phalanx. **A,** Incorrect. **B,** Correct. (From Fess, E.: Splinting for mobilization of the thumb. In Hunter, J.M., et. al., editors: Rehabilitation of the hand, ed. 2, St. Louis, 1984, The C.V. Mosby Co.)

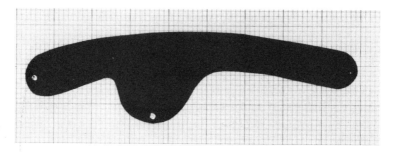

Fig. 12-6. When using elastic traction to mobilize the thumb carpometacarpal joint, this modified Phelps/Weeks sling provides two-directional force application to the first metacarpal. (Courtesy Karen Priest Barrett, O.T.R., Atlanta, GA.)

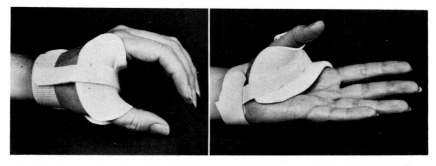

Fig. 12-7. A simple carpometacarpal maintenance splint such as this web spacer allows full range of motion of adjacent metacarpophalangeal joints while exerting rotational force to the distal aspect of the first metacarpal. Straps are designed to prevent distal migration of the splint. (From Fess, E.: Splinting for mobilization of the thumb. In Hunter, J.M., et al., editors: Rehabilitation of the hand, ed. 2, St. Louis, 1984, The C.V. Mosby Co.)

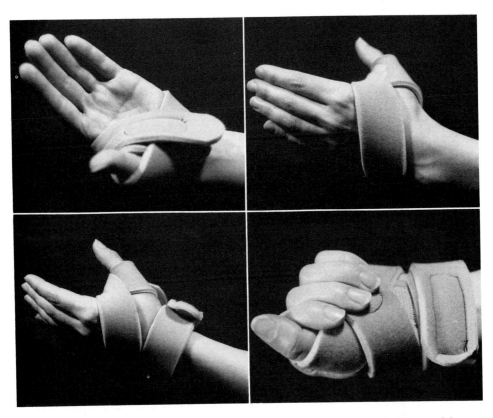

Fig. 12-8. By altering the placement and configuration of wrapping, soft splinting materials may position or immobilize thumb joints. (Courtesy Bobbie-Ann Neel, O.T.R., Opelika, AL. Splint, patent pending.)

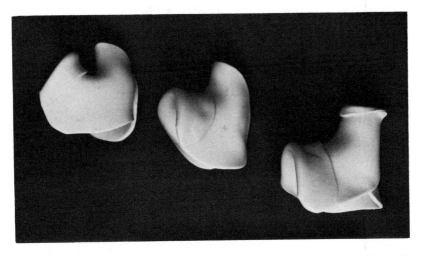

Fig. 12-9. Serial CMC mobilization splints are widened every 2 or 3 days. (From Fess, E.: Splinting for mobilization of the thumb. In Hunter, J.M., et al.: Rehabilitation of the hand, ed. 2, St. Louis, 1984, The C.V. Mosby Co.)

Metacarpophalangeal level

The middle joint in the important thumb chain is the metacarpophalangeal joint. At this level, stability is a more important consideration than mobility.

A wide discrepancy exists in the amount of thumb metacarpophalangeal motion found in the general population, with flexion ranging from only a few degrees to 90 degrees. It is apparent that the functional sequelae of limited or absent metacarpophalangeal motion is negligible if the joint is positioned properly and stable. According to some authors, metacarpophalangeal joint of the thumb, unlike those of the fingers, tend to be more nearly of the ginglymoid, or hinge, type. In mobilizing this joint of the thumb, care should be taken to apply a rotational force perpendicular to the center of the axis of rotation of the metacarpophalangeal joint. If this concept is disregarded, attenuation of either the ulnar or radial collateral ligament may occur with resulting deviation of the proximal phalanx and metacarpophalangeal joint instability. The angle of the mobilizing force should also be 90 degrees to the proximal phalanx.

A simple metacarpophalangeal flexion splint in the form of a wristband with flexion cuff (Fig. 12-10) is one of the least complicated means of facilitating thumb metacarpophalangeal flexion. It must be remembered that this splint affects motion at the thumb carpometacarpal joint, in addition to the metacarpophalangeal joint. Therefore an incorrect force angle may cause medial or lateral rotation of the first metacarpal with stretching of the carpometacarpal ligaments and intraarticular pressure, as well as undue stressing of the metacarpophalangeal collateral ligaments and joint surfaces.

A compound metacarpophalangeal flexion splint allows the application of the full magnitude of the rotatory force on the metacarpophalangeal joint by stabilizing the thumb carpometacarpal joint (Fig. 12-11). Once again, attention must be directed to-

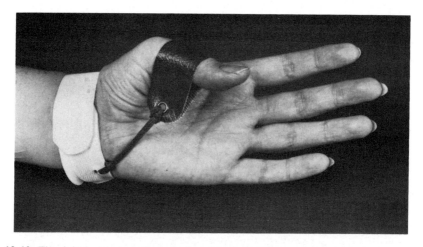

Fig. 12-10. The rigid low-temperature plastic component of the wristband is closely fitted around the ulnar border of the wrist to prevent the entire band from rotating as elastic traction is applied to the metacarpophalangeal joint. (From Fess, E.: Splinting for mobilization of the thumb. In Hunter, J.M., et al., editors: Rehabilitation of the hand, ed. 2, St. Louis, 1984, The C.V. Mosby Co.)

ward ensuring that the force angle of approach is directed 90 degrees to the proximal phalanx and perpendicular to the center of the axis for rotation of the metacarpophalangeal joint.

Secondary wrist immobilization is a definitive characteristic of long thumb mobilization splints. These splints may be fitted dorsally or palmarly, and, as with the long immobilization splints, wrist position through a tenodesis effect influences tension on the extrinsic thumb musculotendinous units. Either the dynamic assist or C bar should apply a 90-degree rotary force to the segment being mobilized; in the case of metacarpophalangeal or interphalangeal mobilization, the traction should also be perpendicular to the axis joint rotation (Fig. 12-12).

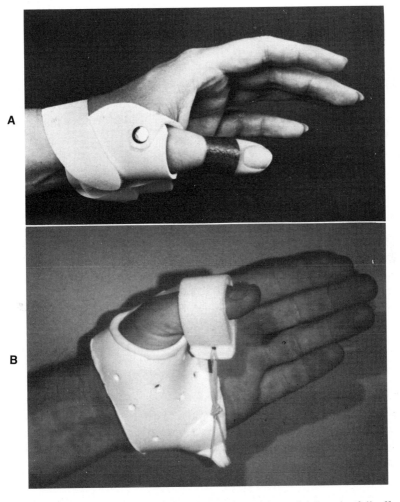

Fig. 12-11. Because of the immobilization of the carpometacarpal joint, the full effect of the traction is focused on the metacarpophalangeal joint in these compound splints. (**A** From Fess, E.: Splinting for mobilization of the thumb. In Hunter, J.M., et al., editors: Rehabilitation of the hand, ed. 2, St. Louis, 1984, The C.V. Mosby Co.; **B** courtesy Susan Emerson, M. Ed., O.T.R., Dover, NH).

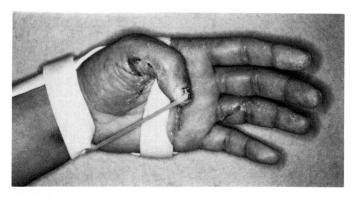

Fig. 12-12. This long thumb flexion splint influences articular motion and extrinsic tendon excursion.

As with metacarpophalangeal joint mobilization in the companion digits, the most carefully designed and constructed splints may totally fail to overcome contracture (usually extension) despite the most vigorous efforts of both therapist and patient. It must be realized at the onset that in many instances this type of fixed deformity has such rigid underlying fibrosis and ligamentous pathologic conditions that no amount of splinting, however well conceived, may be expected to succeed. To avoid frustration, a realistic understanding by all those involved of the possibility of failure is essential when the splinting program is initiated.

Interphalangeal level

Although strong interphalangeal joint motion is valuable to thumb performance, its absence is not critical. In most cases thumb functions are possible if there is a good carpometacarpal joint and perhaps some metacarpophalangeal joint motion. Since the interphalangeal joint of the thumb is a true uniaxial hinge articulation, the mechanical principles previously mentioned regarding mobilization of the thumb metacarpophalangeal joint are applicable to the mobilization of the thumb interphalangeal joint. For optimum results, the angle of approach should be 90 degrees to the distal phalanx of the thumb and perpendicular to the center of the axis of rotation of the interphalangeal joint.

A wristband and a fingernail clip (Fig. 12-13) mobilize the carpometacarpal, metacarpophalangeal, and interphalangeal joints of the thumb. In fitting this simple classification splint, care must be taken to check the angle of force application. The incorporation of all three joints of the thumb into the splint leaves little room for error and may tend to cause or accentuate deformity because of the multiple lever arms. The angle of approach of the rubber band must be perpendicular to the axis of rotation of the metacarpophalangeal and interphalangeal joints without causing transverse rotation of the first metacarpal.

A compound interphalangeal flexion splint (Fig. 12-14) may be employed to stabilize the carpometacarpal and metacarpophalangeal joints of the thumb. This allows for increased magnitude and accuracy of the application of the rotatory force at the inter-

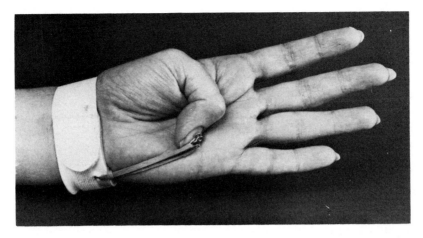

Fig. 12-13. A wristband with rigid ulnar component and fingernail clip enhances passive flexion of the carpometacarpal, metacarpophalangeal, and interphalangeal joints of the thumb. (From Fess, E.: Splinting for mobilization of the thumb. In Hunter, J.M., et al., editors: Rehabilitation of the hand, ed. 2, St. Louis, 1984, The C.V. Mosby Co.)

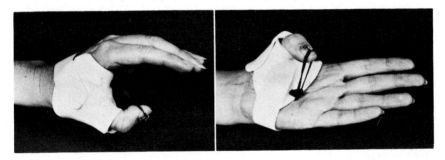

Fig. 12-14. This circumferential compound interphalangeal flexion splint allows the application of the elastic traction to affect only the distal thumb joint. The clip, a dressmaker's no. 2 hook, is attached with ethyl cyanoacrylate glue. (From Fess, E.: Splinting for mobilization of the thumb. In Hunter, J.M., et al., editors: Rehabilitation of the hand, ed. 2, St. Louis, 1984, The C.V. Mosby Co.)

phalangeal joint, by way of a fingernail clip. To decrease the amount of pressure incurred by inhibiting motion at the carpometacarpal and metacarpophalangeal joints, this splint should be extended as far distally as possible along the proximal phalanx without interfering with full interphalangeal flexion. Room for complete flexion of the adjacent digital metacarpophalangeal joints and support of the transverse metacarpal arch should also be provided.

The fingernail clip should be attached to the center and proximal aspect of the thumbnail to eliminate the possibility of transverse rotation of the distal phalanx and to minimize the leverage effect of the nail on the proximal nail bed.

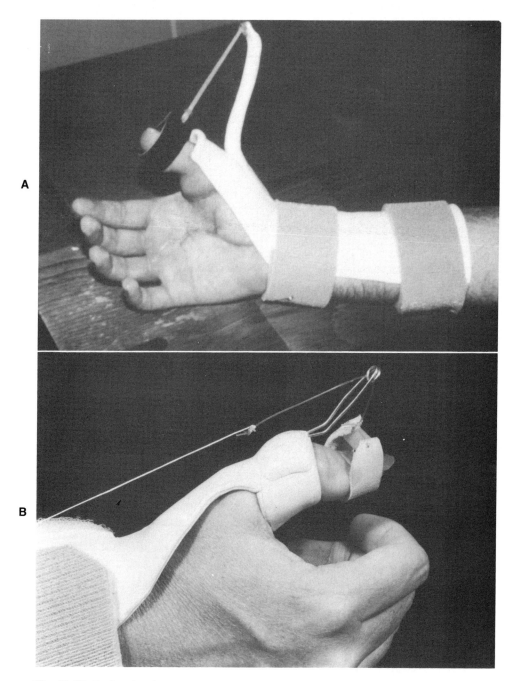

Fig. 12-15. Designed to increase passive interphalangeal joint extension, these splints use elastic traction with different height outriggers. (**A** courtesy Kathryn Schultz, O.T.R., Altamonte Springs, FL; **B** courtesy Kenneth Flowers, R.P.T., Phoenixville, PA.)

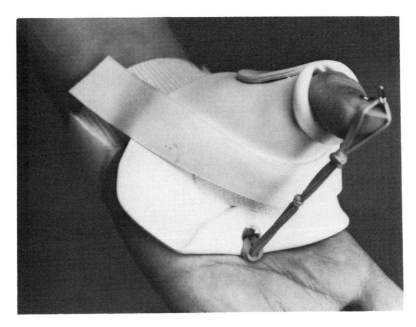

Fig. 12-16. The combination of thumb web spacer and fingernail clip allows for the simultaneous mobilization of carpometacarpal and interphalangeal joints. (From Fess, E.: Splinting for mobilization of the thumb. In Hunter, J.M., et al., editors: Rehabilitation of the hand, ed. 2, St. Louis, 1984, The C.V. Mosby Co.)

Providing fine adjustments to pinch and grasp, both interphalangeal flexion and extension are important to thenar function. By immobilizing the proximal joints of the thumb, a compound interphalangeal extension splint directs the force of the elastic traction to the stiff interphalangeal joint (Fig. 12-15). As with flexion mobilization splinting, the angle of force application must be perpendicular to the axis of joint rotation and 90 degrees to the distal phalanx.

The techniques discussed in this chapter for splinting individual joints may be combined effectively for the simultaneous mobilization of multiple joints of the thumb. A carpometacarpal mobilization splint, combined with a fingernail clip and elastic traction (Fig. 12-16), facilitates motion at both the carpometacarpal and interphalangeal joints. In designing and fitting this splint, it is necessary to be certain that the plastic fully extends around the proximal phalanx of the thumb, thus rendering the metacarpophalangeal joint immobile and diminishing the pressure on the palmar aspect of the phalanx. Once again, the angle of approach of the rubber band should be at a 90-degree angle to the distal phalanx and perpendicular to the center of the axis of rotation of the interphalangeal joint. The metacarpophalangeal joints of the fingers should also be permitted a full range of motion into flexion.

SUMMARY

It is of utmost importance that thumb splints be created to provide functional position, stability, and at least basilar joint mobility. Although careful adherence to the basic design, mechanics, construction, fit, and mobilization principles remains important, the thumb must be considered as a separate, unique unit. Splints should be used to carefully provide a maximum return of thumb participation in the important pinching and grasping activities of the hand. If done properly, the combination of splinting, exercise, and purposeful activity may help to minimize the disabling effect of disease and trauma to the thumb and enhance the results of surgery.

PART FOUR

Special situations

CHAPTER 13

Splinting the arthritic hand

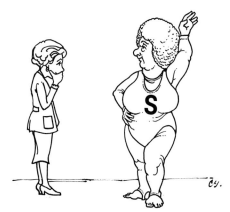

"MRS. GRAHAM, I THINK YOU'RE EXPECTING
TOO MUCH FROM YOUR NEW JOINTS."

PATHOMECHANICS

Before undertaking a splinting program with a patient with rheumatoid arthritis, the therapist must understand the pathomechanics of the disease process.

Rheumatoid arthritis is a chronic disease that not only may affect multiple joints, but also may have systemic manifestations. The course of the disease is unpredictable, but it is often one of exacerbations and remissions. The predominant signs and symptoms are joint swelling, inflammation, and stiffness. There are often associated systemic signs such as generalized malaise, fever, chills, fatigue, and anorexia. In severe cases there can be lung, heart, or vascular involvement.

Early involvement of the hands may show dorsal tenosynovitis of the wrist. The extensor tendons glide in synovial sheaths that extend approximately 1 cm above and 1 cm below the extensor retinaculum. Since rheumatoid arthritis involves synovial tissue, dorsal tenosynovitis follows this anatomic pattern.

The flexor tendons, however, glide in synovial sheaths at the wrist, palm, and digits and may therefore be affected in any of those areas. Palmarly, tenosynovitis at the wrist

309

may compress the median nerve, leading to carpal tunnel syndrome. When the palm and digits are involved, limited active motion or digital triggering or locking may result.

Swelling of the metacarpophalangeal joints is also a sign of early hand involvement. The proximal interphalangeal joints are characterized by fusiform swelling, pain, and limited motion. The distal interphalangeal joints are often not affected to the same extent as are the other joints of the hand, but frequently are involved secondary to musculotendinous imbalance, as seen in swan neck and boutonniere deformities.

In the normal hand there is a fine balance between the bony architecture, the capsuloligamentous system, and the muscle and tendon system. In rheumatoid arthritis both internal and external forces disrupt this intricate relationship. It should be remembered that all rheumatoid deformities have their origin either primarily or secondarily from the synovial hypertrophy that occurs within the joint. This synovitis may stretch out the capsuloligamentous system and invade the tendons that glide in synovial sheaths. This then leads to a compromise in the normal biomechanics of the hand and wrist. A musculotendinous imbalance occurs, as does a disruption of the normal bony architecture, due to stretching of the supporting soft tissue structures. Later erosive bone changes may occur. This leads to the deformities that are often seen in a patient with rheumatoid arthritis.

Deformities at the metacarpophalangeal joints are usually manifested by palmar subluxation and increasing ulnar deviation. The metacarpophalangeal joints allow a wide range of motion and are subjected to greater stresses during functional activities. The extensor tendons are vulnerable to disruption and often sublux ulnarly into the valleys between the metacarpal heads. Forces generated by the flexor tendons during grip and pinch may cause stretching of the collateral ligaments and lead to an ulnar displacement of the flexor tendons. As the normal restraining mechanisms of the metacarpophalangeal joints become attenuated, the intrinsic muscles are placed at an enhanced mechanical advantage and may become a deforming factor themselves. Normally when a fist is made, the metacarpal heads slope in an ulnar direction. As palmar subluxation and ulnar drift occur, the use of the hand in daily activities continues to aggravate this situation. Other factors, including the condition of the wrist, may also affect ulnar deviation at the metacarpophalangeal joints. As the wrist shifts radially, one sees associated metacarpophalangeal joint ulnar deviation in the characteristic zigzag deformity.

At the proximal interphalangeal joint level, synovitis of the joint leads to shortening of the collateral ligaments, and stretching of the joint capsule and the central slip. This results in palmar displacement of the lateral bands and eventually leads to a boutonniere deformity, with flexion of the proximal interphalangeal joint and hyperextension of the distal interphalangeal joint.

The swan neck deformity, which is characterized by hyperextension of the proximal interphalangeal joint and flexion of the distal interphalangeal joint, may have its origin at any of the three digital levels. It may begin when the metacarpophalangeal joints become involved and tight intrinsic muscles develop, leading to a musculotendinous imbalance. Swan neck deformity may also develop when the proximal interphalangeal joint becomes involved, stretching out the palmar plate or causing the lateral bands to become stuck dorsally. Another cause of this deformity is a ruptured superficialis tendon. At the distal interphalangeal joint a mallet deformity may lead to an imbalance resulting in a swan neck deformity.

Wrist involvement in rheumatoid arthritis has a significant effect on overall hand function. Involvement is often seen early in the course of the disease and affects the radiocarpal, intercarpal, distal radioulnar, or any combination of these joints.

INDICATIONS FOR SPLINTING

The patient with rheumatoid arthritis presents numerous treatment challenges to the therapist. Whether to splint is a major decision. A rheumatoid arthritic hand may be splinted for the following reasons: (1) to help decrease inflammation, (2) to rest and support weakened joint structures, (3) to properly position joints, (4) to help minimize joint contractures, or (5) to help improve function through better positioning of the joints by providing increased stability and relieving pain.

Controversy, however, still surrounds this subject. Most agree that splinting has a place, especially in the acute stage, in a total rehabilitation program for the person with rheumatoid arthritis. However, there are few documented or well-established indications for splinting the rheumatoid hand. Therefore, before any splinting program is undertaken for a patient with rheumatoid arthritis, a careful evaluation needs to be done to determine the feasibility of splinting. Each splint fabricated will then fit the individual needs of the patient. Patients with longstanding rheumatoid arthritis and those taking certain medications, such as corticosteroids, may have thin, delicate skin that bruises easily. In these cases special precautions need to be taken to prevent skin breakdown, and more frequent checks of the splint are necessary.

Alexander, Feinberg, Gault, Mills, Partridge, Rotstein, and Stouter (1983, 1981, 1969, 1971, 1963, 1965, 1971) have advocated the use of both hand splints and rest when the joints are inflamed. During periods of inflammation the joints are more vulnerable to damage from both internal and external forces. Splinting has been noted to reduce pain and decrease inflammation and muscle spasm, thus reducing stress to the joints and allowing increased motion and function. A study by Zoeckler and Nicholas (1969) showed that 63% of the patients who responded to their questionnaire found moderate or great relief from pain and morning stiffness by using splints.

IMMOBILIZATION SPLINTS

Resting splints, either for the whole hand or for the wrist, are often recommended for use during acute periods of inflammation. It is suggested that the splints be worn full time except for brief periods of gentle range of motion exercises and to perform necessary self-care tasks. As inflammation subsides, the splints are worn intermittently. The splints should, if feasible, be worn at night for several weeks after resolution of acute inflammation. If bilateral splints are necessary, alternating the use of each splint often seems more reasonable to the patient and leads to better acceptance and compliance. The patient's activities may be gradually increased as tolerated, and joint protection may be taught at this time. In cases where the metacarpophalangeal joints are

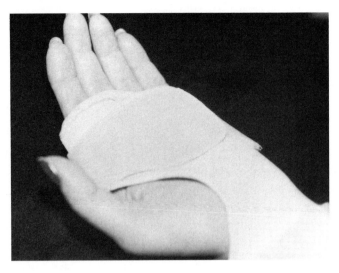

Fig. 13-1. A resting splint for the wrist and metacarpophalangeal joints. This splint may also be used as an exercise splint for the proximal interphalangeal joints.

involved but the interphalangeal joints are not, a resting splint may be fabricated to include the metacarpophalangeal joints but to leave the interphalangeal joints free (Fig. 13-1). This type of splint may also be used as an exercise splint for intrinsic lengthening. For this situation the metacarpophalangeal joints are held in full extension to place the intrinsics on stretch. The patient then puts the splint on for short periods of exercise several times during the day.

When positioning an arthritic hand in a wrist/fingers/thumb immobilization splint, one should keep in mind the pathomechanics of the disease. The tendency, as previously mentioned, is for the metacarpophalangeal joints to sublux palmarly. Therefore the metacarpophalangeal joint should be held in about 25 to 30 degrees of flexion to provide palmar support to those joints and surrounding soft tissue (Fig. 13-2). The proximal interphalangeal joints are then held in approximately 30 degrees of flexion. The wrist should, if possible, be positioned in neutral to 10 degrees of dorsiflexion. Too much dorsiflexion increases pressure on the carpal tunnel and may lead to median nerve symptoms. This is especially significant if there is evidence of flexor tenosynovitis at the wrist, a frequent cause of median nerve compression in rheumatoid arthritis. When the thumb is included in the splint, it should be positioned in abduction and palmar flexion.

The position for resting a rheumatoid hand is different from the safety position for splinting an injured hand. After injury the metacarpophalangeal joints are held in 70 to 90 degrees of flexion with the interphalangeal joints in full extension to protect the collateral ligaments. A rheumatoid hand held in that position would increase palmar subluxation of the metacarpophalangeal joints and stiffness of the proximal interpha-

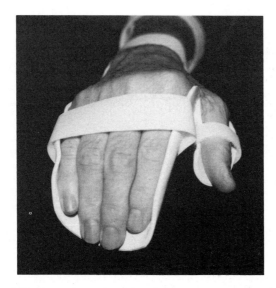

Fig. 13-2. An immobilization splint to position the wrist and hand during a period of acute inflammation.

langeal joints. Metacarpal and interphalangeal joints should be held in only slight flexion.

ELASTIC TRACTION SPLINTS

Elastic traction splints are used to help or minimize a joint contracture, to position joints, or to aid in postoperative positioning. A study of dynamic splinting in 51 nonsurgical patients done by Convery and associates (1967 and 1968) suggested that hand function was not improved and the progression of deformity was not uniformly prevented. They also showed that correction of preexisting deformity was not achieved. The authors felt that there was a greater loss of motion than would have been expected if splints had not been used. Others, however, such as Granger, Young, and Swanson (1965, 1980, 1966), have found a well-designed and properly fitted dynamic splint may help in both preoperative and postoperative management. None suggest, however, that an established deformity may be corrected by splinting. Flatt (1983) stresses the necessity for gentle continuous pull and avoidance of sudden violent force on a joint when any dynamic splinting is used. Forceful manipulation may cause permanent damage to the joints and supporting structures already under stress from the disease process.

POSTOPERATIVE SPLINTING

Another use of splinting is in postoperative management. Either elastic traction or immobilization splints are used. The type of splint is determined by the surgery performed and the status of the patient's soft tissue. Therefore good communication between the therapist and the physician is necessary to design the most effective splint.

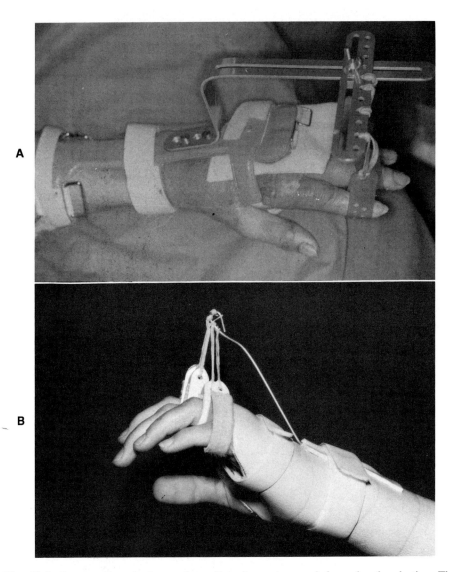

Fig. 13-3. Postoperative elastic traction splints for metacarpophalangeal arthroplasties. These splints maintain proper alignment of the metacarpophalangeal joints and allow guarded motion while the new capsuloligamentous system is forming. Controlled radial extension may be accomplished through an adjustable outrigger **(A)** or progressively longer rubber bands attached to a stationary radially placed extension outrigger **(B). C,** Depending on the extent of the surgical repair, the flexion assists may also be directed radially. A spination outrigger with a Velcro fingernail attachment device **(D),** a supinatory splint **(E),** or a two-sling force couple **(F)** helps prevent the recurrence of a pronation deformity of the index or long finger **(E** and **F** from Swanson, A.B., Swanson, G.G., and Leonard, J.: Postoperative rehabilitation program in flexible implant arthroplasty of the digits. In Hunter, J.M., et al., editors: Rehabilitation of the hand, ed. 2 St. Louis, 1984, The C.V. Mosby Co.)

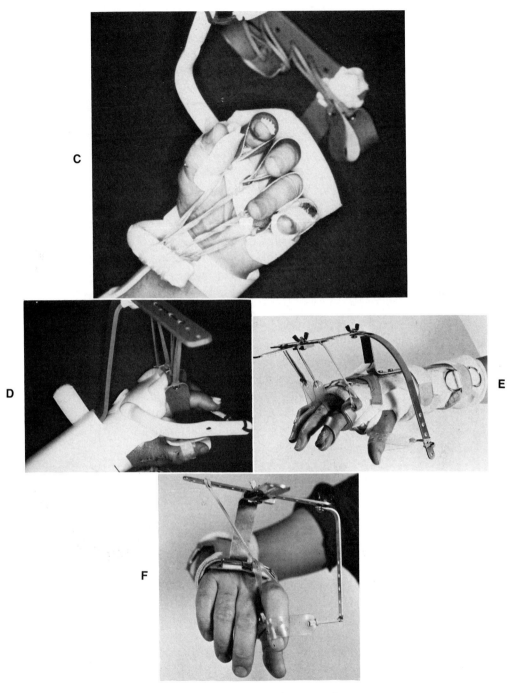

Fig. 13-3, cont'd. For legend see opposite page.

In the postoperative management of metacarpophalangeal joint arthroplasty, the purposes of elastic traction splinting are to maintain alignment of the joints and allow guarded motion while the new capsuloligamentous system is forming (Fig. 13-3). Elastic traction splinting may be supplemented by a static positioning splint at night.

When wrist arthroplasty is done, the goals of the surgery are to provide a stable, pain-free wrist with about a 50-degree arc of motion. Therefore the wrist is placed in an immobilization splint for 4 to 6 weeks. In some cases a controlled mobilization splint is used after the removal of the immobilization splint (Fig. 13-4). It is recommended that the patient always wear a wrist immobilization splint for protection when performing heavier tasks.

Following surgery for correction of a boutonniere deformity, immobilization splinting is used for a while before an exercise program is started. The length depends on the exact nature of the surgery performed. Elastic traction splinting is introduced following discontinuation of the daytime immobilization splinting and is used to maintain surgical correction until the soft tissue has stabilized. Immobilization night splinting may be continued for several weeks in conjunction with intermittent daytime elastic traction splinting. A long-term splinting and exercise program may be necessary to prevent recurrent deformity.

Elastic traction splinting to increase flexion after proximal interphalangeal joint arthroplasty is used when the patient is having difficulty obtaining an adequate range of flexion. In many cases this may be achieved with the use of Coban. The patient holds the finger down in flexion with the Coban for specified periods several times a day (Fig. 13-5). When an extension lag develops, elastic traction splinting for extension may be considered.

Tendon ruptures are a frequent complication of rheumatoid disease. Extensor tendons rupture more frequently than do the flexor tendons. Tendons rupture through attrition caused by the tendon rubbing on a bony spur, through direct synovial invasion into the tendon, and through pressure of the hypertrophied synovium on the tendons. It is often not possible to do an end-to-end repair of the tendons, since frequently the patient does not seek immediate medical attention. Also, the condition of the soft tissue may be poor. Therefore tendon transfer is frequently done to restore function. Determination rests on the number of tendons ruptured and individual patient factors.

When tendon transfers have been performed for extensor tendon ruptures, immobilization splinting with the metacarpophalangeal joints in about 15 to 20 degrees of flexion is used for the first 3 weeks to support the wrist and metacarpophalangeal joints while the transfer heals. Later in the rehabilitation program an elastic traction splint for extension may be used if the patient cannot obtain adequate extension. A helpful exercise in rehabilitating a patient who has undergone tendon transfer is to tape the interphalangeal joints into a clawlike position. This helps to isolate the long extensors. The patient then flexes and extends the metacarpophalangeal joints with the hand in this position (Fig. 13-6, *A* and *B*). With practice, the patient often learns to do this exercise without the tape. The patient needs to be aware that several months of rehabilitation may be required before a final result is obtained. The end result of tendon transfers is determined by the number of tendon ruptures and the condition of the soft tissue.

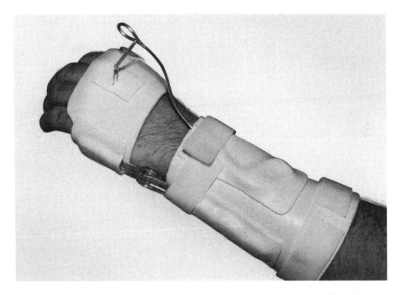

Fig. 13-4. A controlled mobilization wrist splint that may be used to allow protected wrist motion following removal of the immobilization splints when a wrist arthroplasty has been performed.

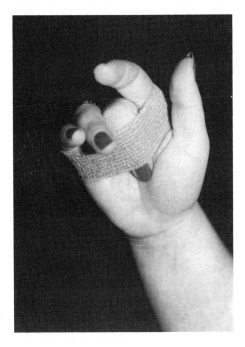

Fig. 13-5. A simple method of flexion/assist splinting with the use of Coban.

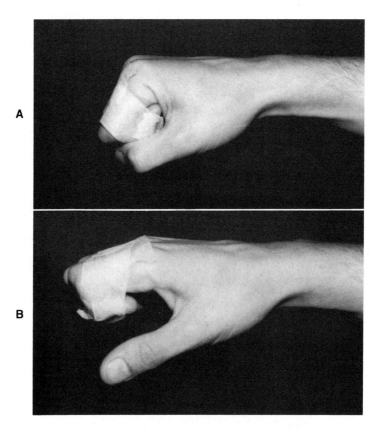

Fig. 13-6. Taping exercise has been found helpful after tendon transfer. **(A)** Inflexion. **(B)** In extension.

FUNCTIONAL SPLINTING

Functional splints for the person with rheumatoid arthritis help a patient who is having difficulty with daily tasks function with more ease and safety. From time to time functional splints are used instead of surgery for patients who for one reason or another are not surgical candidates. When assessing a patient for a functional splint, the therapist should keep in mind that the degree of deformity does not always correlate with loss of function.

The wrist is often a source of pain that interferes with a person's functioning. This is usually manifested in decreased grip strength and inability to perform many routine activities. A simple wrist splint supports the wrist, often increases grip strength, and allows an increase in activities of daily living by relieving wrist pain (Fig. 13-7).

Another common problem seen in rheumatoid arthritis is ulnar deviation of the metacarpophalangeal joints. This may not necessarily cause functional loss and does not routinely require splinting. In some cases, though, a patient expresses a need to have a splint to continue with certain activities. Some patients lose dexterity due to inability to

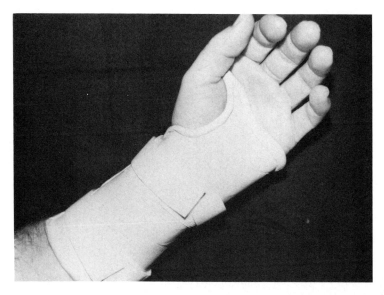

Fig. 13-7. A simple wrist splint used to aid function and protect the wrist.

effectively position thumb, index, and midfingers for pinch. In those cases either an immobilization or an elastic traction splint to help position the metacarpophalangeal joints may benefit the patient (Fig. 13-8). The design should fulfill the individual patient requirements. The splint should provide palmar support to the metacarpophalangeal joints, since palmar subluxation is often a component of ulnar drift. It would be unrealistic, however, to expect this splinting to correct the ulnar deviation. This needs to be explained to the patient before the splint is made.

When the thumb becomes involved in the rheumatoid process, the function of the hand is often significantly compromised. This is especially true with activities requiring fine manipulation. Thumb deformities in rheumatoid arthritis have been classified by Nalebuff (1968).

Type I deformity has its origin at the metacarpophalangeal joint and is characterized by metacarpophalangeal joint flexion and interphalangeal joint hyperextension. This deformity is further accentuated by normal pinch forces in daily activities. This deformity may be referred to as an extrinsic minus deformity, since there is a loss of extrinsic extensor power at the metacarpophalangeal joint level.

Type II deformity has its origin at the carpometacarpal joint and is characterized by flexion at the metacarpophalangeal joint and hyperextension at the interphalangeal joint. It looks similar to the type I deformity except that adduction of the metacarpophalangeal joint occurs due to contracture of the adductor pollicis.

Type III deformity follows the same pattern as type II except that it is characterized by hyperextension of the metacarpophalangeal joint and flexion of the interphalangeal joint. This deformity also has metacarpophalangeal joint adduction.

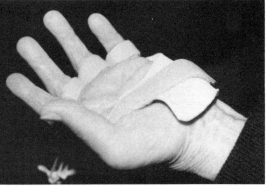

A

B

Fig. 13-8. A small hand-based MP extension radial deviation splint is helpful in increasing function when ulnar deviation is present. **A,** Dorsal aspect of splint. **B,** Volar aspect of splint.

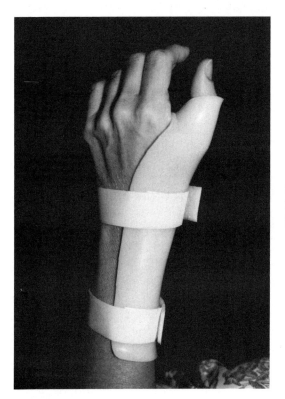

Fig. 13-9. A thumb splint to protect the carpometacarpal joint, relieve pain, and improve thumb function.

Type IV deformity is the result of stretching or rupture of the ulnar collateral ligament. The proximal phalanx deviates laterally at the metacarpophalangeal joint with the first metacarpal secondarily assuming an adducted position.

In type V deformity the major deforming factor is an attenuated palmar plate of the metacarpophalangeal joint. The metacarpophalangeal joint becomes hyperextended and the distal joint assumes a flexed position. Unlike the type III deformity, the metacarpal does not become adducted.

As in all rheumatoid deformities these thumb deformities are the result of muscle and tendon imbalance occurring between the joints of the thumb ray. In each case the alteration of posture at one joint influences the posture at adjacent joints.

Splinting may have particular value for the thumb, both for function, by stabilizing the joints, and in postoperative care. In the postoperative phase of thumb reconstruction extended periods of splinting are necessary to ensure stability for effective pinch.

When the carpometacarpal joint becomes involved, the synovitis stretches out the joint capsule, leading to joint subluxation or dislocation. The metacarpal often assumes an adducted position. The goals of the therapist at this point are to prevent an adduction contracture and to maintain a functional range of motion. A long carpometacarpal/metacarpophalangeal immobilization splint may be fabricated to protect and stabilize the joint and maintain the web space (Fig. 13-9). The splint should extend two thirds up the forearm and distally to the interphalangeal joint crease. The interphalangeal joint should be left free to move. A "short opponens" splint is sometimes made for this problem, but in many cases this proves ineffective. The short splint often does not provide the needed support when the carpometacarpal joint is involved. The longer forearm splint

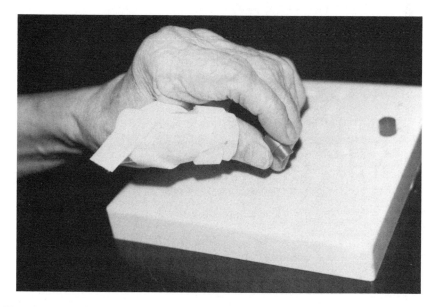

Fig. 13-10. Another splint designed to support the metacarpophalangeal joint of the thumb.

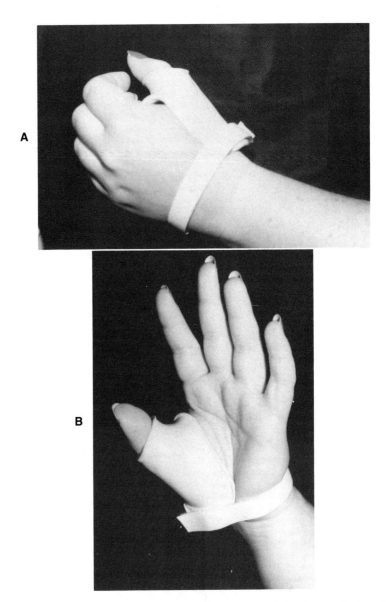

Fig. 13-11. A splint to protect the metacarpophalangeal joint of the thumb. **A,** Dorsal aspect of splint. **B,** Volar aspect of splint.

ensures good carpometacarpal protection while helping to maintain the metacarpal in the corrected position. Patients generally wear the splint during the day when performing functional activities and at night for positioning. Patients should be instructed to remove the splint several times a day for light range of motion.

When the metacarpophalangeal joint is involved, the goals are to prevent the deformity from becoming fixed, to improve function, and to help protect the joint from external forces that could produce further joint damage and deformity. One way to accomplish this is to use a small splint that will protect the metacarpal joint. In this case, neither the carpometacarpal nor the interphalangeal joints need to be immobilized. The exception to this is if there is also deformity or involvement at the adjacent joints. The metacarpophalangeal joint may be immobilized with a small aluminum and foam splint or a splint made from thermoplastic (Figs. 13-10 and 13-11). Immobilizing the metacarpophalangeal joint often improves function by providing a more stable base for pinching, thus also protecting the joints from external forces. The interphalangeal joint also may be immobilized with the use of an aluminum and foam splint (Fig. 13-12) or a small splint fabricated from thermoplastic, providing both stability and protection of this joint. Continued pinching activities may lead to stretching of the supporting soft tissue, leaving the joint unstable and pinching difficult. If the joint becomes unstable, splinting may improve the patient's functional level.

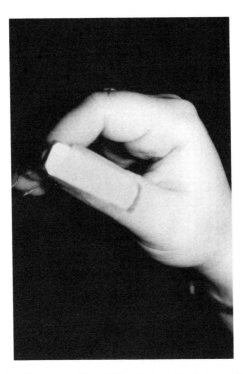

Fig. 13-12. A small splint to provide stability to the interphalangeal joint of the thumb.

Postoperative immobilization of the thumb is maintained for approximately 4 to 6 weeks to ensure good capsular healing and joint stability. During the immobilization period the patient should be encouraged to perform range of motion of the fingers several times a day to prevent stiffness. After discontinuation of splinting, therapy is geared toward the functional use of the thumb. The goal of the therapy program is to obtain a stable, pain-free, and functional pinch, and any exercise and splinting program should be directed toward the end.

Once a splint has been made, it is necessary to monitor the patient periodically for proper fit and any change in status. When embarking on a functional splinting program for a patient with rheumatoid arthritis it is important to remember that splinting one area places more stress on adjacent areas. Therefore the patient should be monitored for signs of inflammation in surrounding joints. Since the patient does have a chronic disease, splints are used for a long time and will need adjustments or replacement from time to time. Since the disease is unpredictable, the patient's needs often change and should be reassessed. Splinting should be only a part of a well-coordinated rehabilitation program.

SUMMARY

In summary, splinting the rheumatoid hand is controversial but may often be beneficial in both medical and surgical management along with a well-planned rehabilitation program. Knowledge of the biomechanics of the disease process, good communication with the physician and other team members, and careful assessment of the patient's individual situation and functional status all help the patient to derive maximum benefit from the splinting program.

CHAPTER 14

Exercise and splinting for specific problems

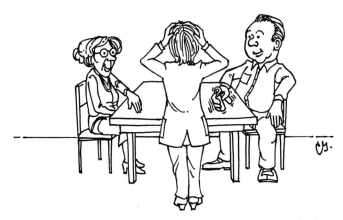

"OH NO, MRS. MILLER, PLEASE DON'T
SHARE YOUR EXERCISES WITH OTHER PATIENTS."

Encompassing a number of frequently encountered clinical hand conditions, this chapter suggests an appropriate splinting approach to each problem. Although there may be considerable variation in the individual presentation of a particular hand problem, certain common features must be dealt with in each situation. Consideration of the underlying pathologic condition of each of these problems is given, as well as an integrated program with emphasis on splinting provided to help restore the afflicted extremity to its best functional level.

Although specific splint designs illustrate this chapter, it should be noted that these do not represent the only solutions for the problems described. The important concept is to understand how a splint functions in relation to the pathologic condition presented. As has been emphasized throughout this book, there are often several different splint configurations, all of which function in a similar manner, that may be used to treat a given hand problem. It is up to the hand specialist to decide which design is most applicable on an individual, patient-by-patient basis.

325

Additionally, it should be clearly understood that in most cases it is necessary to use splinting as a part of a more comprehensive rehabilitation program directed by a knowledgeable physician-therapist team. It is therefore appropriate to include general exercise concepts in this chapter.

EXERCISE

To produce optimum results during hand rehabilitation, splinting and exercise must be carefully integrated. All too often splinting is erroneously viewed as an isolated treatment technique. Splints are used to improve passive range of motion, or in the supple hand they may provide control or substitute for absent active motion. Infrequently they are even designed to provide resistance to weakened muscles. However, the application of an external device such as a hand splint will do little to enhance the critically important active range of motion that must be provided by voluntary use of strong forearm and hand muscles whose tendinous extensions have adhesion-free excursion and smooth gliding beds. Active motion through exercise and purposeful activity is the true key to establishing and maintaining the functional capacity of a hand (Fig. 14-1).

The maximum passive range of motion of a joint must be realized before a corresponding range of active motion may be achieved. Splinting, therefore, is frequently employed as one of the initial treatment modalities when exercise alone is insufficient to attain an acceptable level of motion. A combination of appropriate hand splinting

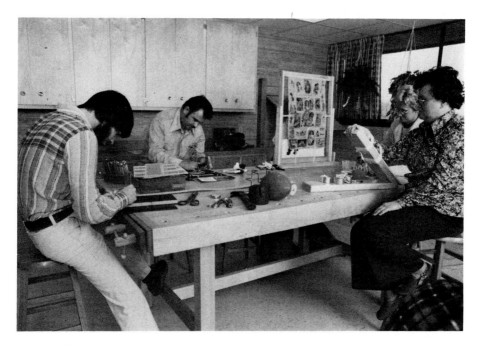

Fig. 14-1. Group interaction helps maintain enthusiasm and interest during the rehabilitation process. Patients are encouraged to use their afflicted hands in functional activities as soon as it is medically feasible.

augmented with a structured and individualized exercise program may best provide for the restoration of the maximum functional potential in a given hand problem.

Since entire books are available that deal solely with the subject of exercise, the purpose of this chapter is not to compete with these works, but rather to review the fundamental concepts of exercise to produce a common framework of terminology and theory that may then be related to the clinical use of splinting of the upper extremity.

Basically, there are three types of exercise: (1) passive exercise, in which a joint is moved through an arc of motion by an external force without the assistance of active muscle contraction; (2) active exercise, in which joint movement is the result of physiologic muscle contraction; and (3) resistive exercise, in which an external opposing force is applied against the mobile segment of the joint as active motion is attempted. The focus of each type of exercise is centered on different anatomic structures, and the respective objectives and methods of implementation of each are significantly different.

Passive exercise

Passive exercise produces gliding of the articular surfaces and excursion of tendons and capsular structures through the use of externally applied forces such as manipulation techniques or traction devices. Hand splinting is an effective conservative means of attaining passive mobility and, when used appropriately, produces a gradual rearrangement or lengthening of the pericapsular structures and an elongation of adhesions through directed gentle traction. The small joints of the hand, with their delicate pericapsular ligamentous arrangement, are uniquely susceptible to stiffening and deformity resulting from direct trauma or chronic edema. Overzealous attempts to improve passive range of motion of a hand joint by overly tight elastic traction or poorly applied manual techniques (Fig. 14-2) may not only fail to improve motion, but may actually create

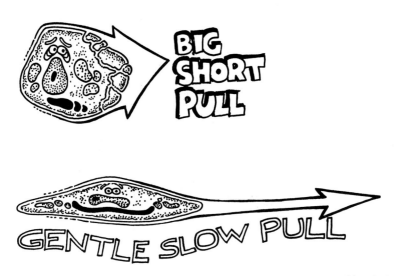

Fig. 14-2. Forceful passive range of motion may tear delicate structures, resulting in increased inflammatory response and additional scar formation.

further tissue damage and edema. Any passive method of joint mobilization should be carefully monitored with specific attention to patient discomfort, hand edema, skin temperature, and changes in the range of motion.

Active exercise

Active exercise through purposeful activity and individualized exercise routines produces joint motion effected by muscle contraction and resultant tendon excursion. Achievement of a functional level of active motion depends on the presence of adequate muscle strength and passively supple joints. Active range of motion may be considerably benefited by correctly implemented passive motion and splinting techniques that are designed to mobilize arthrofibrosed joints and adherent tendons or lengthen myostatically shortened muscles or tight pericapsular structures. For joints whose diminished range of motion is secondary to an extrinsic tenodesis effect from tendon adhesion or muscle shortening rather than a pericapsular pathologic condition, the active improvement from passive mobilization efforts may be substantial. Since the application of traction has little effect on motion at the musculotendinous level once the full passive mobility of a joint is established and the tenodesis effect minimized, splinting should not be used exclusively to increase active motion. However, an active exercise program may be augmented by an appropriately applied splint designed specifically to supplement prescribed exercises. Allowing greater function than would otherwise take place, this type of splint often supports weaker muscles, stabilizes adjacent (usually proximal) joints, particularly the wrist, maximizes tendon amplitude at a given joint, or uses or negates a tenodesis effect (Fig. 14-3).

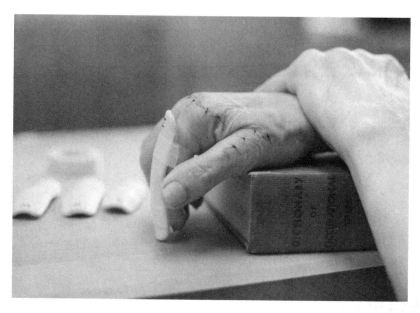

Fig. 14-3. Splinting distal interphalangeal joints allows the effects of active extrinsic tendon glide to be concentrated on mobilizing the metacarpophalangeal joint. (Courtesy Jolene Eastburn, O.T.R./L., Scranton, PA.)

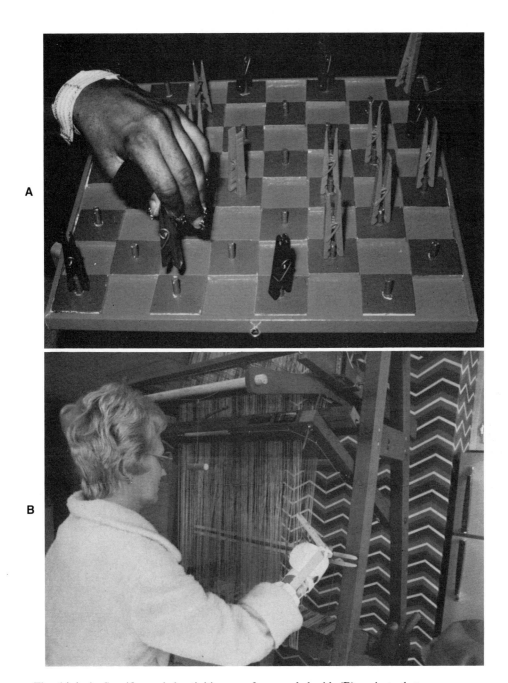

Fig. 14-4. A, Specific graded activities are often coupled with **(B)** projects that encourage gross motion of the entire extremity. (**A** courtesy Joan Farrell, O.T.R., Miami, FL.)

Repetitive attempts at active motion in the form of specific structured exercises and the use of the extremity in functional adapted and graded activities are the most productive means for increasing and maintaining strength and amplitude at the musculotendinous level (Fig. 14-4).

Resistive exercise

The purpose of resistive exercise is to produce sufficient muscle strength to allow maximum tendon excursion, full joint motion, and the execution of normal daily activities. This may be accomplished through purposeful graded activities and progressive resistive exercises. An external splinting force applied to a wrist or hand joint has little appreciable effect on improving muscle strength, since strengthening requires voluntary effort of muscles to enhance power. In addition to strengthening muscles, resistive exercises may be used to provide a type of biofeedback to the patient, allowing increased awareness of the position and function of key muscle groups (Fig. 14-5). Resistive exercises may be used at many stages of rehabilitation but should not be relied on solely to increase the passive range of motion of stiffened joints. Mechanically, because of the angle of approach of a tendon to a given joint, the strength of a muscle is often lost in translational force when attempting active mobilization of a stiff joint (Fig. 14-6). From a physiologic viewpoint, the musculotendinous unit cannot provide the long-term tension on the joint needed to cause pericapsular readjustment. Splinting will effect a more advantageous and sustained angle of pull because of its external position, producing better results with less force.

· · ·

These three basic exercises may be effectively merged to meet the needs of the individual situation. For example, active assistive exercise is a combination of active and passive exercises in which the involved joint is moved actively as far as possible with passive completion of the remaining arc of motion.

A sequential program employing these basic types of exercise in a logical order eliminates for the patient many hours of well-intentioned but nonproductive exercise. The achievement of passively supple joints is a prerequisite to the establishment of active range-of-motion and resistive exercises. It must be recognized that the active motion of a joint cannot be greater than its existing passive range of motion, and, regardless of the strength or amplitude of the involved musculotendinous unit, the absence of satisfactory passive joint motion will negate its functional effect. Adequate active joint motion depends on a minimum of fair grade muscle strength. In the presence of resistance-producing tendon adhesions the involved musculature should be functioning on a good or normal level to effect excursion change.

Muscle atrophy, with or without myostatic contracture, will have a profound effect on the ultimate performance of a joint after it has been successfully mobilized. Therefore, it is extremely important to develop and maintain muscle strengthening exercises early in the rehabilitation process, often well in advance of the ability of the muscle to effect appreciable motion at the joints it crosses. It is also important that these strengthening exercises be carried out in all extremity muscle groups, not only in those whose weakness or atrophy is obvious.

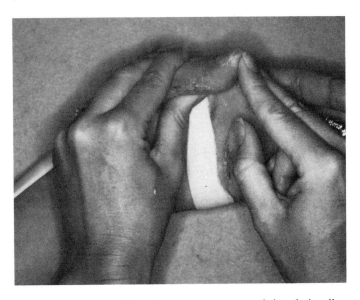

Fig. 14-5. Manual application of mild resistance to a segment as it is volutionally moved through its arc of motion may be used as a type of biofeedback.

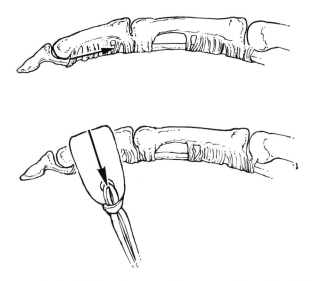

Fig. 14-6. Because extrinsic digital tendons normally run parallel to the phalanges, their force angle of approach to the joints they cross is not as mechanically advantageous as that which may be achieved by an externally positioned splint.

Timing and type of exercise

Exercise, like splinting, should be adapted to abide by the physiologic concepts of wound healing. Knowledge of the inflammatory process and the reparative schedule of the various tissue types found in the hand is paramount in successful therapeutic intervention. Individual factors such as structures involved, etiology, surgical procedures, medications, age, intelligence, motivation, and prognosis all influence the timing and type of exercise used. For example, although tension may be applied to some cutaneous and soft tissue repairs within a few hours postoperatively, the use of active exercise is often contraindicated for tendon or ligament repairs until the third or fourth postoperative week or longer. Resistive exercises are frequently delayed 8 to 12 weeks after repair. Some exercise routines, such as early passive mobilization of tendon repairs, are used for adults, but they are inappropriate for young children or those whose motivation or abilities are limited. And, although full active motion may be attained quickly, unrestricted use of the hand may not be permitted at 12 weeks in a flexor tenolysis patient who has a history of previous rupture.

Throughout the rehabilitative period care should be taken to ensure that the adopted splinting and exercise program is truly effective. Range of motion measurements provide numeric verification of the progress being made and assessment of volume; skin color, and skin temperature ensure that detrimental ramifications such as local inflammation or increased hand edema are prevented.

Coordination of exercises and splinting schedules

The coordination of exercise and splinting schedules is dictated by individual patient requirements. Although general guidelines based on diagnosis must be followed, the rigid adherence to a predetermined routine without consideration of specific patient factors produces less than desired results. It is important to remember that, although they may have similar diagnoses, no two patients respond to therapeutic intervention exactly alike. The astute hand specialist has an overall concept of the course of treatment to pursue, but this is guided, refined, and adapted to meet the unique needs of the patient.

Before a schedule is devised, splinting and exercise parameters must first be defined with measurements obtained from precise and accurate assessment instruments. Some schedules are straightforward and fairly routine; many others require experience and open-minded creativity on the part of the hand specialist. For example, it is noted that 3 weeks after proximal interphalangeal joint capsulectomy a patient has greater limitation in active and passive extension than in flexion. To emphasize the extension problem, the patient may be instructed to wear the extension splint twice as long as the flexion splint but to continue his active flexion and extension exercises on an hourly basis (Fig. 14-7, *A*). If after a week, routine goniometric measurements indicate that passive and active flexion have improved considerably but passive extension has plateaued. The patient is instructed to increase the amount of time in the extension splint, and the flexion splint time and frequency of active exercise are relatively decreased (Fig. 14-7, *B*).

SPLINT-EXERCISE SCHEDULE

Wear *EXTENSION* splint *0* hour, *50* minutes.

Exercise *10* minutes.

Wear *EXTENSION* splint *0* hour, *50* minutes.

Exercise *10* minutes.

Wear *FLEXION* splint *0* hour, *50* minutes.

Exercise *10* minutes.

Repeat schedule throughout day. Sleep in ___*NIGHT*___ splint.

Call Hand Rehabilitation Center if you have questions.

A

SPLINT-EXERCISE SCHEDULE

Wear *EXTENSION* splint *1* hour, *50* minutes.

Exercise *12* minutes.

Wear *EXTENSION* splint *1* hour, *50* minutes.

Exercise *10* minutes.

Wear *FLEXION* splint *0* hour, *50* minutes.

Exercise *10* minutes.

Repeat schedule throughout day. Sleep in ___*NIGHT*___ splint.

Call Hand Rehabilitation Center if you have questions.

B

Fig. 14-7. By increasing the periods of extension splinting while decreasing flexion splinting and exercise times, passive proximal interphalangeal joint extension is emphasized.

Assessment data provide guideposts for coordinating splinting and exercise programs. Without evaluation, splinting and exercise programs are directionless and limited in their effectiveness. Each tied to the other, assessment, splinting, and exercise play unique and critical roles in the rehabilitation process of a diseased or injured hand.

AMPUTATION

Unfortunately, amputation of portions of a digit or hand frequently occurs after hand injury. From both a psychologic and functional standpoint it is important that all efforts be devoted to rapidly restoring the amputation victim to a productive status.

Splinting a hand that has undergone amputation of a part may be directed toward (1) the maintenance of motion of uninvolved joints, (2) protective splinting to the area of amputation, and (3) functional splinting to improve prehensive patterns. Emphasis is placed on prevention of adhesions and the return of maximum function commensurate with the particular loss. The unnecessary stiffening of unaffected digital joints after amputation usually reflects a failure to establish motion programs at an early stage. The patient with a digital amputation is often reluctant to remove bandages and resume hand motion because of self-consciousness and fear of pain. The hand specialist must be especially supportive, while reinforcing constantly the need to use the extremity and to resume social contacts.

Amputation often results in generalized edema of the hand, increasing the risk of stiffness in the remaining adjacent joints. Splinting therefore may be required to augment exercise programs. In the early postamputation phase, joints in adjacent digits readily respond to uncomplicated traction devices (Fig. 14-8), such as wide rubber bands and glove rubber bands for flexion and three-point fixation splints for extension. Joints proximal to the site of amputation may be more resistant to the establishment and maintenance of good passive and active range of motion, requiring more complicated splints to attain an acceptable level of motion.

To encourage early use of the hand in purposeful activity, a temporary protective splint may be designed to fit over the distal aspect of the remaining digit. This prevents unintentional bumping of the tender stump and allows more uninhibited use of the hand as healing progresses. These splints are frequently fitted over dressings and should be removed during inactive periods for cleaning and to allow ventilation. Care should be taken to prevent wound maceration from an improper splint-wearing schedule and poor skin hygiene.

The potential for dependence on a protective splint should be acknowledged, and measures taken to gradually wean the patient from the splint as self-confidence increases and area sensitivity decreases. The initiation of a desensitization program is often instrumental in hastening unprotected hand use (Fig. 14-9). Persistent hypersensitivity at the healed site of amputation may indicate unresolved problems such as retained terminal neuromas, and evaluation by a physician should be requested.

Functional splinting of a partially amputated hand permits accomplishment of special occupational tasks (Fig. 14-10). Splint designs range from relatively simple to extremely

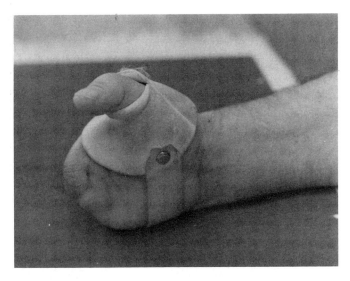

Fig. 14-8. This simple thumb carpometacarpal maintenance splint helps prevent joint contracture and loss of thumb motion in a hand that has sustained a partial amputation. (Courtesy Jolene Eastburn O.T.R./L., Scranton, PA.)

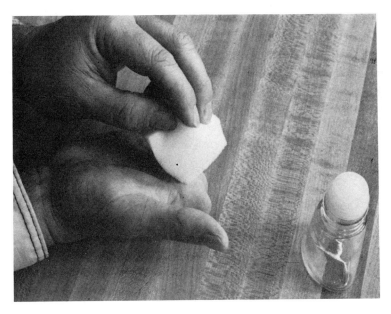

Fig. 14-9. Initiation of an early desensitization program often facilitates functional use of the hand after amputation.

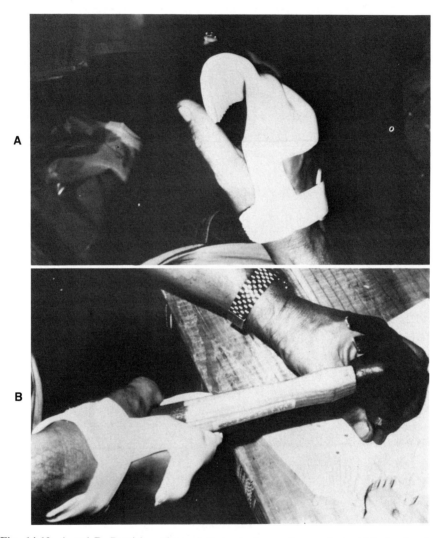

Fig. 14-10. A and **B,** Provision of an adapted gripping surface against which the thumb could oppose allowed this patient to grasp and use a hammer. **C,** Prosthetic thumb post provides a stable surface against which normal fingers can oppose for pinch and grasp activities. (**A** and **B** courtesy Joan Farrell, O.T.R., Miami, FL; **C** courtesy of Jolene Eastborn, O.T.R./L., Scranton, PA.)

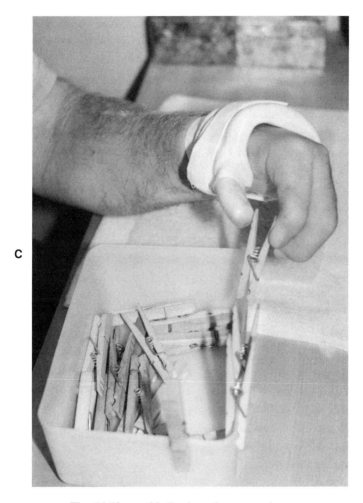

C

Fig. 14-10, cont'd. For legend see opposite page.

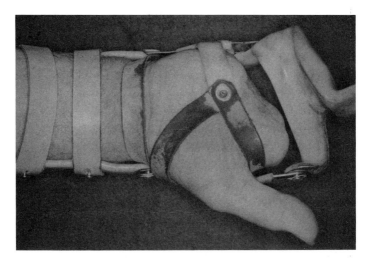

Fig. 14-11. Because this man required splint durability that could not be attained with routine splinting materials, he was referred to an orthotist who specializes in metal hand braces.

complicated, depending on specific anatomic loss and patient requirements. Durability of the splint is often a key factor and may necessitate collaboration with an orthotist (Fig. 14-11).

It is important that an excellent rapport is established with the hand amputation patient. The loss of a body part is a severe psychologic blow, regardless of the level, and the patient must be gently brought to understand the importance of accepting the loss and devoting efforts toward maintaining and restoring maximum function in the remaining hand.

CAPSULOTOMY/CAPSULECTOMY

Capsulectomy involves the surgical division (capsulotomy) or excision (capsulectomy) of a portion of the collateral ligaments of a digital joint with normal articular surfaces but limited passive motion because of contracted periarticular ligamentous structures. Although a substantial improvement of motion may be reliably anticipated at the metacarpophalangeal level, the results of a capsulectomy procedure at the proximal interphalangeal joint are less predictable. Mobilization efforts are usually initiated within 1 to 7 days postoperatively. These efforts should involve aggressive splinting and exercise programs for the patient which are carefully monitored.

Preoperative splinting and exercises are designed to attain as much passive joint motion as possible, enhancing the postoperative arc of motion and assuring adhesion-free tendon excursion essential to the active maintenance of passively improved post-operative motion. Splints should be adapted to meet individual patient variations. The decision as to the type of splint to be applied depends on the presence or absence of wrist-produced tenodesis effect. If the limitation is purely articular, simple or compound splints will suffice (Fig. 14-12). Long splints with adjunctive wrist immobilization are

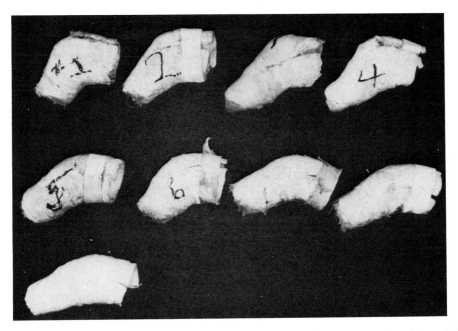

Fig. 14-12. Serial cylinder casts, which are changed every two or three days, may be used to enhance passive interphalangeal joint motion before a capsulotomy/capsulectomy procedure is undertaken. Cylinder casts are also effective in maintaining postoperative motion once the initial edema subsides and the incision is healed.

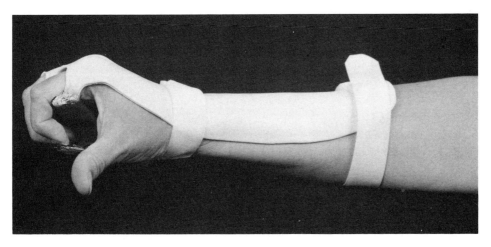

Fig. 14-13. Splint designs that incorporate the wrist eliminate compensatory tenodesis effect as traction is applied to more distal joints.

required to control the effects of wrist position on distal joints in the presence of extrinsic tendon adhesions or poor postural habits that unfavorably affect digital joint mechanics (Fig. 14-13).

Splinting of a joint that has undergone a capsulectomy procedure maintains the motion gained from the combined preoperative and operative efforts. Because of the potential recurrence of extension contractures, the metacarpophalangeal joints are usually splinted to encourage joint flexion. Extension is often more difficult to regain than is flexion in the capsulectomized proximal interphalangeal joint. For this reason extension splinting, which is interspersed with frequent exercise periods and limited flexion splinting, may need to be prolonged to prevent recurrence of deformity. It is important that postcapsulectomy splinting and exercise programs be frequently reevaluated by members of the hand rehabilitation team during the first 2 or 3 postoperative months, and appropriate changes be instigated to ensure optimum results. One should emphasize to the patient undergoing these difficult joint mobilization procedures that the tendency of recurrent stiffening of the involved joints is great and that splinting may be necessary for many months.

CRUSH, BURN, AND COLD INJURIES

Although of dissimilar etiologies, extensive soft tissue damage resulting in crush, burn, and frostbite injuries often requires similar conservative treatment. Hand splinting requirements after these injuries depend on the site and extent of tissue damage. When a major portion of the hand is involved, early use of a safe position splint (long metacarpophalangeal flexion, interphalangeal extension immobilization splint) alternated with exercise facilitates preservation of collateral ligament length by maintaining joint postures that place these ligaments at near-maximum tension (Fig. 14-14).

Philosophies regarding optimum thumb position in a safe position splint differ. Full thumb abduction is advocated by some, whereas full extension is preferred by others. The key concept involved, however, is to maintain maximum passive range of motion at the first carpometacarpal joint and to adapt the splint to meet the individual requirements of the patient. To prevent the occurrence of additional arthrofibrotic changes in a hand already predisposed to swelling and stiffness, the use of this long immobilization splint must be accompanied by frequent periods of passive and active exercises to the wrist and digital joints. As the extent of the injury becomes more apparent and additional splinting is required to maintain passive motion of specific joints, a safe position splint may be alternated with mobilization splints or used only at night in deference to daytime exercise and mobility splinting.

Splints fitted on hands with soft tissue loss or damage must be altered at the design stage to adapt for the presence of surface defects, skin grafts, and draining areas. Underlying fractures are often present in this type of injury, and protruding internal fixation wires may require adjustments in the basic splint design. To enhance cleanliness and decrease the chance of tissue maceration from the presence of excessive moisture, splints are fitted over several layers of light bandage. To ensure consistent and contiguous splint application, care must be taken to keep these dressings to a minimum. Padding is usually considered inappropriate in splints used on hands that have sustained

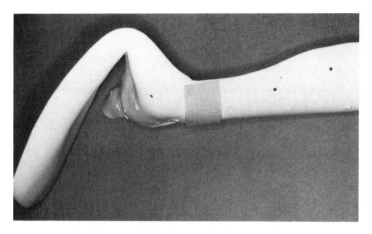

Fig. 14-14. Safe position splints are frequently used during the early stages of burn, crush, or frostbite injuries.

extensive soft tissue damage because it tends to become contaminated with tissue exudate. The use of wide straps or overlapping rolled gauze or ace wrap diminishes the possibility of circumferential constriction with the resultant propagation of increased edema.

FRACTURES

Trauma resulting in fracture of the small bones of the hand is one of the most commonly encountered injuries of the upper extremity. Fractures of the distal phalanx occur most frequently, followed by metacarpal, proximal phalangeal, and finally middle phalangeal fractures. The potential functional loss from this type of injury may be underestimated. Even if fracture healing occurs uneventfully, residual joint stiffness may become a serious factor in limiting composite hand function.

It has been shown by Strickland and associates (1979) that fracture immobilization beyond 4 weeks has a dramatically unfavorable effect on digital performance, although no clear-cut evidence is available to indicate that mobilization before the third week has any profound effect on the final range of motion. A patient age of over 50, fracture comminution, and, perhaps most important, associated tendon injuries also have a strongly detrimental effect on the final outcome of digital motion following fracture.

In the presence of a fracture, it is important to maintain the mobility of adjacent joints and digits to prevent magnification of the original injury through the development of secondary periarticular pathology (Fig. 14-15). Internal fixation of the fracture with Kirschner wires or small compression plates often eliminates the need to immobilize uninvolved joints and allows early mobilization of the hand, which is the key to preventing residual joint stiffness.

Splints should be designated to forestall the insidious development of deformity caused by edema and accompanying arthrofibrosis. Because the mechanical and physiologic repercussions of a fracture differ according to the severity of the injury, site of

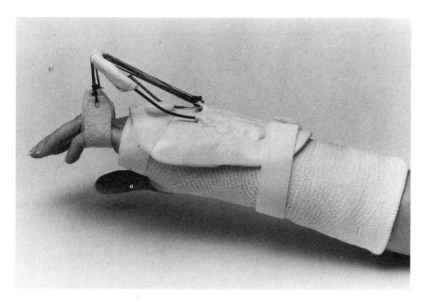

Fig. 14-15. A detachable outrigger allows this fracture patient, who is being treated with a fore-arm cast, to begin early motion of distal finger joints. Note that because the cast is rigid and distributes pressure evenly, the need for a longer base of attachment of the outrigger is negated. (Courtesy Barbara Allen, O.T.R., Oklahoma City.)

the fracture, quality of reduction, and method of immobilization used, each patient must be objectively evaluated and splint and exercise program created to meet the specific needs. The splint(s) should also be adapted to support the fractured segment and avoid protruding fixation pins. Pressure on pins may lead to pin-site irritation or possible infection. Long splints with adjunctive wrist immobilization usually are not required in treating stable phalangeal fractures but may be of use with metacarpal fractures or unstable finger fractures where wrist control may lessen deforming tendon forces. It is not uncommon to splint for both flexion and extension of adjacent joints of a segment that has sustained a fracture.

Tendon injuries associated with phalangeal fractures have a particularly prejudicial effect because of the tendency for the tendon to become strongly adherent to the site of fracture healing. This obligatory loss of tendon amplitude, most often involving the extensor mechanism or flexor superficialis over the proximal phalanx or profundus over the middle phalanx, severely limits distal joint excursion by virtue of its check-rein effect. In these instances it is extremely dangerous to rely on strong manipulative or mobilization traction techniques to improve digital joint motion because the restrictive adhesions may be so strong that tendon rupture or attenuation occur, resulting in irreparable consequences. More gentle range-of-motion techniques are indicated here with consideration for early surgical lysis with or without capsulectomy when a strong tendon-bone bond is apparent.

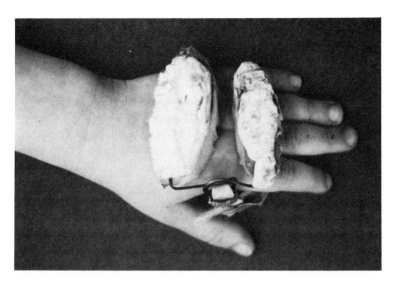

Fig. 14-16. Splinting materials used in children's splints should be durable and nontoxic. The plastic portion of this Orthoplast and spring-wire splint is almost unrecognizable because of the patient's habit of chewing on it.

The presence of associated ligament or neurovascular injury considerably alters the mode of conservative treatment. Consultation among members of the hand rehabilitation team is of paramount importance to establish goals and guidelines for postreduction management.

PEDIATRICS

In addition to the basic splinting principles, other variables should be taken into consideration when working with pediatric patients. These variables are incorporated and adapted according to the specific age and capabilities of the child being treated.

Because of the seemingly limitless physical activity of growing children, their splints must be solidly constructed of highly durable materials that are nontoxic and easily cleaned (Fig. 14-16). They should also be designed to remain in place on the extremity, and in case of an infant or young child, the splint should be difficult to remove except by an adult.

Parents must be instructed as to proper splint care and wearing procedures. It may also be helpful to share this information with teachers and others who are frequently responsible for the child's care. Experience has shown that a combination of verbal and written guidelines produces less confusion than do verbal instructions alone.

During the fitting phase of splint fabrication, the child's anxiety may be diminished by allowing him to play with material scraps or by making up games or stories to promote cooperation. Drawing a face or design on the completed splint is also a successful enticement to encourage the child's acceptance of the splint (Fig. 14-17).

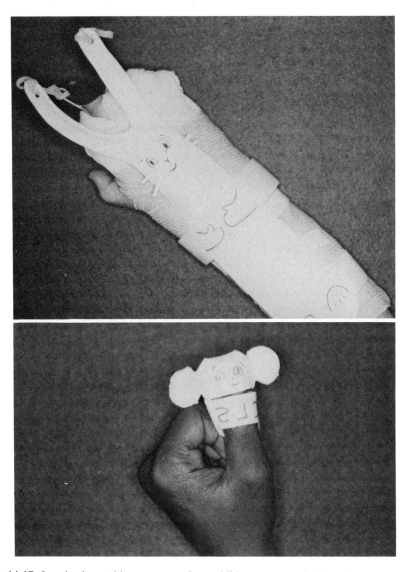

Fig. 14-17. Imagination and humor can entice a child to cooperate in the splinting program.

Although these "extras" may be initially time consuming, they ultimately result in the production of a more effective splint and improved results because of a cooperative patient and well-informed family.

PERIPHERAL NERVE INJURIES

The potential for the restoration of optimum hand function after peripheral nerve injuries of the upper extremity depends on the preservation of good passive joint motion. It is also necessary to protect periarticular structures and denervated musculature by avoiding improper positioning of the partially paralyzed extremity. In the presence of existing deformity, splints may be designed to restore passive mobility to digital joints. Adapted to the individual requirements of the patient, these splints range from uncomplicated rubber bands to complex multifunction splints. Once free gliding of articular surfaces has been established, maintenance and positioning splints may be used until reinnervation occurs or until tendon transfer procedures are carried out to restore balance to the hand. These positioning splints should be used in conjunction with a good exercise program. They serve to prevent deformity that results from the unopposed antagonists of the paralyzed muscles as well as to position the hand for use while awaiting nerve regeneration. The splints may assume predictable configurations based on the nerve(s) involved and must be light, without excessive components, and easily applied or they will not be worn.

In the supple hand, the need for protective splinting varies according to the type of lesion and the inherent laxity of the ligamentous structure of the individual hand. Not all patients who have sustained ulnar nerve injuries proceed to develop the classic claw hand posture of hyperextension of the fourth and fifth metacarpophalangeal joints and concomitant interphalangeal flexion. Some have unusually firm palmar plate restraint at the metacarpophalangeal joints and are not predisposed to hyperextension deformities, despite the lack of intrinsic opposition to the long extensor muscles. It is important, however, that these patients be monitored throughout rehabilitation to ensure that late-blooming deformity does not occur. All patients with total loss of radial nerve innervation to the wrist and digital extensors will develop a wrist drop and require external support to properly position the hand, both to avoid deformity and allow function.

Splinting requirements for each type of nerve loss are fairly predictable and will be considered.

Median nerve

The median nerve provides the critical sensory perception to the palmar surface of the hand with the exception of the small finger and half of the ring. This nerve is also responsible for innervation of the pronator muscles, the radial wrist flexor, the superficial flexors of all digits, profundus flexion of the index and long fingers, and the long flexor of the thumb. At a more distal level the median nerve innervates the thenar muscles, whose function is abduction and opposition. High median nerve lesions, therefore, are more disabling than is interruption at the wrist level, with the former affecting extrinsic as well as intrinsic digital function. However, the main disability with a median nerve lesion is the loss of sensibility.

Splinting of median nerve injuries depends on the level of lesion. Emphasis is placed on maintenance of passive mobility of the involved joints and enhancement of function. High interruption may require splints that assist finger flexion as well as opposition of the thumb (Fig. 14-18). Emphasis may be reduced to the prevention of thumb web contractures after more distal loss (Fig. 14-19). An understanding of each patient's functional capacity and substitution patterns is important before a splint design is initiated. For example, many patients whose long thumb flexor or short abductor and opponens action has been lost achieve adequate thumb use through substitution of the abductor pollicis longus, flexor pollicis brevis (deep head), and adductor pollicis.

Radial nerve

A high-level radial nerve injury results in loss of active wrist, thumb, and finger extension and a weakening of supination and thumb abduction. Because the wrist provides the key to hand function at the digital level, the loss of the ability to properly position the hand in extension markedly weakens grasp and diminishes coordination. The coexisting deficit of metacarpophalangeal extension presents a less significant problem because the intrinsic muscles provide active extension of the interphalangeal joints.

The most important objective in splinting a high radial nerve injury is to support the wrist in extension, enhancing hand function and preventing overstretching of the extensor muscle groups. For most patients the use of a simple wrist extension splint is sufficient to allow satisfactory hand use (Fig. 14-20). Long finger and thumb extension splints with extension outrigger attachments are sometimes considered excessive and

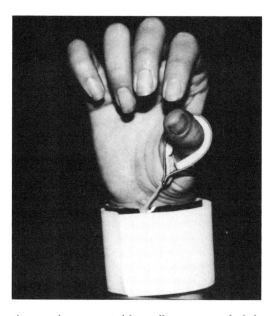

Fig. 14-18. Thumb motion may be augmented in median nerve paralysis by a simple carpometacarpal opposition splint. (Courtesy Gretchen Maurer, O.T.R., Virginia Beach, VA.)

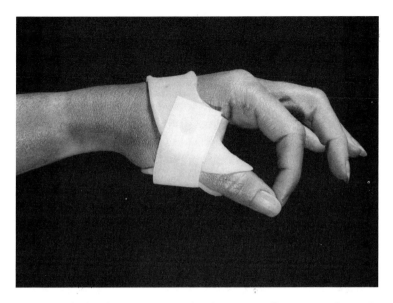

Fig. 14-19. This simple thumb carpometacarpal maintenance splint prevents first web space contracture in a median nerve injury. (Courtesy Sharon Flinn-Wagner, M.Ed., O.T.R./L., Cleveland, OH.)

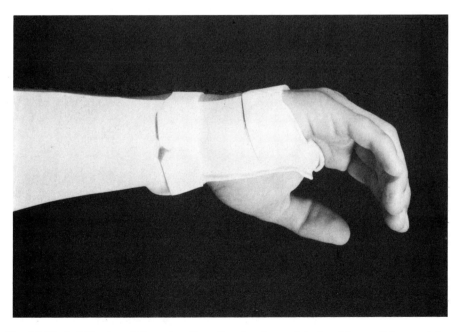

Fig. 14-20. Stabilization of the wrist allows functional use of the hand in a radial nerve injury.

should be used in situations in which full digital extension is required for successful accomplishment of given tasks. Since these are substitution rather than correction splints, low profile outrigger configurations are preferable (Fig. 14-21).

Ulnar nerve

The ulnar nerve, with its important intrinsic innervation, is largely responsible for delicate coordinated movements of the hand. In addition, it also influences flexion of the ring and small fingers and ulnar deviation and flexion of the wrist. Disruption of the ulnar nerve may result in the development of a claw deformity with metacarpophalangeal joint hyperextension and interphalangeal joint flexion of the fourth and fifth digits. Loss of small finger abduction and opposition and adduction of the thumb with the resultant weakness of pinch also accompanies ulnar paralysis.

The goals of splinting a hand that has sustained an ulnar nerve lesion are directed toward the attainment and maintenance of full passive motion and the improvement of hand function. Existing joint limitations, often at the proximal interphalangeal joint of the ring or small finger, must be corrected before maintenance or substitution splinting programs may be initiated. Splints designed to correct deformity should be specifically created to meet individual needs and should be changed to maintain optimum mechanical purchase as joint motion improves. When full passive motion has been established, or if the hand is supple at the time of initial examination, preventive splinting may commence.

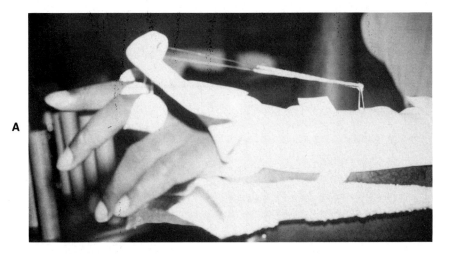

Fig. 14-21. In special circumstances it may be necessary to mechanically assist full finger extension (**A, C,** and **D**) or wrist and finger extension (**B**) for a patient who has sustained a radial nerve injury. (**A** courtesy Robin Miller Wagman, O.T.R., Fort Lauderdale, FL; **B** courtesy Linda Tresley, O.T.R. and Joanne J. Zitter, O.T.R./L., Chicago; **C** and **D** courtesy Christine Heaney, B.Sc., O.T., Ottawa, Ontario.)

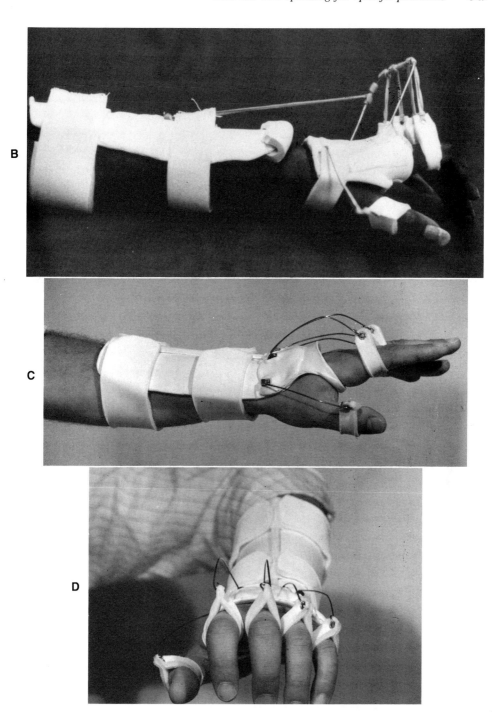

Fig. 14-21, cont'd. For legend see opposite page.

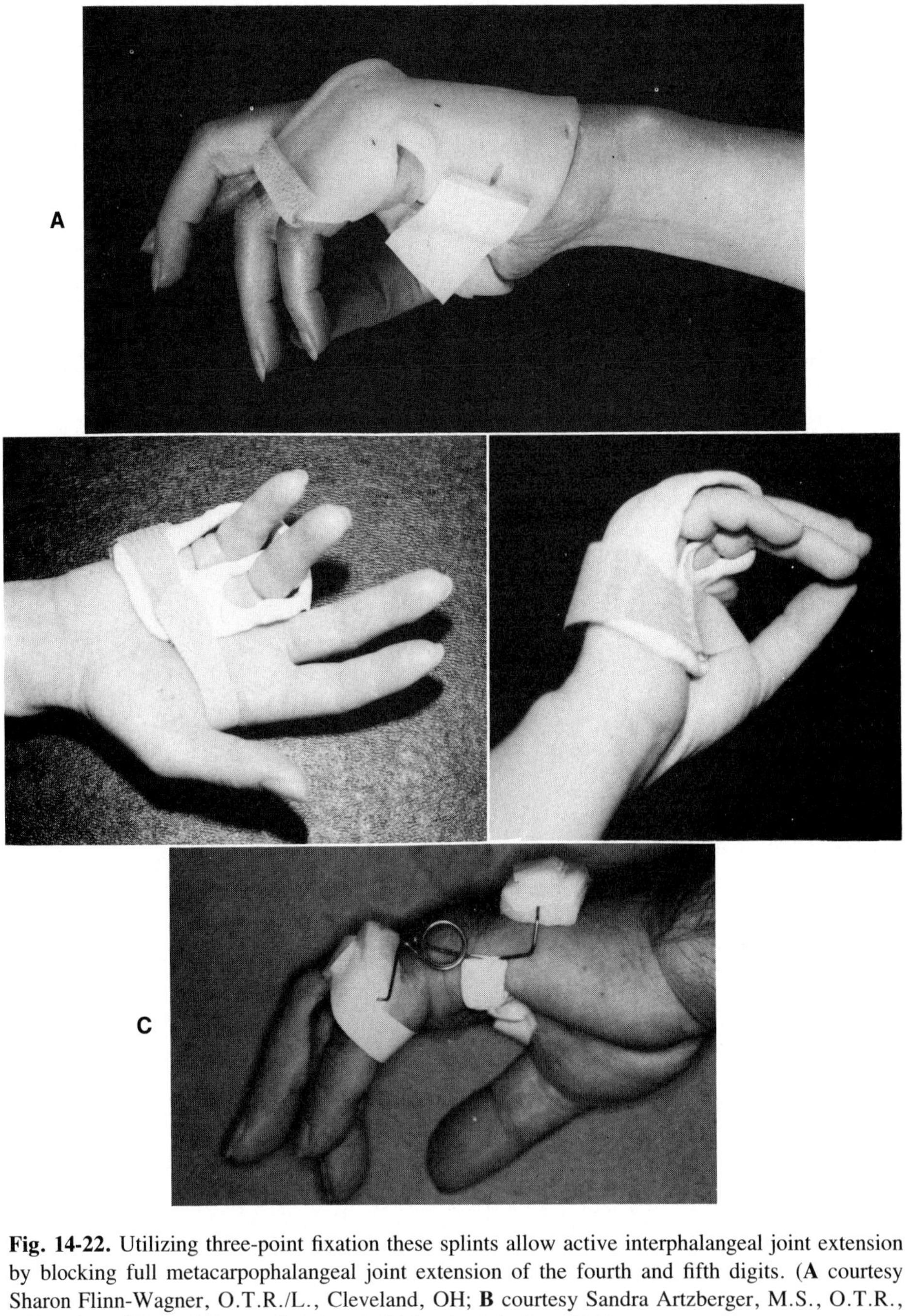

Fig. 14-22. Utilizing three-point fixation these splints allow active interphalangeal joint extension by blocking full metacarpophalangeal joint extension of the fourth and fifth digits. (**A** courtesy Sharon Flinn-Wagner, O.T.R./L., Cleveland, OH; **B** courtesy Sandra Artzberger, M.S., O.T.R., Milwaukee, WI. and Bonnie Fehring, L.P.T., Fond du Lac, WI.)

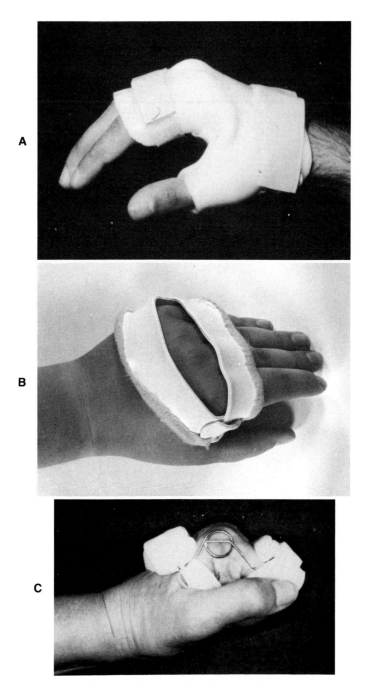

Fig. 14-23. These splints prevent metacarpophalangeal hyperextension of the second through fifth metacarpophalangeal joints while allowing partial to full digital flexion. They may be used with combined ulnar and median nerve lesions. (**A** courtesy Gretchen Maurer, O.T.R., Virginia Beach, VA; **B** courtesy Ruth Coopee, O.T.R., Easthampton, PA.)

Positioning the fourth and fifth metacarpophalangeal joints in slight flexion allows the amplitude of the extrinsic digital extensor muscles to act effectively on the interphalangeal joints. Numerous splint designs accomplish this objective (Fig. 14-22). One of the most acceptable is a three-point piano wire splint described by Wynn Parry (1973). Adaptation of this splint to the use of low-temperature materials for the dorsal and palmar metacarpal bars and dorsal phalangeal bar makes construction and fitting easier (Fig. 14-22, *C*). Substitution splints may be used until nerve regeneration is complete, or until tendon transfer procedures are done.

Combined nerve injuries

Damage to multiple nerves of the upper extremity is not uncommon, and the resulting potential for the development of deformity is, of course, magnified. Splinting programs should continue to incorporate the concepts previously mentioned for each individual injury, with even more care taken to monitor progress and make necessary adaptations as changes occur (Fig. 14-23).

The splinting of peripheral nerve injuries should be augmented with individually designed exercise programs that promote the maintenance of active and passive motion and enhance hand dexterity. Although the goals of these two programs are almost identical, each brings a unique contribution to minimizing the resultant disability, and in conjunction with one another they provide an integrated and practical approach to hand rehabilitation. Each splint and exercise routine should also be interspersed with periodic objective reevaluation sessions, which allow for program modification and continued patient progress.

QUADRIPLEGIA

Splinting of the quadriplegic hand depends on the level of the spinal cord lesion. Extremities that lack innervation above the seventh cervical nerve (C7) level often require the development of a passive or active tenodesis function for grasp, whereas those at C7 have active gross grasp and release through innervated extrinsic flexors and extensors. The intrinsic muscles of the hand are usually innervated at the first thoracic nerve level, allowing normal hand function.

Fifth cervical nerve

Patients with lesions at this level usually have active elbow flexion and deltoid shoulder movements, allowing gross positioning of the forearm and hand. Paralyzed wrist and hand musculature necessitates external wrist support in the form of a simple wrist immobilization splint to provide distal stability of the extremity. Accommodation of the splint to serve as the basis of attachment for adapted equipment is important to establishing independence in activities of daily living (Fig. 14-24). Thumb carpometacarpal position and passive motion may be maintained through web spacers that alternately position the thumb in abduction and extension. Wrist and thumb splints are often combined (Fig. 14-25).

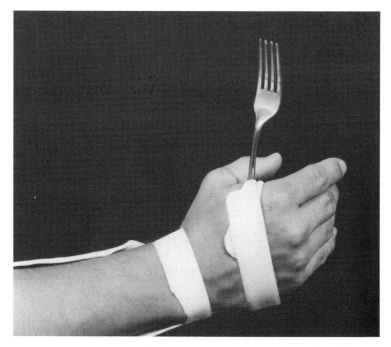

Fig. 14-24. To help patient independence, splints may be designed to hold ADL, homemaking, or work-related equipment.

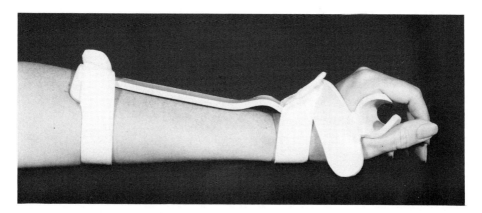

Fig. 14-25. A long thumb CMC/MP positioning splint is one of several designs that may be used to stabilize the wrist and maintain the first web space of a C5 spinal cord lesion patient.

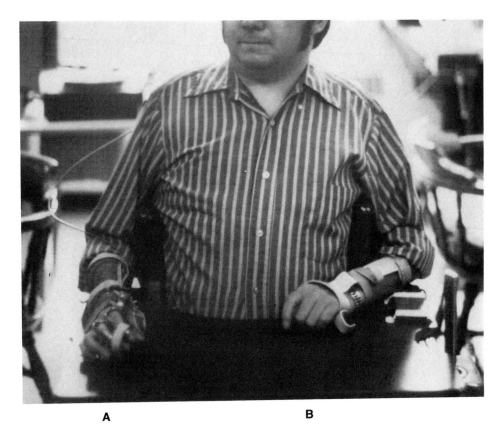

A   **B**

Fig. 14-26. A, A battery-powered external orthosis allows this C5 quadriplegic patient to grasp and release objects. **B,** The orthosis is triggered when the patient touches his watch-band to the copper plate mounted on his lap board. (United States patent No. 3967321: Ryan, Fess, Babcock, et al.)

If the patient is a candidate for an externally powered splint, the development of a passive tenodesis hand may be considered (next section). Most externally powered splints create a gross grasp or pinch by providing a power source to drive a conventional wrist-operated tenodesis splint. Power sources vary, as do triggering mechanisms (Fig. 14-26).

Sixth cervical nerve

In spinal cord lesions at this level, shoulder and elbow motions are stronger, resulting in more coordinated extremity positioning, but active elbow extension is absent. The important wrist extensors are spared, permitting a tenodesis hand in which grasp is achieved through an active wrist extension–passive finger flexion pattern. Tenodesis hands can be maximally developed through carefully supervised exercise and splinting programs. Exercises are oriented toward allowing controlled extrinsic flexor tightness to occur while maintaining passive range of motion of the wrist and digits. Finger exten-

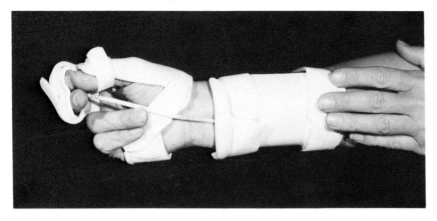

Fig. 14-27. This tenodesis splint produces passive approximation of the index and long fingers to the thumb through active wrist extension.

sion exercises are performed with the wrist in flexion, and finger flexion exercises are carried out with the wrist in extension. Splints designed to augment these patterns are used to reinforce the tenodesis motion in functional activities (Fig. 14-27). As habit patterns become established, gradual weaning from the splint is encouraged, allowing increasingly independent tenodesis hand use.

Moberg (1975) describes a method for using the wrist extensors to enhance flexor hinge key grip of the thumb. Splinting for this procedure involves maintaining passive motion of the thumb carpometacarpal and metacarpophalangeal joints preoperatively and protecting splinting of the transfer during the early postoperative mobilization phase. A small web spacer may occasionally be required to maintain carpometacarpal motion as postoperative time increases.

Seventh cervical nerve

Patients with lesions at this level usually have gross active finger flexion and extension but lack the intrinsic musculature that allows fine hand coordination and dexterity. Splinting and exercise programs are directed toward maintenance of passive joint range of motion with emphasis on thumb carpometacarpal mobility and prevention of extension deformities at the metacarpophalangeal joints. Splinting to position the thumb in opposition may be used to enhance prehension of small objects.

• • •

As a result of severe muscle imbalance and limited active motion, many quadriplegic hands have a tendency to become slightly edematous and to assume a resting posture of metacarpophalangeal extensions, proximal interphalangeal flexion, and thumb adduction. These factors may lead insidiously to stiffness and eventually to severe joint contractures, which are correctable only through surgical intervention. In anticipation of these problems, preventive measures should be initiated within the first week after injury, since joint stiffness and contractures severely limit rehabilitative potential. As with hand injuries, it is important to position the resting quadriplegic hand in a posture of antideformity to prevent shortening of digital ligaments. So-called functional position splints do not provide sufficient metacarpophalangeal flexion and proximal interphalangeal extension to prevent collateral ligament shortening. With the wrist in neutral position, the metacarpophalangeal joints should be splinted in 70 to 90 degrees of flexion; interphalangeals in 0 to 10 degrees of flexion; and the thumb carpometacarpal in abduction or extension (safe position). Although a vigil for early deforming forces must always be maintained, the need for safe position splinting during periods of rest diminishes as the patient increases the use of his hands in functional compensatory patterns and the potential for edema subsides.

REPLANTATION

The splinting program employed with patients who have undergone replantation procedures emphasizes the attainment and maintenance of motion in adjacent uninvolved digits and in the replanted segment. Because of the obligatory immobilization of repaired structures to promote healing, the interval between the initiation of each type of splinting is often several weeks.

Depending on the level of severance, viability status of the replant, and size of the postoperative dressing, splinting and exercises may be carried out on joints not included in the dressing within the first postoperative week, provided that the mobilization does not stress repaired structures.

Splinting of the replanted segment may begin as early as 3 weeks after replantation. With immobilization splints providing external support to internally fixated fractures, gentle mobilization traction designed according to individual requirements may be initiated. Because of lack of sensation and the potential damaging effect of edema, careful

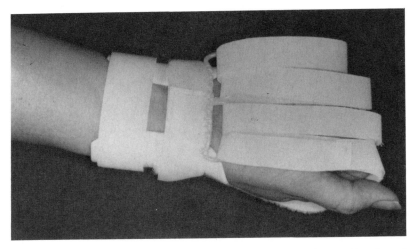

Fig. 14-28. The wristband of this simple finger flexion splint has been widened to decrease pressure from the splint on the distal forearm.

attention must be directed to obtaining a congruous splint fit that does not produce pressure, obstruct venous return, or impair arterial flow. Straps and splint components may be widened to alleviate undue pressure on underlying soft tissue (Fig. 14-28). Splints that apply small areas of three-point pressure or are circumferential in design are contraindicated during the early mobilization of a replanted segment. Careful monitoring of the replant is essential after splint application. An alteration of digital color or increase in edema of the replanted segment necessitates immediate removal of the splint. As the vascular status of the implant becomes less tenuous, its sensitivity to pressure decreases, allowing the use of more conventional splint designs.

SPASTICITY

Historically, the subject of splinting the hypertonic hand has been riddled with controversy. Based on an extensive literature review encompassing 125 years, Neuhaus and associates (1981) identified two basic treatment theories: the biomechanical approach, which emphasizes mechanical techniques to combat deformity, and the neurophysiologic approach, which uses movement and handling techniques to reduce spasticity. In many of the early neurophysiologic theories rigid, nonarticulated splinting was either omitted or contraindicated. More recently splints that use the effects of textured, elastic, or articulated components have been recommended for use in conjunction with established facilitation treatment techniques.

Some physicians and therapists feel strongly that the hypertonic extremity should not be splinted, whereas others are equally adamant that splinting has beneficial results. Even among proponents of splinting, numerous disagreements exist concerning splint design, surface of splint application, wearing times and schedules, joints to be splinted, and specific construction materials for splints and splint components.

Although numerous splints have been advocated to combat the effects of deforming forces to the upper extremity from upper motor neuron lesions, few, if any, have been shown to produce consistently satisfactory results. The literature abounds with treatises on the technique and ramifications of splinting the spastic hand, but close examination reveals a surprising paucity of supporting data based on solid scientific research design and statistically significant analysis. Problems include weak or limited research design, extremely small population samples, invalid and unreliable methods of measuring hypertonicity, lack of variable control, and lack of consistent methodology.

Aside from the inadequacy of research data, one of the most glaring omissions seems to be a fundamental lack of understanding that the upper extremity is an open-ended intercalated articular chain. Some of the most frequently used splints are designed to position spastic digits in extension without controlled wrist position; or they influence the wrist without affecting the fingers and thumb. These splints produce a consistent sequence of events that are both predictable and immediately evident. Either the wrist assumes a compensatory flexed attitude as the fingers and thumb are brought into extension, or the unsplinted digits assume a greater attitude of flexion as the wrist is extended. This compensatory chain of events occurs because the tendons of the extrinsic finger flexors cross and affect not only the digital joints but the wrist as well.

With prolonged progressive plaster serial casting of both the digital and wrist joints, a spastic hand may be slowly brought into a more functional position, and hypertonicity seems to decrease. However, when corrective splinting is discontinued, if the source of the deforming forces has not been altered, the hand and wrist will gradually return to a position of deformity. To date no study has shown through good research design and appropriate statistical analysis that splinting will *permanently* control or diminish hypertonicity in the upper extremity.

For purely hygienic reasons, a cone or other device may be used prophylactically to prevent skin maceration from prolonged immobilization in a fisted attitude and to stop fingernails of severely hypertonic digits from becoming embedded in the palmar surface of the hand.

TENDON GRAFTS

Tendon grafting involves the bridging of a gap in tendon with an autogenous donor tendon from the same or a separate extremity. Commonly used donor tendons include the palmaris longus, the plantaris, and on occasion a toe extensor. One of the most important criteria for a successful tendon graft procedure is the establishment and maintenance of good passive motion of the disabled segment and adjacent rays. Splinting may be effectively employed for creating and preserving supple digits, both preoperatively and during the postoperative course.

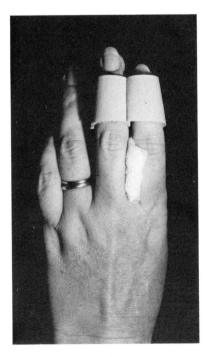

Fig. 14-29. The use of a "finger trapper" facilitates the maintenance of passive motion during the preoperative phase of a tendon graft procedure.

Preoperative splinting should be designed to meet the individual problems presented. If wrist position does not influence passive motion, simple and compound splints such as compound proximal interphalangeal extension splint, simple proximal interphalangeal extension splint, simple finger flexion splint, or simple thumb carpometacarpal maintenance splint are usually efficient devices for maximizing passive joint motion. If, however, significant wrist-produced tenodesing of the extrinsic flexor or extensor tendons is present, the wrist must be incorporated into the splint to control its influence at digital levels. Once passive motion is reestablished, the splinting program is directed at maintaining joint status. This often involves uncomplicated night splinting and a routine exercise program during the day (Fig. 14-29).

The philosophy of postoperative management to which one subscribes dictates the type of splinting program employed after surgical attachment of the tendon graft. Some authors advocate immobilization for 3 weeks to promote tendon healing before initiating splinting and conservative therapy, whereas others begin early controlled passive motion in hopes of diminishing scar formation between the sutured graft and its gliding bed. It appears, however, that many of the adhesion-modifying benefits of early controlled motion after primary flexor tendon repair are not as applicable to tendon grafting, and results following the application of these techniques to grafts have been disappointing. The splinting programs differ considerably and should not be undertaken without knowledge of the postoperative management plan for each patient and without a thorough understanding of the concepts involved. (See also the section of postoperative splinting of tendon repairs.)

Staged flexor tendon grafts

The general concepts employed in the management of single-stage tendon grafts may be applied to the treatment of two-stage flexor tendon grafting procedures, except that the pregraft time period is expanded to allow the development of a pseudosheath around a flexible tendon implant that is removed at the time of grafting. As with the one-stage grafts, a supple hand is a prerequisite to surgical procedures. Once this is established, a flexible tendon implant is inserted with its distal end anchored to the tendon stub or to bone. Postoperatively the hand and wrist are immobilized in flexion posture for approximately 3 weeks, during which time the pseudosheath forms, providing a smooth gliding bed for the second-stage autogenous graft. Early splinting may be required to reestablish preoperative passive motion levels. Finger taping, frequent conscientious exercise periods, and individualized splinting are the keys to maintaining good passive motion during the first stage of the postoperative phase.

Once the implant is removed and the tendon graft connected, the two-stage procedure is treated similarly to the single-stage tendon graft (see the following section).

Active tendon implant

A relatively new concept, the active tendon implant designed by Hunter et al. (1986) allows controlled active motion during stage one postoperative phase. With a preoperative stage similar to those for tendon grafting and the two-stage tendon implant, stage one postoperative management of the active tendon follows a regime similar to that of early passive mobilization of a tendon graft with some modifications. While in the long dorsal protective splint with elastic flexion traction, "passive hold" exercises are begun in addition to the active extension-passive flexion with elastic band exercises. At 6 to 8 weeks the dorsal splint is replaced with a wrist band with elastic flexion traction for continued protection. Active exercises are begun at 8 to 10 weeks and at 10 to 11 weeks postoperatively graded resistive exercises may be initiated. As with the passive two-stage implant, the active implant is removed and replaced with a tendon graft at stage two surgery. Since this is a new technique, before embarking on a treatment regime for an active tendon implant, it is recommended that those involved in the rehabilitation process familiarize themselves with the specific protocols outlined by the Hand Rehabilitation Center, Philadelphia, PA.

FLEXOR TENDON REPAIRS

Splinting involved in tendon repairs falls into two categories: splints used in the early passive mobilization techniques for flexor tendon repairs in zones one and two and those used to protect or to enhance motion once active motion of the repair has been initiated.

Traditionally tendon repairs have been immobilized from 3 to 5 weeks before motion is permitted. However, it is been well demonstrated by Mason (1941) that there is little or no tensile strength at a flexor tendon repair site until it is subjected to stress. Kleinert and associates (1975) and Duran (1978) have developed methods for early passive mobilization of repaired flexor tendons in "no-man's-land" that seem to lessen the effect of amplitude-limiting adhesions on the repaired tendon. The method of Kleinert and colleagues is based on use of antagonistic active extension, whereas Duran advocates passive motion at the interphalangeal joints. Both methods require careful adherence to specific splinting and exercise routines, and neither should be undertaken without a thorough understanding of the concepts involved. Although splints developed to be used with these early mobilization techniques differ in configuration, similarities exist. Each requires a posture of wrist flexion to decrease tension on the repair and some method of eliminating active digital flexion and passive digital extension while permitting periods of limited passive excursion of the flexor tendon repair (Fig. 14-30).

When designing a splint for early passive mobilization, one should consider the effect of integrated motion of the flexor tendons, which to some degree limits independent digital action. Because the index finger and the thumb are considered the only truly independent digits, repair of the long, ring, or small flexor tendons necessitates inclusion of all three digits in the splint.

Early passive mobilization concepts may be used for repairs of tendons other than those in zones one and two (Fig. 14-31). Again, it is important that all members of the rehabilitation team be included during the initial planning stages for poor communication or misunderstandings may seriously jeopardize the patient's ability to reach his full rehabilitative potential.

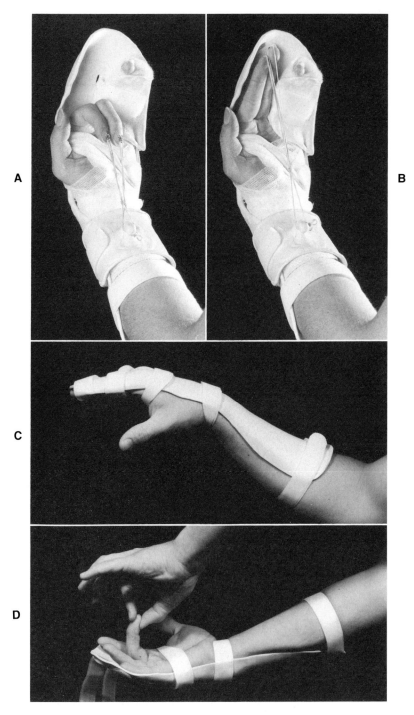

Fig. 14-30. A and **B,** While immobilizing the fourth and fifth digits, this splint permits the Kleinert technique (passive flexion and active extension) of early passive mobilization of flexor tendon repairs to the index and long fingers. **C** and **D,** Passive flexion and extension are used with the Duran technique. (**A** and **B** courtesy Joanne Kassimir, O.T.R., Plainview, NY; photography by Owen Kassimir.)

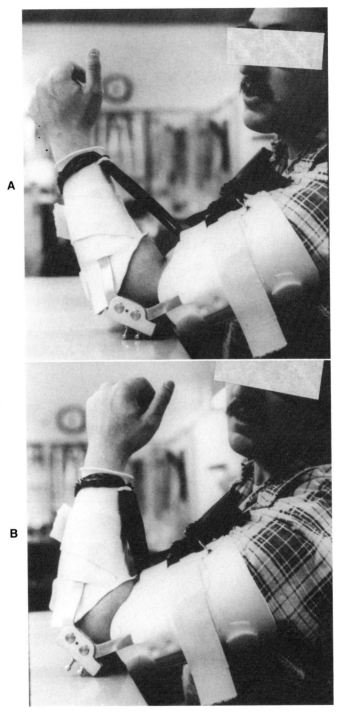

Fig. 14-31. Designed for modified early passive mobilization of a biceps tendon repair, this splint allows active elbow extension **(A)** with passive flexion **(B)** provided by a dynamic assist of Theraband©. The amount of elbow extension is controlled by an adjustable hinge component which may be changed to allow greater motion as healing permits. (Courtesy Linda Tresley, O.T.R./L., and Barbara Sopp, O.T.R./L., Chicago, IL.)

EXTENSOR TENDON REPAIR

Traditionally extensor tendon repairs have been treated by immobilizing the wrist and digital joints in extension. Problems of adhesions between the repair site and the gliding bed are not as limiting to extensor tendons as they are to flexor tendons because of the relatively long fibroosseous canals through which the flexor tendons course. However, with severe extensor injuries in which periosteum, retinaculum, or soft tissues are involved, adhesions can significantly restrict active motion and limit the patient's potential for rehabilitation.

Based on physiologic concepts similar to those used with early mobilization of flexor tendon repairs, Evans and Burkhalter (1986) reported an average total active motion of 210.4 degrees using a method of early mobilization of extensor tendon repairs which they devised. Incorporating the wrist in approximately 45 degrees extension and allowing 5 mm extensor tendon glide, a long finger extension assist/finger flexion block splint (Fig. 14-32) is fitted 2 to 5 days after repair. On a predetermined daily protocol, the patient is instructed to flex the metacarpophalangeal joints until the fingers touch the flexion block portion of the splint, and to allow the wire dynamic assists to passively return the digits to 0 degrees. Prescribed passive interphalangeal joint exercises are done with the wrist and metacarpophalangeal joints in extension to avoid stress to the repair. The authors emphasized the need to calculate extensor tendon excursion in relation to metacarpophalangeal joint motion to obtain the appropriate motion allowed by the splint.

· · ·

Repaired flexor or extensor tendons that have been treated with initial immobilization may require a period of protective splinting to prevent undue accidental stress to the repair site between controlled exercise periods. Flexion of the wrist and digital joints decreases tension on flexor repairs; conversely, extensor repairs are protected with extension positioning (Fig. 14-33). It should be remembered, however, that these positions require greater active excursion of the tendon to effect joint motion, and active exercises done in these splints may be less effective than with reverse positioning to increase tension. The patient should thoroughly understand the exercise and splinting programs before being allowed to proceed with an unsupervised course of self-therapy. As tensile strength increases, the protective positioning is gradually changed and ultimately discarded. If joints that have become stiffened during the period of immobilization do not respond to exercises, mobilization splinting, splinting that does not impart stress to the tendon repair, may be required. Gentle mobilization splinting in a direction that stresses the tendon repair site may be applied concomitant with the initiation of light resistive exercises about 6 to 8 weeks after surgery.

TENDON TRANSFERS

In developing a rehabilitation program for the patient with a partially paralyzed hand who is a candidate for the transference of muscle power, it is imperative that the therapist work closely with the physician to understand the exact deficit and the specific

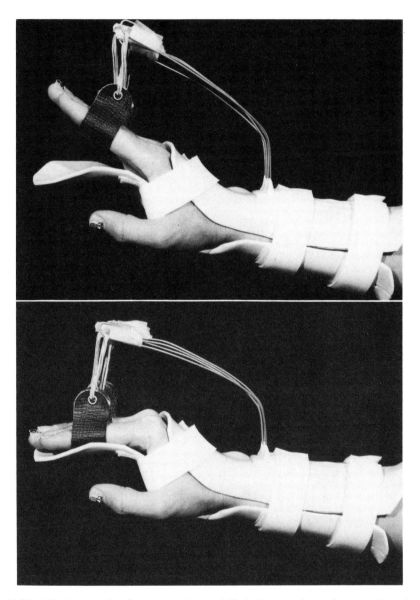

Fig. 14-32. Allowing passive finger extension and limited active finger flexion, this splint was designed for use with early passive mobilization of complex extensor tendon injuries. (Courtesy Roslyn Evans, O.T.R., Vero Beach, FL.)

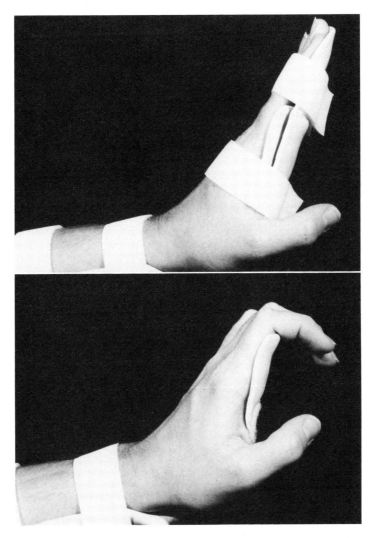

Fig. 14-33. While protecting extensor tendon repairs by positioning the wrist and metacarpopha-langeal joints in extension, the distal portion of this splint can be removed to permit interphalan-geal joint exercises. (Courtesy Roslyn Evans, O.T.R., Vero Beach, FL.)

plans for surgical restoration. Postoperatively it is equally important to gain a thorough appreciation of the transfers used, their course, and realistic functional goals. Without this understanding the patient may be subjected to ineffective and unreasonable exercise and splinting programs that often diminish the benefit of the tendon transfers.

The splinting and exercise program used with tendon transfers is divided into three chronologic subcategories: (1) preoperative phase, (2) early postoperative phase, and (3) late postoperative phase. Each phase is characterized by distinctly different purposes for exercise and splinting.

It is important that exercise programs be implemented at an early stage in the management of the patient who has developed paralysis secondary to the interruption or disease of a major peripheral nerve. When tendon transfers are anticipated, the strengthening of donor muscles is helpful, particularly if testing indicates that weakness has developed secondary to disuse. Predictable patterns of paralysis are seen after median, ulnar, or radial nerve loss, and consultation with the hand surgeon provides valuable information regarding anticipated functional return, potential tendon transfers, and the therapeutic needs of a specific patient.

To obtain maximum benefit from tendon transfer procedures, a hand must be supple. During the preoperative phase, emphasis is placed on attaining and maintaining maximum passive range of motion of wrist and digital joints. If a hand exhibits restricted passive motion, splints must be designed and fitted to correct the specific joint limitations. However, when full passive motion is present and maintenance of this mobility is the indication for splint application, substitution splints may be considered. Manual muscle test data and active range-of-motion measurements govern the designing of a splint used to prevent the development of joint stiffness while allowing improved functional use of the partially paralyzed hand. Splints employed to prevent deformity from occurring in some of the more common types of peripheral upper extremity paralyses are described in the section of this chapter on peripheral nerve injury.

Early postoperative splinting encompasses three facets: (1) protection of the transfer after dressing removal, (2) correction of stiffness secondary to the immobilization necessitated by surgery, and (3) controlled increase of tension on the transferred musculotendinous unit(s).

Splinting may be used to protect tendon transfer during the earliest stages of mobilization. These splints are designed to decrease tension on the transfer and are used before and during exercise periods and at night (Fig. 14-34). They are usually discarded within the first week of mobilization.

Since a period of immobilization is required to promote healing after surgical intervention, adjacent uninvolved joints may become stiff. In some cases splinting is required to regain diminished passive motion. Joints whose stiffness originates from this relatively brief period of immobilization usually respond quickly to splinting efforts and require little more than exercise to maintain motion once it has been regained.

The third reason for employing splinting in the early postoperative phase is to gradually increase the tension on transferred tendons to help lengthen any adhesion that may have formed and to allow for the initiation of mechanically advantageous active motion. Careful control of splint traction techniques during this phase can allow the splinted

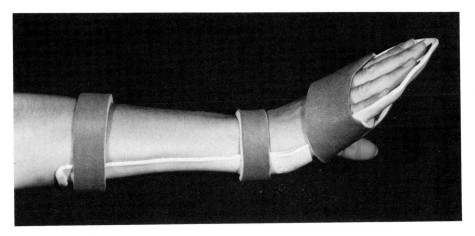

Fig. 14-34. This long wrist and finger immobilization night splint eliminates tension on an extrinsic transfer that runs dorsal to the wrist axis of rotation.

joints to regain the desired range of motion without the unfavorable reverse deformity that sometimes accompanies tight transfers. Since some lengthening may occur as function returns, care must be taken not to place too much tension on a transfer, or muscle imbalance may recur. Timing of this type of splinting may correspond with the initiation of light resistive exercises and activities.

Altering the position of joints crossed by the specific musculotendinous combination of a given transfer permits an increase or decrease in the tension stress on the tendon. Immobilizing the wrist in a direction opposite to the side in which the tendon transfer was routed effectively tightens the transfer and maximizes its function. An example of this tenodesis effect may be seen in the tension imparted to a donor motor tendon that passes volarly to the wrist axis by placing the wrist in extension. Similarly, a posture of wrist flexion would intensify the pull on the dorsally placed extrinsic donor (Fig. 14-35). In cases of tendon transfers designed to function across multiple digital joints, the splint may be extended distally to position consecutive joints in attitudes that will effectively control tension. As the amplitude and tensile strength increase and active motion of the involved joints improves, the use of splints may be gradually eliminated to permit unassisted use of the transfer.

Splinting in the late postoperative phase involves the conversion of learned substitution patterns by gradually eliminating the mechanically advantageous use of wrist tenodesis and requiring greater excursion of the donor musculotendinous unit(s). The wrist may now be gradually positioned in an attitude opposite to that used in the early postoperative phase with active contraction of the motor tendon replacing the tension impaired by the splint. The concept now is to decrease the postural tension on the donor musculotendinous unit and force greater tendon excursion to accomplish segmental motion.

It is important to note that the requirement for splinting during the postoperative phase of tendon transfers may be extremely variable, depending heavily on the specific

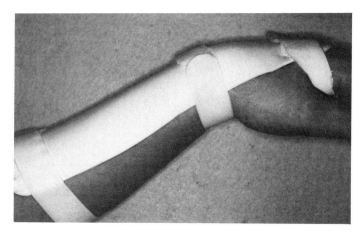

Fig. 14-35. Wrist flexion increases the tension on a dorsally placed extrinsic donor tendon and mechanically facilitates active digital extension.

transfer procedure used, the expertise of the surgeon, and the inherent adaptability of the patient. Many patients require only initial instruction at the time of dressing removal, readily accommodating to the altered kinetic and kinematic effects of the transfer procedure. This is particularly true in patients whose tendon transfers have been synergistic with wrist flexors used for finger extension and wrist extensors for finger flexion. Others, often with "out-of-phase" transfers, require considerable assistance in the form of splinting, exercise, and guidance to attain acceptable tendon transfer performance. Synergy, however, is not considered to be a major factor in choosing a muscle for transfer; the direction of pull of the transfer is far more important.

TENOLYSIS

Tenolysis involves the surgical freeing of adhesions around a tendon to improve tendon gliding and excursion. Active range-of-motion exercises and splinting are usually initiated within 24 hours after surgery.

A tenolysis program employs splinting to achieve and maintain passive motion preoperatively and to maintain passive range of motion postoperatively. Preoperative splints are designed to correct specific joint limitations and may be used at night to sustain passive motion once it has been achieved. The most common types of splints used to augment postoperative motion are of the simple and compound classifications. Alteration of both flexion and extension splints may be required, and, despite the involvement of extrinsic tendons, the need to immobilize the wrist is unusual. However, if the patient consistently assumes a protective wrist posture that is unfavorable to use of maximum tendon amplitude, a long splint that favorably positions the wrist as an adjunctive measure to digital mobilization should be applied. For instance, after flexor tenolysis, if the patient uses an inefficient wrist flexion posture when flexing the digits, a long splint that immobilizes the wrist in extension will encourage flexor tendon excursion.

Because active motion is paramount after a tenolysis procedure, splint wearing times must be interspersed with frequent exercise periods. Depending on individual circumstances, patients are often instructed to exercise 15 minutes of every hour and to alternate splints every 1 to 2 hours during the day. In addition, patients are usually instructed to sleep in the splint which imparts either dynamic or static positioning to correct problem motion.

Often delayed for 6-8 weeks, resistive exercises should be initiated only after consultation with the surgeon. Since tenolysis causes interruption in the blood supply, resistance applied too early may lead to tendon rupture. This is especially true if previous surgical procedures have been done on the tendon. To decrease the chance of rupture, it is important for the surgeon to inform those who are responsible for postoperative management of the condition of the tendon at the time of the tenolysis.

Exercise and splinting programs must be continuously reevaluated and adapted as changes in motion status occur. As active motion improves, the splinting program is gradually curtailed to permit progressively longer durations of unassisted functional hand use. Night splinting is continued until the patient is able to consistently maintain active passive motion through exercise alone.

SUMMARY

From these sections one can see that special problems relating to hand injury and disease and the appropriate surgical management of these conditions present somewhat predictable splinting requirements. Although broad generalization with regard to the splinting of these problems may be offered, it is obvious that wide variations occur in the clinical presentation of each problem and its therapeutic approach. Armed with an appreciation of the potential peculiarities of each of these general categories, one may become familiar with the individual circumstances and subsequently initiate the most applicable splinting and exercise program.

PART FIVE

Application

CHAPTER 15

Analysis of splints

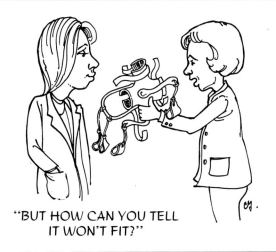

"BUT HOW CAN YOU TELL
IT WON'T FIT?"

Generally speaking, most of the mistakes made in hand splinting are caused by inattention to detail. The types of splints chosen are correct according to the circumstances presented. However, they fail to be effective because of relatively minor design or adjustment flaws that cause discomfort, mechanical inefficiency, or poor appearance. Each splint fitted on a patient must be thoroughly evaluated according to the principles of design, construction, fit, mechanics, immobilization/mobilization and dynamic assists concepts, and kinesiologic impact. Failure to do so may not only produce poor results but may compound or cause additional deformity.

The purpose of this chapter is to provide the reader with an opportunity to apply the theoretical material presented in the previous chapters and to allow for immediate independent assessment through self-evaluation techniques. Although there is no substitute for actual practical learning, it is hoped that this chapter will initiate, facilitate, and strengthen sound analytical thinking in regard to splint design and fabrication.

On the following pages illustrations of improperly constructed splints are presented and analyzed according to classification, purpose of application, clinical problems, and solutions to the problems. The splints, although generally constructed correctly, incorporate one or more common mistakes that clinically produce diminished results. The reader is asked to assess these illustrations using the information in the preceding chapters of this book as a theoretical framework. Comparison of one's results with those presented here will provide a standard for self-evaluation.

So that the reader may more easily adapt this chapter to a personal level of expertise, the format of splint illustrations and their accompanying assessments is presented consistently (Fig. 15-1). Selected sections may be blocked out to reduce the amount of background information given about each splint illustrated (Figs. 15-2 to 15-19), making analysis more or less difficult. For example, the novice may choose not to block any of the sections, allowing open comparison of the classification, purposes, problems, and solutions of each example, whereas someone with intermediate experience may identify the blocked-out problems and solutions knowing only the classification and purpose of application of the splints. Finally, the blocking of all four sections and the "incorrect/correct" drawings requires the reader to independently identify the classification, purposes, problems, and solutions of each splint picture. Use of the splint checkout form (Appendix C) may be helpful in providing an organizational basis for splint analysis. For immediate feedback, we recommend that readers compare their conclusions with those accompanying each illustration before proceeding to the next splint picture. Red indicates areas of changes in the correct drawings.

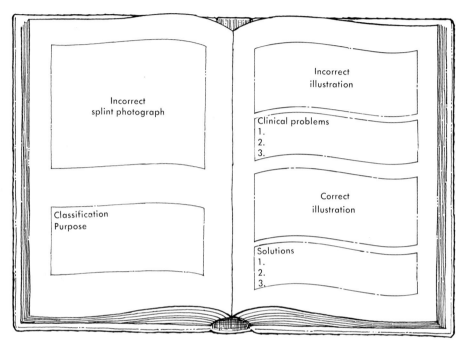

Fig. 15-1. Each splint analysis unit is presented in a consistent order: incorrect splint photograph, classification and purpose, incorrect drawing, clinical problems, corrected drawing, and solutions to clinical problems.

Fig. 15-2

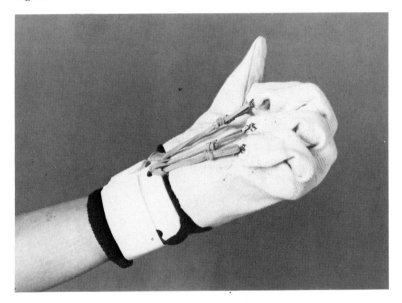

Classification
Simple finger flexion splint
Purpose
To flex the metacarpophalangeal and interphalangeal joints of the fingers.

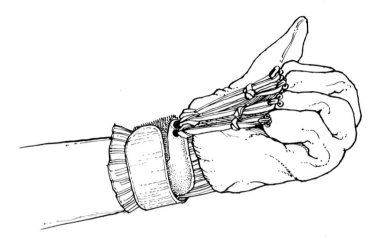

Clinical problems
1. The traction does not adequately affect the stiffer metacarpophalangeal joints.
2. The glove decreases sensory feedback, is bulky and hot, and retains moisture and dirt.

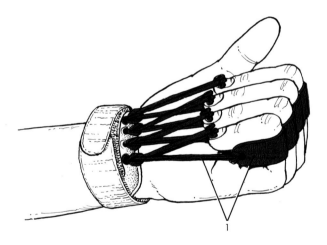

Solutions
1. Add dynamic traction to individual joints such as finger cuff for metacarpophalangeal flexion, fingernail clip for proximal interphalangeal flexion, or glove rubber band for distal interphalangeal flexion.
2. A wrist cock-up with volar outrigger may be necessary to provide a 90-degree angle of pull of the traction device (see Fig. 15-14, solutions).

Fig. 15-3

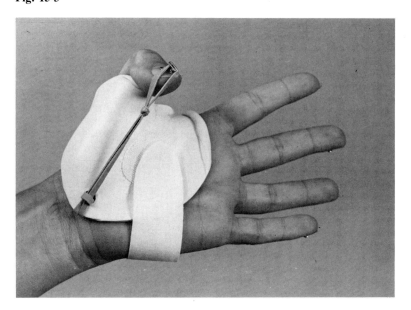

Classification
Compound thumb IP flexion splint
Purposes
1. To flex the interphalangeal joint of the thumb.
2. To maintain the thumb web space.
3. To immobilize the metacarpophalangeal joint.

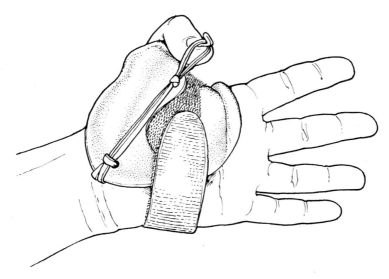

Clinical problems

1. Because the angle of the dynamic traction is not perpendicular to the axis of rotation of the interphalangeal joint, unequal stress is applied to the collateral ligaments and may result in ulnar collateral ligament attenuation.
2. The distal end of the splint inhibits index and long metacarpophalangeal flexion.

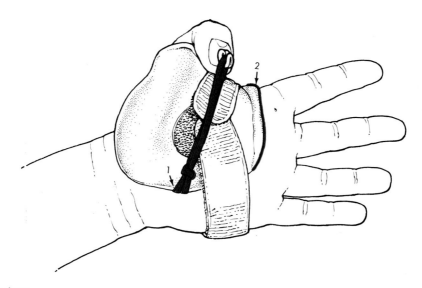

Solutions

1. Adjust the elastic traction to provide a perpendicular angle of approach to the interphalangeal joint axis of rotation.
2. Roll the distal edge of the splint proximally. It should not extend beyond the distal palmar flexion crease.

Fig. 15-4

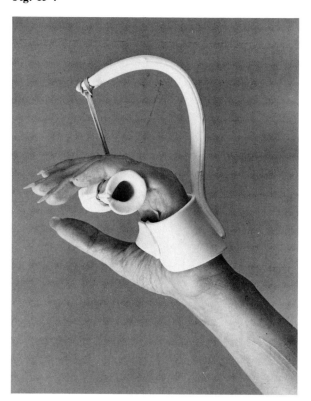

Classification
Simple MP extension splint
Purpose
To extend the metacarpophalangeal joints.

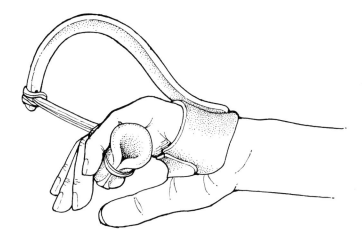

Clinical problems
1. The distal aspect of the dorsal metacarpal bar is causing pressure on dorsum of hand.
2. Flexion of ring and small proximal interphalangeal joints is limited by palmar phalangeal bar.
3. The transverse arch is not supported at the phalangeal level.
4. Second to fifth metacarpophalangeal joints are mobilized in unison.
5. The 60-degree angle of elastic traction to proximal phalanges causes the palmar phalangeal bar to slip distally.

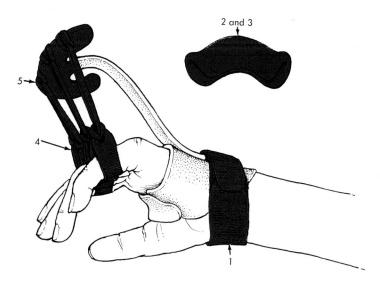

Solutions
1. Add a wrist strap to the proximal aspect of the dorsal metacarpal bar.
2. Adjust the phalangeal bar to allow for differences in the lengths of the digital rays.
3. Adjust the phalangeal bar to support the transverse arch at the proximal phalangeal level.
4. Add individual metacarpophalangeal extension finger cuffs.
5. Design and adjust the extension outrigger to provide a 90-degree pull of the elastic traction to proximal phalanges that also provides a perpendicular force to the flexion/extension axis of motion of each joint. (NOTE: Use either 2 and 3; or 4.)
6. Wrist may need to be included in some cases.

Fig. 15-5

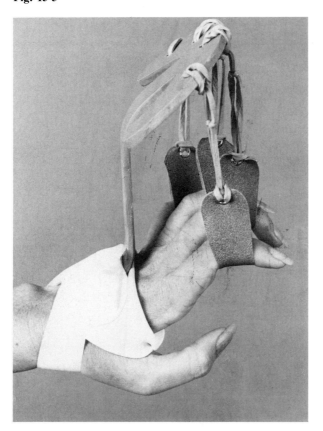

Classification
Simple finger extension splint
Purpose
To extend the proximal interphalangeal joints.

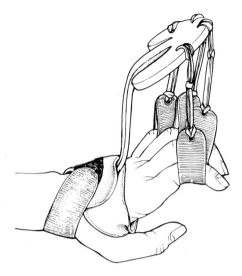

Clinical problems

1. The more mobile metacarpophalangeal joints are hyperextended.
2. The angle of elastic traction to the proximal phalanges enhances metacarpophalangeal joint hyperextension.
3. The finger cuffs prevent full interphalangeal joint flexion.
4. The uncovered Velcro hook fastener is abrasive to clothing.

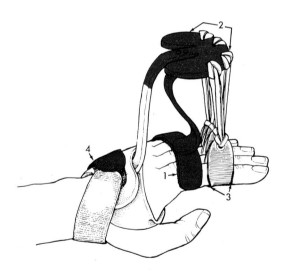

Solutions

1. Add a dorsal phalangeal bar to prevent metacarpophalangeal hypertension. NOTE: Classification changes to compound PIP extension splint.
2. Adjust outrigger to provide a 90-degree angle of the elastic traction to middle phalanges.
3. Trim the proximal and distal edges of the finger cuffs to interphalangeal joint flexion.
4. Lengthen the wrist strap to provide full closure.
5. Wrist may need to be immobilized in some instances.

Fig. 15-6

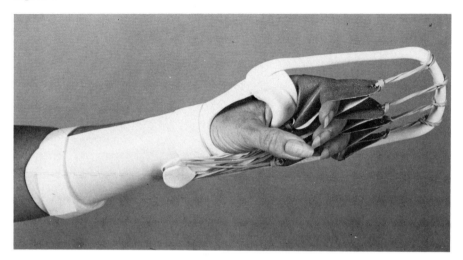

Classification
Long MP flexion/PIP extension splint
Purposes
1. To flex the metacarpophalangeal joints.
2. To extend the proximal interphalangeal joints.
3. To immobilize the wrist joint.

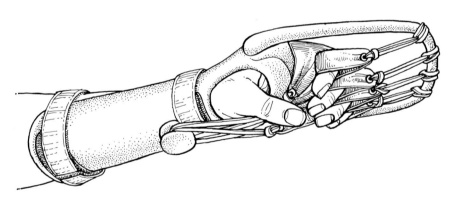

Clinical problems
1. The antagonistic elastic traction on consecutive joints results in diminished flexion and extension forces.
2. The distal end of the splint inhibits flexion of the metacarpophalangeal joints.
3. The acute angle of approach of elastic flexion traction to the proximal phalanges results in metacarpophalangeal joint compression.
4. The angle of elastic extension traction to the middle phalanges results in diminished rotational force and may cause metacarpophalangeal hyperextension.
5. The finger cuffs inhibit interphalangeal joint flexion.
6. The ends of the straps have sharp corners.

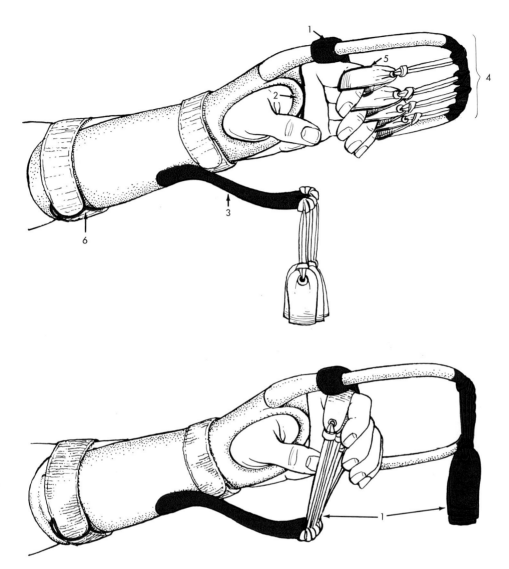

Solutions

1. If the metacarpophalangeal joints exhibit full flexion, add an immobile dorsal phalangeal bar to stabilize the proximal phalanges and to prevent hyperextension. If the metacarpophalangeal joints lack flexion, separate wearing times for metacarpophalangeal flexion and proximal interphalangeal extension, and add a dorsal phalangeal bar to prevent metacarpophalangeal hyperextension while in the extension cuffs.
2. Adjust the distal end of the splint to be proximal to the distal palmar flexion crease.
3. Add a palmar outrigger to provide a 90-degree angle of approach of the elastic traction to the proximal phalanges.
4. Adjust the outrigger to provide a 90-degree angle of approach of the elastic traction to the middle phalanges.
5. Contour the extension finger cuffs.
6. Round the ends of the straps.

Fig. 15-7

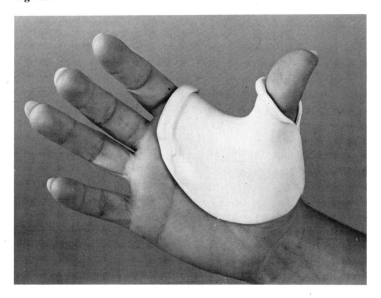

Classification
Simple thumb CMC extension/abduction splint
Purpose
To increase or maintain the thumb web space.

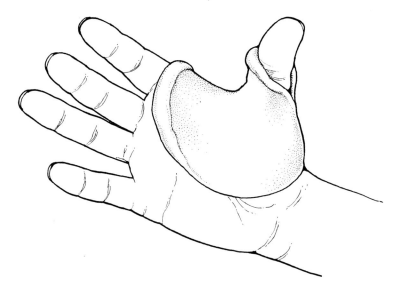

Clinical problems

1. Flexion of the index and long metacarpophalangeal joint is inhibited by the distal end of the splint.
2. Thumb interphalangeal flexion is limited by the distal end of the thumb post.
3. Distal migration of the splint results in application of the rotational force to the proximal phalanx of the thumb with potential stretching of the metacarpophalangeal ulnar colateral ligament.
4. Pressure at wrist.
5. Pressure in palm.

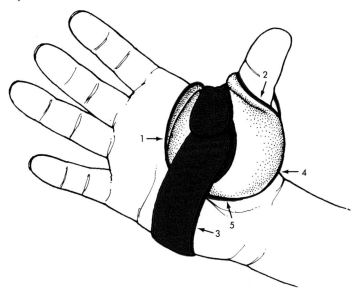

Solutions

1. Adjust the distal edge of the splint to end proximal to the distal palmar flexion crease.
2. Adjust the distal edge of the thumb post to the end proximal to the flexion crease of the thumb interphalangeal joint.
3. Add a strap for stabilization of the splint in the web space.
4. Roll back proximal edge of splint to prevent pressure at the wrist.
5. Trim ulnar border.

Fig. 15-8

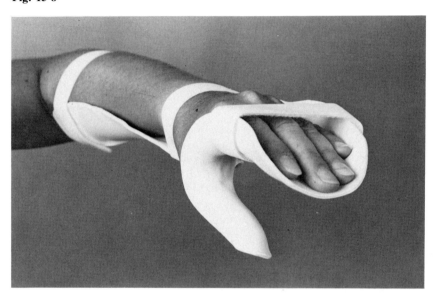

Classification
Long finger and thumb immobilization splint
Purposes
1. To immobilize the finger metacarpophalangeal and interphalangeal joints in slight flexion.
2. To immobilize the thumb in abduction.
3. To maintain the thumb web space.
4. To immobilize the wrist joint in slight extension.

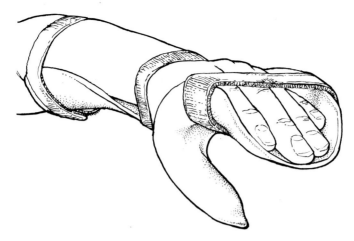

Clinical problems

1. Elbow flexion is limited by the proximal end of the splint.
2. The transverse arch is not supported at the phalangeal level.
3. The high deviation bars of the finger pan prevent finger positioning by the distal strap.
4. The distal end of the thumb post is too long.

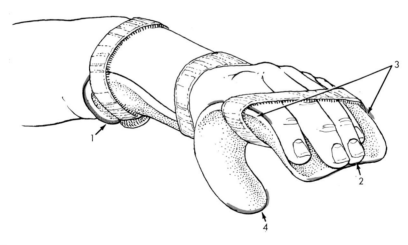

Solutions

1. Shorten the forearm trough to two thirds of "inside elbow" length and flange the proximal end.
2. Continue the transverse arch the length of the finger pan.
3. Decrease the lateral and medial borders to provide continuous contact of the strap across the dorsal aspect of the fingers.
4. Decrease the distal length of the thumb post.

Fig. 15-9

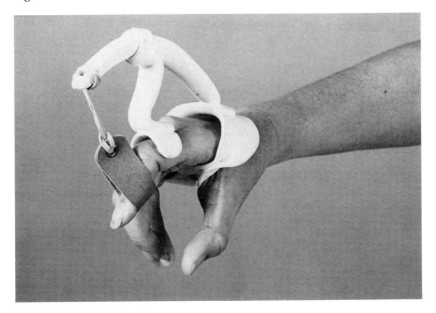

Classification
Compound PIP extension splint
Purpose
To extend the index proximal interphalangeal joint.

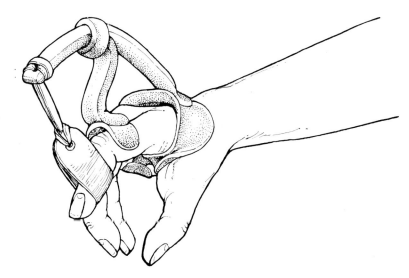

Clinical problems

1. The dorsal and palmar metacarpal bars are loose and allow the splint to rotate.
2. The proximal edge of the dorsal phalangeal bar creates pressure on the dorsum of the proximal phalanx.
3. The angle of the elastic traction to the middle phalanx diminishes the magnitude of the rotational force and compresses the proximal interphalangeal joint surfaces.
4. The finger cuff inhibits interphalangeal joint flexion.

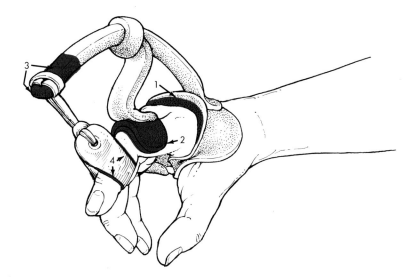

Solutions

1. Adjust the dorsal and palmar metacarpal bars to provide continuous circumferential contact.
2. Adjust the dorsal phalangeal bar to provide equal pressure on the dorsum of the phalanx. To further disseminate pressure, add foam padding to the palmar aspect of the dorsal phalangeal bar.
3. Adjust the outrigger to provide a 90-degree angle of elastic traction to the middle phalanx. This traction should also be perpendicular to the axis of the joint rotation.
4. Trim the proximal and distal edges of the finger cuff.

Fig. 15-10

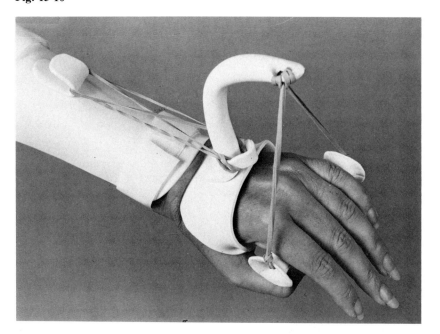

Classification
Simple wrist and MP extension splint
Purposes
1. To increase passive wrist extension.
2. To extend the metacarpophalangeal joints.

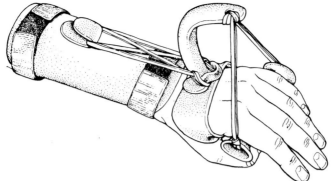

Clinical problems

1. Distal migration of the forearm trough causes pressure on the dorsum of the wrist and on the ulnar styloid process.
2. The 20-degree angle of elastic wrist traction to the metacarpals creates joint compression at the carpal level.
3. The ring and small proximal interphalangeal joint flexion is limited by the palmar phalangeal bar.
4. The transverse arch is not supported at the phalangeal level.
5. The metacarpophalangeal joints are mobilized in unison.
6. The angle of approach of elastic traction to the proximal phalanges results in decreased magnitude of the rotational force.
7. The Velcro hook is abrasive to clothing, and the strap corners are sharp.

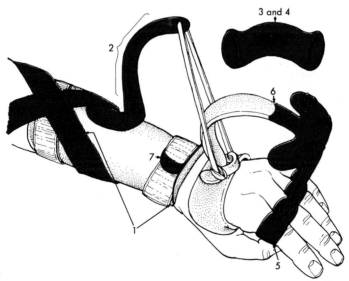

Solutions

1. Flange the distal edge of the forearm trough, and add an elbow strap or cuff.
2. Add a dorsal outrigger to provide a 90-degree pull of the elastic traction to metacarpals.
3. Adjust the phalangeal bar to allow for differences in longitudinal lengths of digital rays.
4. Revise the phalangeal bar to support the transverse arch at the proximal phalangeal level.
5. Add individual metacarpophalangeal extension finger cuffs.
6. Adjust the outrigger to provide a 90-degree angle of the elastic traction to the proximal phalanges. The traction devices should also be perpendicular to the sagittal axis of rotation of each metacarpophalangeal joint.
7. Round the strap corners, and lengthen the straps to complete closure.
   (NOTE: Use either 3 and 4; or 5.)

Fig. 15-11

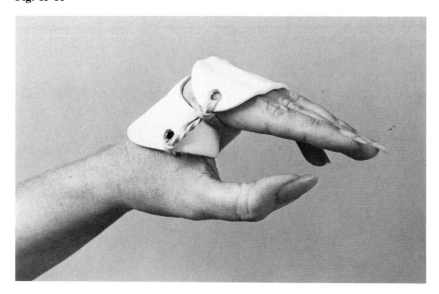

Classification
Simple MP flexion splint
Purpose
To flex the metacarpophalangeal joints.

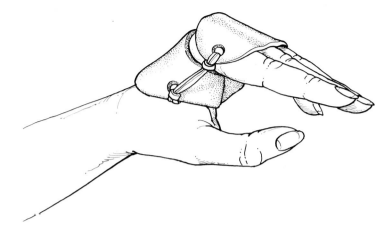

Clinical problems

1. Pressure exists in the thumb web space from the palmar metacarpal bar.
2. The dorsal phalangeal bar migrates proximally.
3. The metacarpal bars migrate distally.
4. The acute angle of approach of elastic traction to the proximal phalanges results in diminished rotational force on the metacarpophalangeal joints.
5. The metacarpophalangeal joints are mobilized in unison.

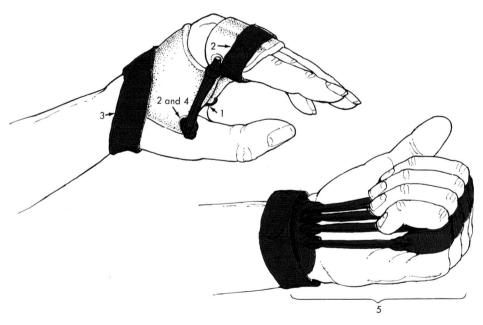

Solutions

1. Flange the proximal aspect of the palmar metacarpal bar edge.
2. Correct the angle of rotational traction to a perpendicular pull, and add a phalangeal strap.
3. Add a wrist strap.
4. Design the splint to provide a 90-degree angle of the elastic traction to proximal phalanges, which is also perpendicular to the axis of sagittal rotation.
5. Use either a wristband with metacarpophalangeal flexion cuffs or a simple wrist immobilization splint with volar outrigger (Fig. 15-14) instead of the splint illustrated.

Fig. 15-12

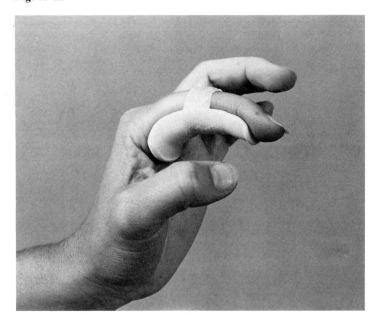

Classification
Simple PIP flexion block splint
Purpose
To prevent index proximal interphalangeal joint flexion beyond 30 degrees.

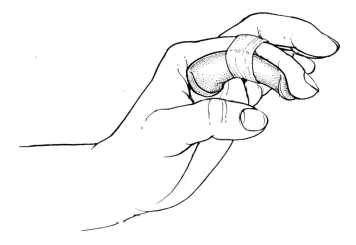

Clinical problems
1. The distal end of the splint limits distal interphalangeal joint flexion.
2. The splint is unstable on the finger.

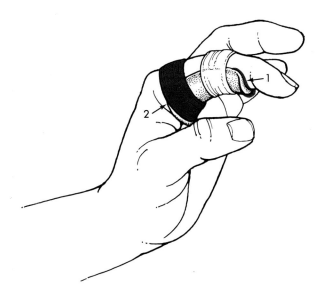

Solutions
1. Shorten the distal splint edge to end proximal to the distal interphalangeal joint flexion crease.
2. Add proximal strap.

Fig. 15-13

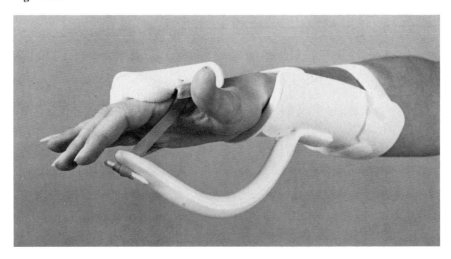

Classification
Simple wrist flexion splint
Purpose
To increase passive wrist flexion.

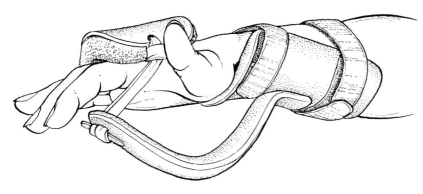

Clinical problems

1. The distal aspect of the forearm trough is too wide.
2. The lateral and medial borders of the dorsal metacarpal cuff may cause pressure areas on the dorsum of the hand.
3. The dorsal metacarpal cuff migrates distally.
4. The angle of approach of the elastic traction to the metacarpals diminishes the magnitude of the rotational force.
5. Pressure exists under the proximal strap.

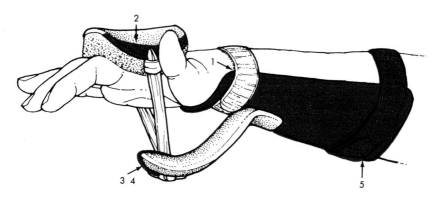

Solutions

1. Decrease the radial border to half the width of the forearm.
2. Widen the dorsal metacarpal cuff.
3. and 4. Adjust the outrigger to provide a 90-degree angle of the elastic traction to the metacarpals.
5. Lengthen the forearm trough and move the strap proximally.

Fig. 15-14

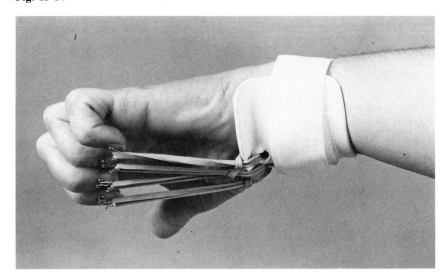

Classification
Simple finger flexion splint
Purpose
To flex the metacarpophalangeal joints.

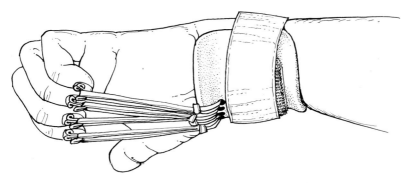

Clinical problem

Because of the difference in the mobility of the metacarpophalangeal and interphalangeal joints, the magnitude of the traction is dissipated at the level of the normal interphalangeal joints.

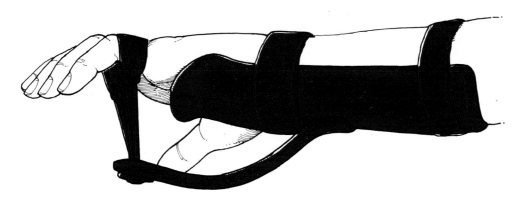

Solution

Change the design of the splint to a volar wrist immobilization splint with an outrigger with individual metacarpophalangeal flexion cuffs. NOTE: Classification changes to long MP flexion splint.

Fig. 15-15

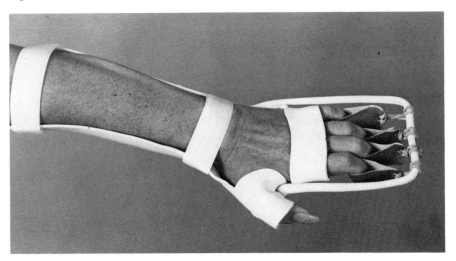

Classification

Long compound PIP extension splint with thumb CMC and MP immobilization

Purposes

1. To extend the proximal interphalangeal joints.
2. To immobilize the thumb carpometacarpal and metacarpophalangeal joints.
3. To immobilize the wrist joint.
4. To prevent hyperextension of 2-5 metacarpophalangeal joints.

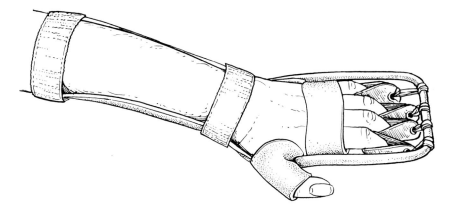

Clinical problems

1. The ulnar aspect of the forearm trough is causing pressure on the ulnar border of the forearm.
2. Thumb interphalangeal flexion is limited by the distal edge of the thumb post.
3. The finger metacarpophalangeal joints are hyperextended.
4. The angle of approach of elastic traction to the middle phalanges causes the finger cuffs to migrate distally.
5. The outrigger is too short to allow satisfactory application of the elastic traction.
6. The radial aspect of the wrist bar is not fitted closely.

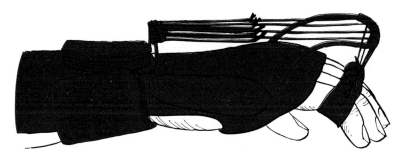

Solution

Change the design of the splint to a dorsal based low profile PIP extension splint with dorsal phalangeal bar and with thumb CMC abduction/MP extension.

Fig. 15-16

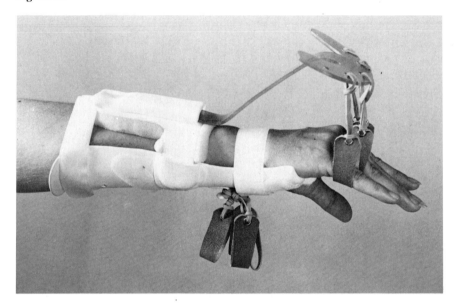

Classification
Long MP extension/flexion splint
Purposes
1. To extend the metacarpophalangeal joints.
2. To flex the metacarpophalangeal joints.
3. To immobilize the wrist.

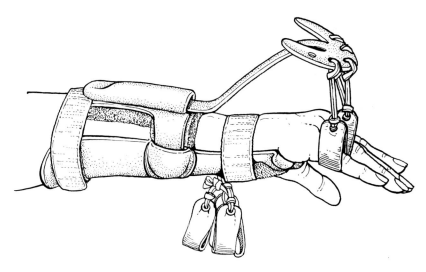

Clinical problems

1. The wrist is not fully immobilized.
2. The outrigger does not provide a rigid basis of attachment for the traction devices.
3. The angle of approach of the elastic traction to the proximal phalanges causes the finger cuffs to cut into the finger webs and decrease the magnitude of the rotational force.
4. It is possible that the angle of pull of the flexion elastic traction to proximal phalanges is incorrect.

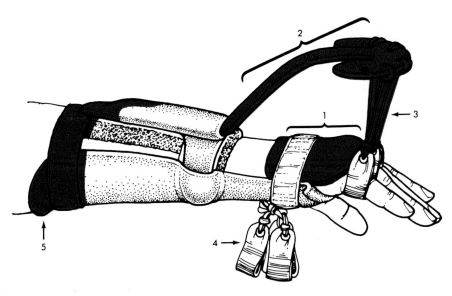

Solutions

1. Add a dorsometacarpal strap or cuff to prevent wrist extension.
2. Construct the outrigger from a stronger material.
3. Adjust the outrigger to provide a 90-degree angle of approach of elastic traction to the proximal phalanges.
4. If the angle of the flexion traction is incorrect, add a volar outrigger, and adjust to allow a 90-degree angle of the dynamic assists to the proximal phalanges.
5. Lengthen the splint proximally.

Fig. 15-17

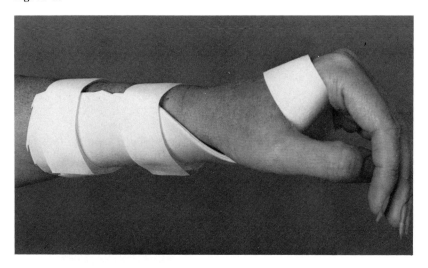

Classification
Simple wrist immobilization splint
Purpose
To immobilize the wrist.

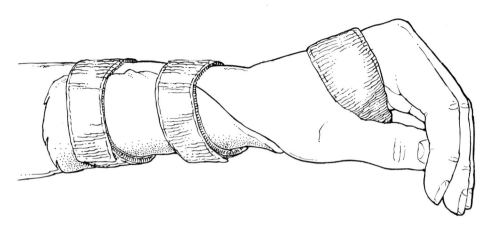

Clinical problems

1. The proximal edge of the splint causes pressure on the forearm.
2. The wrist is not fully immobilized.
3. The strap in the thumb web space causes discomfort.
4. The appearance of the splint is poor.

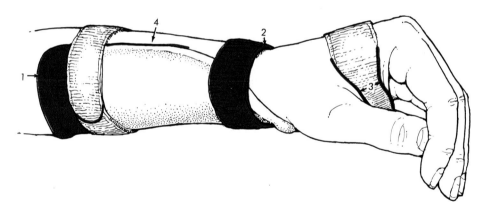

Solutions

1. Increase the length of forearm trough to two thirds the length of the forearm, and flange the proximal end.
2. Position the wrist strap distal to the ulnar styloid process.
3. Contour the distal edge of the strap in the thumb web space.
4. Cut splint edges smoothly, and round the strap ends.

Fig. 15-18

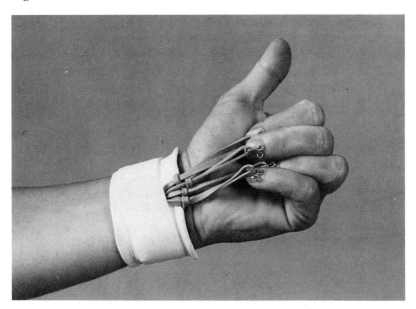

Classification
Simple finger flexion splint
Purpose
To flex the fingers.

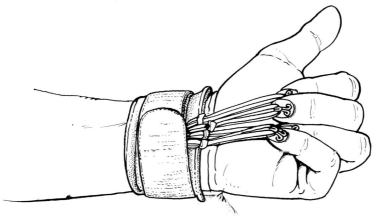

Clinical problem
The single hole causes fingers to "bunch" when flexed simultaneously.

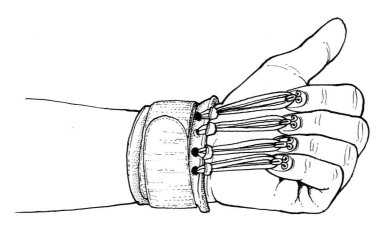

Solutions
1. Design the splint to allow the dynamic traction to arise from three or four separate, slightly radial holes.
2. May need to immobilize the wrist in certain instances.

Fig. 15-19

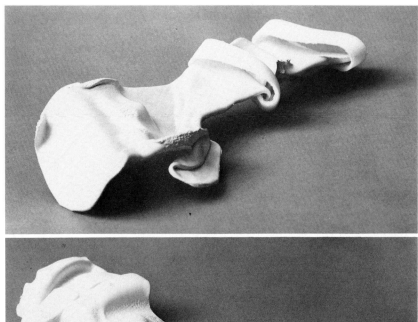

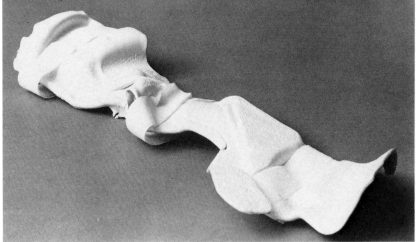

Classification
Long finger/thumb immobilization splint
Purposes
1. To immobilize the finger metacarpophalangeal and interphalangeal joints in slight flexion.
2. To immobilize the thumb in abduction.
3. To maintain the thumb web space.
4. To immobilize the wrist joint in slight extension.

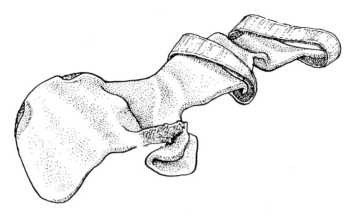

Clinical problem
The splint was left in a closed car on a hot day, which resulted in numerous fit problems.

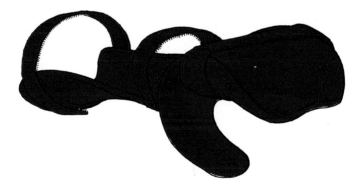

Solution
Start over.

PART SIX

Technique

CHAPTER 16

Patterns

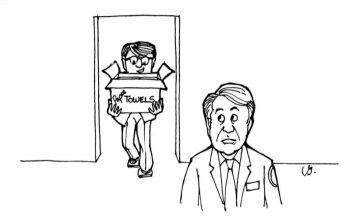

"HEY, ISN'T THIS THE EXPENSIVE PATTERN
MATERIAL YOU ORDERED LAST WEEK?"

The transition from the cognitive design process to the actual construction of tangible splint patterns is facilitated by the progression through the hierarchy of design principles. Once the design process has been traversed, the construction of a workable pattern becomes simplified. Assembly and connection of the various splint parts may then be carried out until the ultimate configuration of the splint becomes apparent. This allows alterations of shape and size to be governed by individual specifications of the extremity being splinted before actual fabrication of splint materials has commenced.

In the pattern stage, simple splints with uncomplicated objectives allow for rather routine application of design principles, whereas in the presence of unusually difficult problems a more innovative approach is required. Nevertheless, a progression through the design principles facilitates a more efficient, organized thought process from which practical variations may be made.

The rigid use of standard, commercially available patterns is not recommended because it may result in the preparation of a splint without the appropriate adaptation necessary to accommodate individual anatomic variations. With experience comes the knowledge of where and how to incorporate changes in these dye patterns, and the potential hazards are diminished considerably (Fig. 16-1). All patterns, whether individually constructed or adapted from a commercial design, should be fitted and checked on the patient before construction of the splint begins, since a poorly conceived or fitted pattern almost always leads to frustration and failure during the subsequent stages of construction, fit and use.

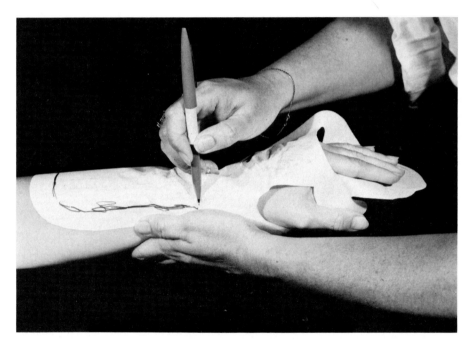

Fig. 16-1. A commercial pattern must be adapted to the variations of the individual hand before it is used.

SPLINT PATTERN FABRICATION

The fabrication of splint patterns is defined according to the construction methods employed: (1) the combining of individual splint parts, (2) the outlining of the total splint configuration, or (3) the taking of specific measurements to form a general pattern shape.

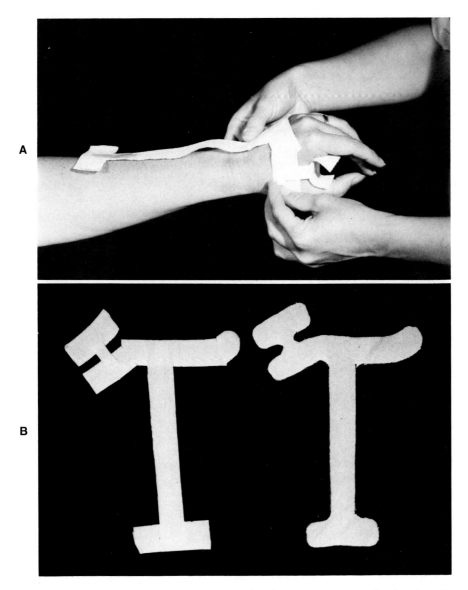

Fig. 16-2. A, A component pattern allows piece-by-piece pattern construction based on the specific requirements of the hand being splinted. **B,** Once the basic form is established, the outside configuration of the pattern is smoothed and refined.

All patterns, like the splints they represent, consist of individual parts that, when combined, form a whole. For the beginner or for the experienced individual attempting to translate a difficult splint design into pattern form, taping and combining cut-out paper splint parts on the patient's extremity may ease pattern construction (Fig. 16-2). An alternative technique of pattern fabrication, the drawing of an outline of a splint, is more efficient when dealing with familiar, uncomplicated splint designs. The uncut pattern material is first applied to the extremity, and the configuration of the proposed splint outlined according to anatomic landmarks and mechanical considerations (Fig. 16-3). These two methods of pattern construction may be effectively combined to blend the efficiency of the outline method with the specificity of the parts technique (Fig. 16-4). The third method of pattern construction is appropriate only when a stretchable splinting material is to be used. This less exacting technique of pattern preparation results in a pattern that bears little resemblance to the finished splint. Length and width measurements are frequently the only requirements for this type of pattern construction because the splint material is stretched, molded, and trimmed during the fitting phase of fabrication (Fig. 16-5).

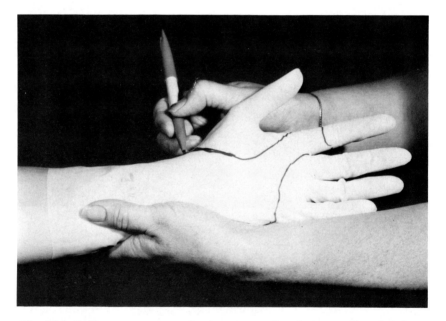

Fig. 16-3. Outline pattern construction is more expedient for uncomplicated designs.

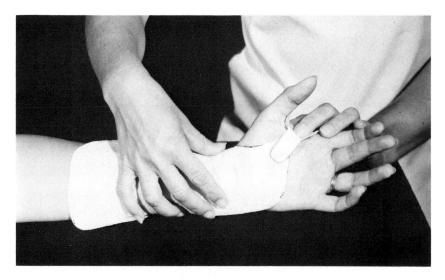

Fig. 16-4. Individual components may be added to a basic outline pattern.

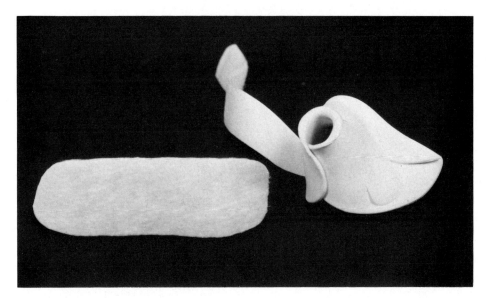

Fig. 16-5. A, As seen in this simple CMC immobilization pattern design by Kay Carl, O.T.R., Indianapolis, measurement patterns often bear little resemblance to the final splint configuration.

Continued.

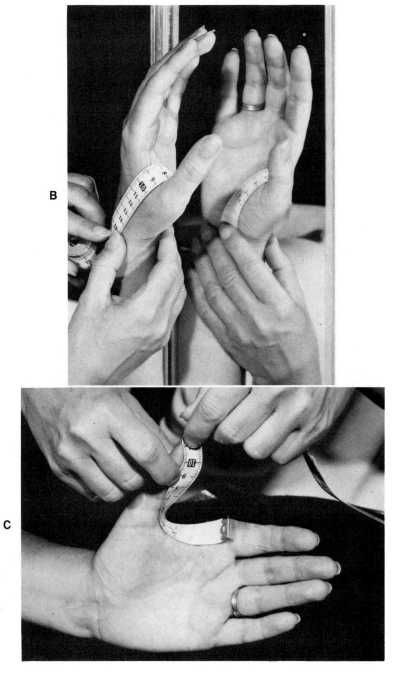

Fig. 16-5, cont'd. B, The length between dorsal and volar wrist flexion creases through the first web space is the pattern length. **C,** The length from the index proximal interphalangeal joint to the thumb interphalangeal joint equals the width.

PATTERN MATERIALS AND EQUIPMENT

Although pattern materials are of seemingly infinite variety, they possess some common properties. They should be readily available, inexpensive, flexible, clean, and allow for marking, taping, and cutting. Examples are paper towels, typing paper, cloth, light cardboard, cellophane, plastic wrap, clear plastic bags, and surgical gloves. The choice of pattern material may be influenced by the splint design, pathologic condition of the extremity, material accessibility, or environmental factors. A pattern for a splint requiring contour would be difficult to make from light cardboard because of its mildly rigid properties, whereas a bar type of splint pattern out of plastic wrap would be flimsy and could allow alteration of the splint form during transfer to the final splint material. Paper towels are available in most medical offices and therapy departments and are flexible enough to allow contouring. Cellophane, plastic bags, and plastic wrap provide the unique property of transparency, giving full visibility to underlying anatomic structures, and a surgical glove allows three-dimensional perspective. The paper towels that are provided with sterile surgical gloves also make excellent pattern materials when working in isolation conditions.

Positioning devices (Fig. 16-6) have been advocated in some circumstances when making a single plane pattern proves to be difficult. These devices allow the various segments of the extremity to be placed in the desired position, theoretically making tracings more accurate. In our experience, however, the final configurations of patterns made with and without a positioning device are similar enough that the addition of the extraneous piece of equipment is usually unwarranted (Fig. 16-7).

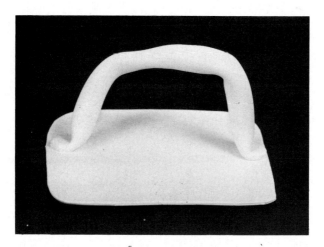

Fig. 16-6. A positioning device may be used to support a paralyzed hand during pattern construction.

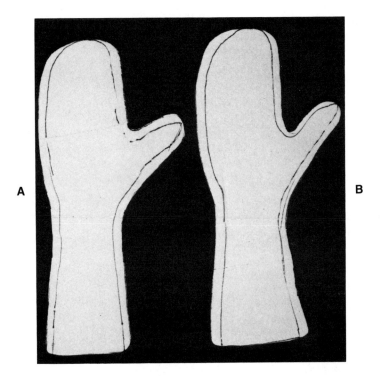

Fig. 16-7. Long finger/thumb immobilization splint pattern made with (**A**) and without (**B**) a positioning device.

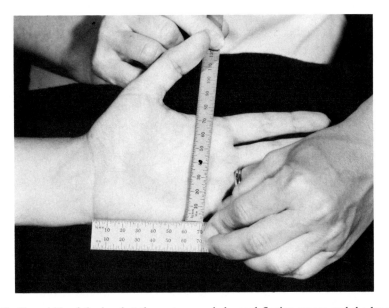

Fig. 16-8. The width of the hand at the metacarpophalangeal flexion crease and the length from the wrist flexion crease to the metacarpophalangeal flexion crease on the ulnar aspect of the palm are the two most important measurements to take when attempting to locate a similar-sized hand for pattern construction.

If it appears that the amount of hand movement required to construct a pattern will be poorly tolerated by the patient, a pattern may be traced from the opposite, unaffected hand, allowing for individual variations such as edema or amputation. This pattern should then be reversed and checked for fit on the injured extremity. If the pathologic condition disallows pattern construction on either extremity, longitudinal and horizontal measurements may be taken (Fig. 16-8), and a hand of similar size located on which a pattern may be made.

SPECIFIC PATTERNS

Although exceptions exist, patterns are generally employed when constructing those major sections of a splint which directly contact the extremity. These constituent elements may function independently or they may form the foundation for attachment of other splint components. With experience hand specialists develop individualized methods of constructing patterns and preferences for certain pattern materials. While no two specialists may make patterns exactly alike and designs for hand splints are seemingly endless, the process of constructing patterns depends on a thorough knowledge of anatomy, an understanding of the principles of mechanics, design, and fit, and familiarity with the physical properties of available splinting materials.

Many patterns for hand splints are derived from one of three basic configurations consisting of specialized components which provide transverse or longitudinal positioning: (1) metacarpal shell, (2) dorsal metacarpal/wrist/forearm shell, and (3) volar metacarpal/wrist/forearm shell. Although inclusion of all the potential variations is impractical, descriptions of these three basic patterns and some of their more common adaptations are briefly outlined and illustrated in this chapter. It is important to remember that although these patterns reflect basic configurations, they must be specifically adapted to individual patients before being used in the clinic setting. Rote application without consideration of the variations in patient anatomy and pathology would be shortsighted and is definitely contraindicated.

BASIC PATTERNS
Metacarpal shell

PURPOSES (Fig. 16-9, *A* and *B*)
1. Supports the transverse metacarpal arch via dorsal and palmar metacarpal bars and hypothenar bar.
2. Provides a base of attachment for finger or thumb phalangeal bars and for outrigger components.

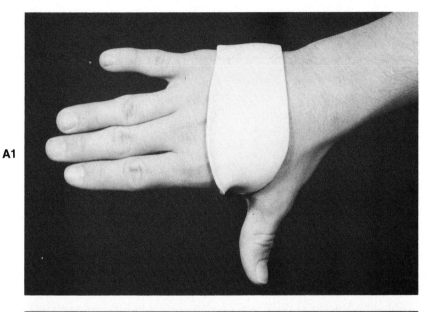

A1

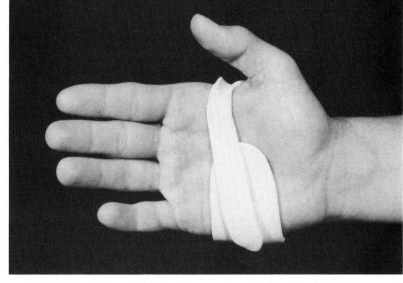

A2

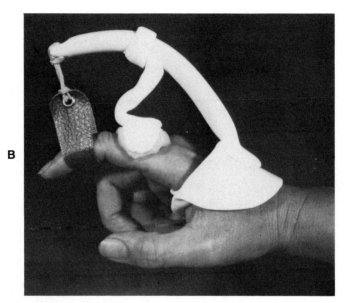

B

Example of completed splint.

ANATOMIC LANDMARKS

1. Dorsal (Fig. 16-9, *C*)
   a. 2-4 metacarpophalangeal joints
   b. First web space
   c. Extensor pollicis longus tendon
   d. Distal wrist extension crease

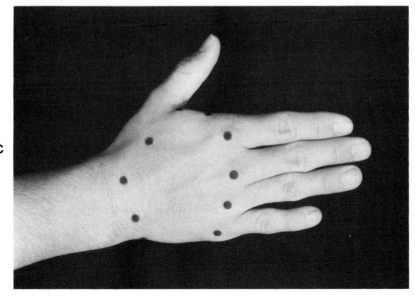

C

BASIC PATTERNS—cont'd
Metacarpal shell—cont'd

ANATOMIC LANDMARKS—cont'd
2. Palmar (Fig. 16-9, *D*)
   a. Distal palmar flexion crease
   b. Opponens crease
   c. Distal ulnar wrist flexion crease

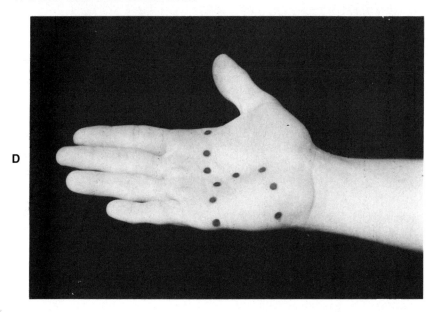

COMPLETED PATTERN (Fig. 16-9, *E*)

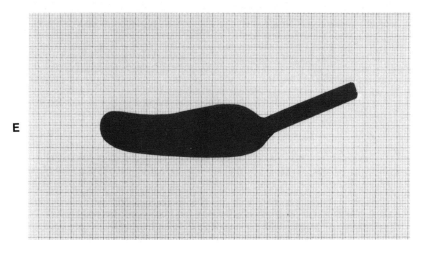

Dorsal metacarpal/wrist/forearm shell

PURPOSES (Fig. 16-10, *A* and *B*)
1. Supports the transverse metacarpal arch via dorsal and palmar metacarpal bars.
2. Positions the wrist.
3. Provides a base of attachment for finger or thumb phalangeal bars and for outrigger components.

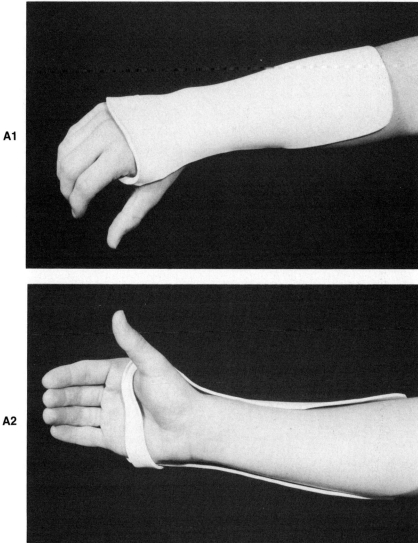

A1

A2

BASIC PATTERNS—cont'd
Dorsal metacarpal/wrist/forearm shell—cont'd

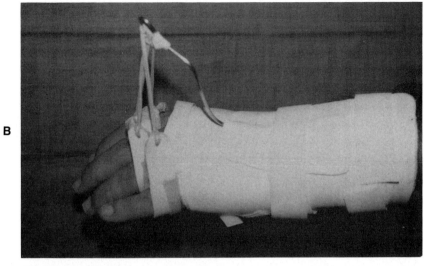

B

Example of completed splint.

ANATOMIC LANDMARKS
1. Palmar (Fig. 16-10, *C*)
    a. First web space
    b. Distal palmar flexion crease

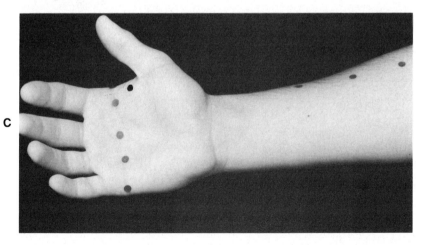

C

2. Dorsal (Fig. 16-10, *D* and *E*)
    a. 2-4 metacarpophalangeal joints
    b. First web space
    c. ⅔ distal length of forearm
3. Medial and lateral (Fig. 16-10, *D* and *E*)
    a. Half thickness fifth metacarpal
    b. Half thickness ulnar and radial wrist
    c. Half thickness ulnar and radial forearm

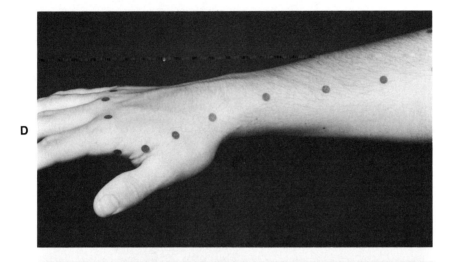

D

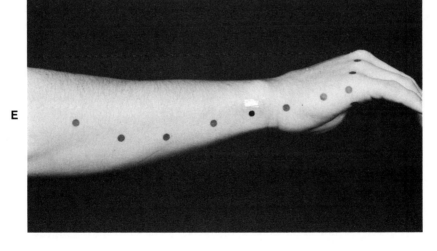

E

BASIC PATTERNS—cont'd
Dorsal metacarpal/wrist/forearm shell—cont'd

COMPLETED PATTERN (Fig. 16-10, *F*)

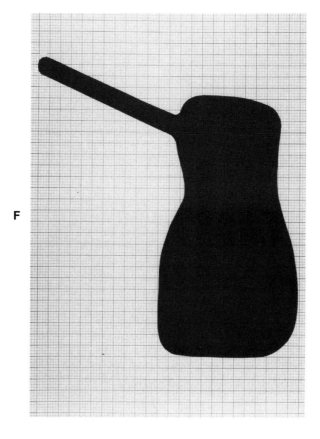

F

Volar metacarpal/wrist/forearm shell

PURPOSES (Fig. 16-11, *A* and *B*)
1. Supports the transverse metacarpal arch via palmar and dorsal radial metacarpal bars.
2. Positions the wrist.
3. Provides a base of attachment for finger or thumb phalangeal bars and for outrigger components.

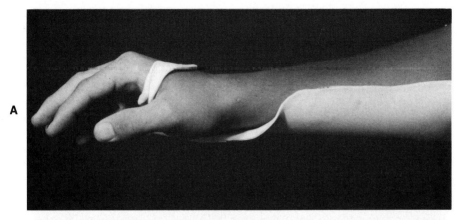

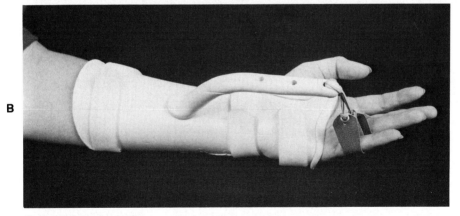

Example of completed splint.

BASIC PATTERNS—cont'd
Volar metacarpal/wrist/forearm shell—cont'd

ANATOMIC LANDMARKS
1. Volar (Fig. 16-11, *C*)
   a. Distal palmar crease
   b. Opponens crease
   c. First web space
   d. Two thirds distal length of forearm
2. Medial and lateral (Fig. 16-11, *C* and *D*)
   a. Half thickness fifth metacarpal
   b. Half thickness ulnar and radial wrist
   c. Half thickness ulnar and radial forearm
3. Dorsal
   a. First web space
   b. Third metacarpal

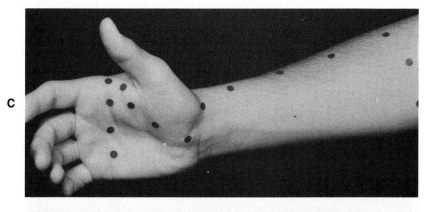

C

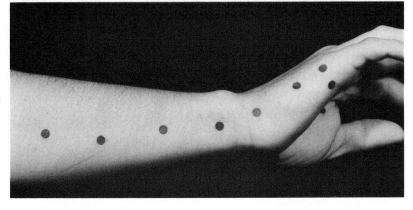

D

COMPLETED PATTERN (Fig. 16-11, *E*)

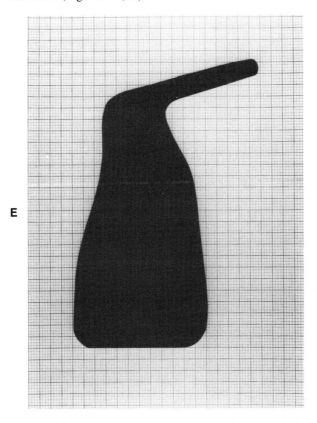

E

CONTIGUOUS ADAPTATIONS OF BASIC PATTERNS
Dorsal proximal phalangeal/metacarpal/wrist/forearm shell

PURPOSES (Fig. 16-12, *A* and *B*)
1. Positions 2-4 metacarpophalangeal joints in predetermined amount of flexion.
2. Supports the transverse metacarpal arch via dorsal and palmar metacarpal bars.
3. Positions the wrist.
4. Provides a base of attachment for thumb phalangeal bar and for outrigger components.

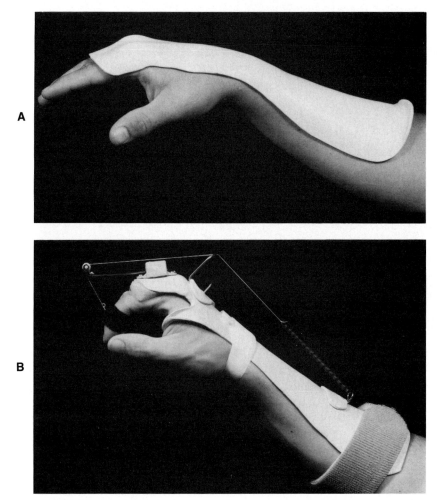

Example of completed splint.

ANATOMIC LANDMARKS

1. Dorsal (Fig. 16-12, *C* and *D*)
   a. 2-4 proximal interphalangeal joints
   b. First web space
   c. Two thirds distal length of forearm
2. Medial and lateral (Fig. 16-12, *C* and *D*)
   a. Half thickness second and fifth proximal phalanges
   b. Half thickness fifth metacarpal
   c. Half thickness ulnar and radial wrist
   d. Half thickness ulnar and radial forearm

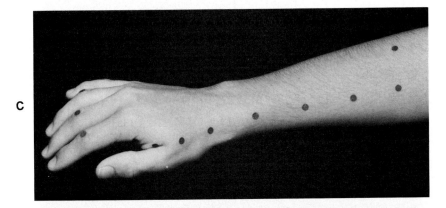

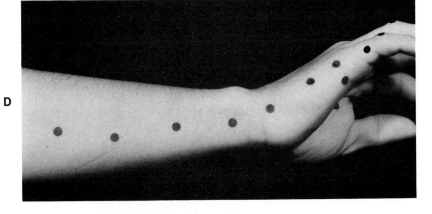

CONTIGUOUS ADAPTATIONS OF BASIC PATTERNS—cont'd
Dorsal proximal phalangeal/metacarpal/wrist/forearm shell—cont'd

ANATOMIC LANDMARKS—cont'd
3. Palmar (Fig. 16-12, *E*)
   a. First web space
   b. Distal palmar flexion crease

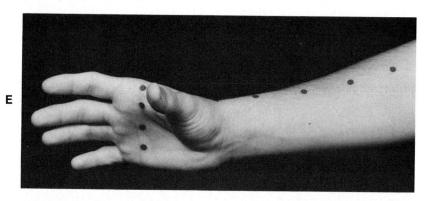

COMPLETED PATTERN (Fig. 16-12, *F*)

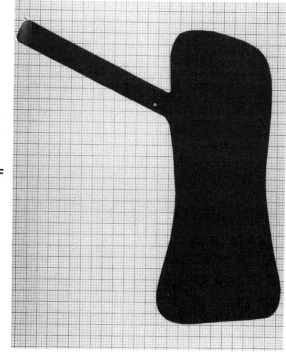

Dorsal finger/metacarpal/wrist/forearm shell

PURPOSES (Fig. 16-13, *A* and *B*)
1. Positions interphalangeal and metacarpophalangeal joints of index, long, ring, and small fingers.
2. Supports the transverse metacarpal arch via dorsal metacarpal bar.
3. Positions the wrist.

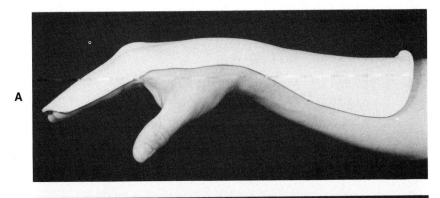

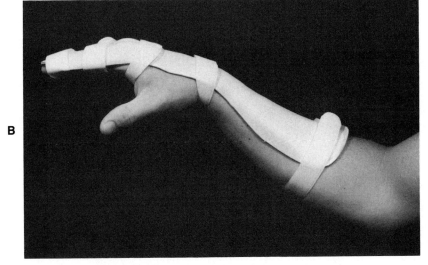

Example of completed splint.

CONTIGUOUS ADAPTATIONS OF BASIC PATTERNS—cont'd
Dorsal finger/metacarpal/wrist/forearm shell—cont'd

ANATOMIC LANDMARKS
1. Dorsal (Fig. 16-13, *C*)
   a. Distal ends of fingers
   b. First web space
   c. Two thirds distal length of forearm
2. Medial and lateral (Fig. 16-13, *C*)
   a. Half thickness second and fifth rays
   b. Half thickness ulnar and radial wrist
   c. Half thickness ulnar and radial forearm

C

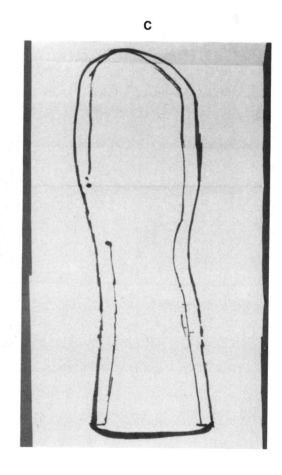

COMPLETED PATTERN (Fig. 16-13, *D*)

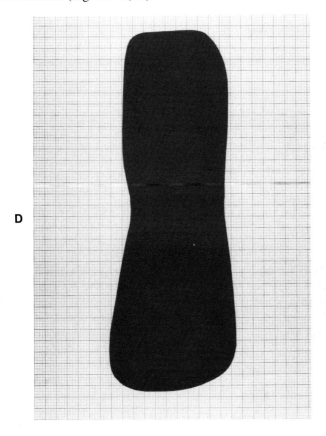

CONTIGUOUS ADAPTATIONS OF BASIC PATTERNS—cont'd
Palmar finger/thumb/metacarpal/wrist/forearm shell

PURPOSES (Fig. 16-14, *A* and *B*)
1. Positions interphalangeal and metacarpophalangeal joints of thumb and fingers.
2. Supports the transverse metacarpal arch via palmar metacarpal bar.
3. Positions the wrist.

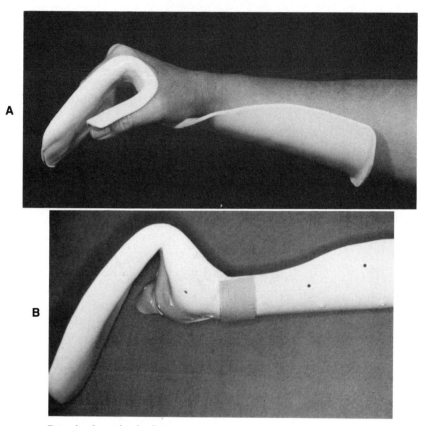

Example of completed splint.

ANATOMIC LANDMARKS

1. Dorsal (Fig. 16-14, *C*)
   a. Distal ends of fingers and thumb
   b. First web space
   c. Two thirds distal length of forcarm
2. Medial and lateral (Fig. 16-14, *D*)
   a. Half thickness second and fifth rays
   b. Half thickness ulnar and radial thumb
   c. Half thickness ulnar and radial wrist
   d. Half thickness ulnar and radial forearm

C

D

CONTIGUOUS ADAPTATIONS OF BASIC PATTERNS—cont'd
Palmar finger/thumb/metacarpal/wrist/forearm shell—cont'd

COMPLETED PATTERN (Fig. 16-14, *E*)

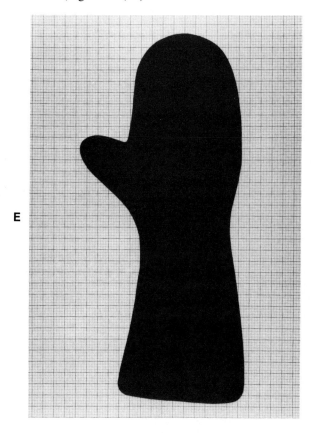

E

SEPARATE COMPONENT PATTERNS
Dorsal phalangeal bar

PURPOSES (Fig. 16-15, *A* and *B*)
1. Positions metacarpophalangeal joints in predetermined amount of flexion.
2. Prevents hyperextension of metacarpophalangeal joints.
3. Maintains transverse metacarpal arch.

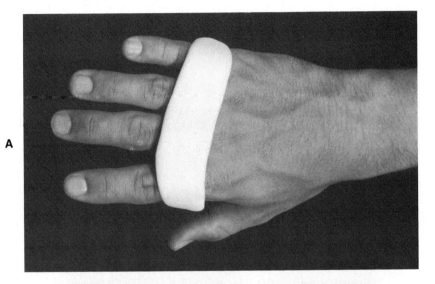

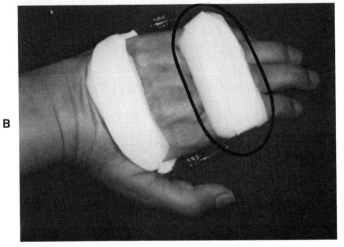

Example of completed splint.

SEPARATE COMPONENT PATTERNS—cont'd
Dorsal phalangeal bar—cont'd

ANATOMIC LANDMARKS
1. Dorsal (Fig. 16-15, *C* and *D*)
   a. 2-5 metacarpophalangeal joints
   b. 2-5 proximal interphalangeal joints
2. Medial and lateral (Fig. 16-15, *C* and *D*)
   a. Half thickness second proximal phalanx
   b. Half thickness fifth proximal phalanx

C

D

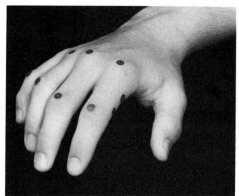
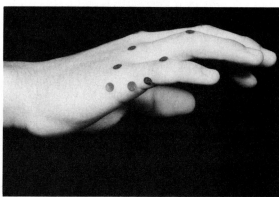

COMPLETED PATTERN (Fig. 16-15, *E*)

E

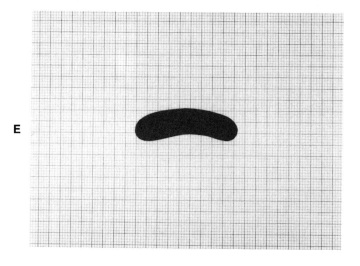

Four-finger outrigger

PURPOSE (Fig. 16-16, *A* and *B*)

Provides a base of attachment or fulcrum for dynamic assist component.

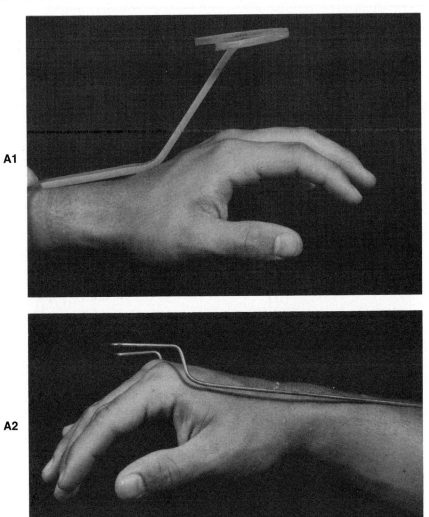

SEPARATE COMPONENT PATTERNS—cont'd
Four-finger outrigger—cont'd

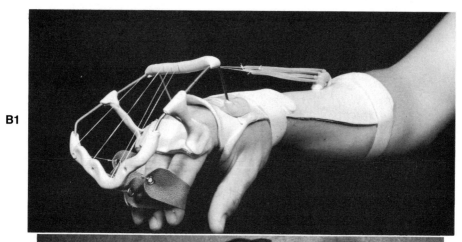

B1

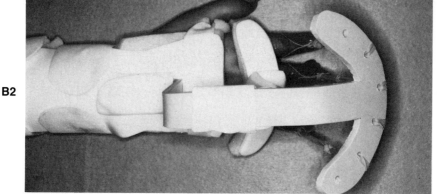

B2

ANATOMIC LANDMARKS

1. For metacarpophalangeal joint motion (Fig. 16-16, *C*)
    a. 2-5 metacarpophalangeal joints
    b. 2-5 proximal interphalangeal joints

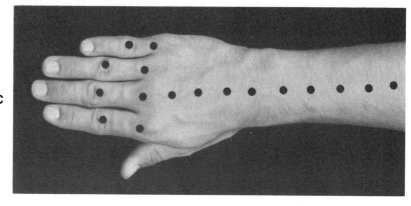

C

2. For proximal interphalangeal joint motion (Fig. 16-16, *D*)
   a. 2-5 proximal interphalangeal joints
   b. 2-5 distal interphalangeal joints

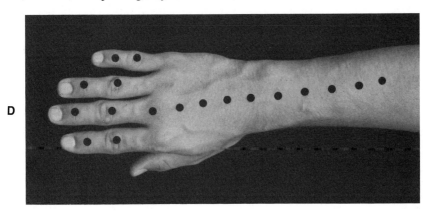

COMPLETED PATTERN (Fig. 16-16, *E*)

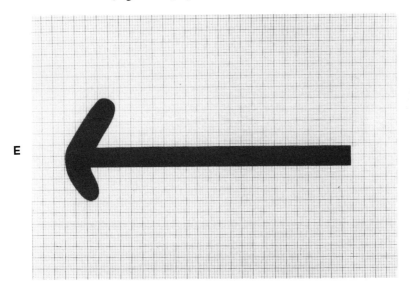

SUMMARY

Constructed to meet anatomic variations and to comply with basic splinting principles, patterns provide visual guidelines during the initial stages of splint fabrication. Employment of patterns diminishes chances for design error and facilitates optimum use of materials and time. Generally speaking, patterns are constructed by assembling separate components, by outlining the configuration of the shell or splint, or by taking specific measurements. Even though all patterns must be adapted to individual patient requirements, many splint designs originate from one of three basic patterns.

CHAPTER 17

Plaster casting for the remodeling of soft tissue

Judith Bell

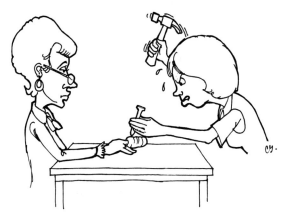

"NOW, DON'T PANIC, MRS. GOLDSBLOOM.
I'M SURE WE CAN GET THIS OFF."

STATIC SPLINTS

While the grouping of splints into those which are static and those which are dynamic may be helpful for splint design, new insight into the biomechanics of hand function has made it necessary to redefine the concept of a static splint. A static splint is not always "static" in its function. It can function dynamically to transfer additional force on joint movement to another joint or joints when the hand is used. For example, a splint that immobilizes the proximal interphalangeal joint of a finger transfers force exerted through the flexor tendons proximally to the metacarpophalangeal joint, and

Clinical Research Therapist and Chief of Hand Therapy, Rehabilitation Research Department, U.S. Public Health Service Hospital, Carville, Louisiana

distally to the distal interphalangeal joint. Similarly, an arthrodesis of the proximal interphalangeal joint transfers additional force of the flexor tendons primarily and distally and can result in an increased range of motion of the two free joints over time (Fig. 17-1).

Static splints, then, can provide or augment dynamic functions, even if they do not have moving parts. Therapists have long used static stabilization or immobilization of one joint or joints for the mobilization of other stiff joints and to increase action of scarred tendons. This is what happens when a therapist blocks one joint with his/her hand while encouraging free movement of another. One step further is to apply this concept of splinting, and in this particular instance to static splinting with plaster of Paris.

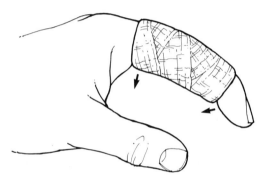

Fig. 17-1. Static dynamic splint. A static splint is not always ''static'' in its function, but can function dynamically to transfer additional force on joint movement to another joint(s) when the hand is used.

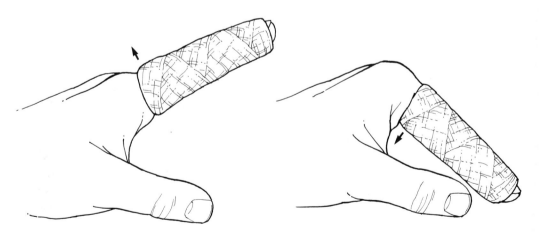

Fig. 17-2. Proximal transfer of force. The stabilization of the finger's interphalangeal joints transfers extension and flexion forces proximal to the metacarpophalangeal joint.

A therapist using plaster splinting must ask not only what will be the action of the cast at the immobilized joint(s), but also what will be the action of the cast at those not casted. The answers to these questions will help make the decision as to where and how the cast is used.

When the proximal interphalangeal joint of the finger is casted, the distal interphalangeal joint is often included in the cast. It may be intentionally left out for exercise if adhesions of the flexor profundus prevent full flexion of the distal interphalangeal joint. It would most certainly be included if, in addition to a joint contracture at the proximal interphalangeal joint or distal interphalangeal joint, there was a musculotendinous contracture of the superficialis or profundus. The casting would not only reduce the interphalangeal joint contracture(s) but would also encourage lengthening of the musculotendinous contacture when the hand is used, particularly during full extension of the wrist and fingers. The stabilization of the interphalangeal joints would transfer the force of the extensor digitorum communis and the intrinsic muscles more proximally to the metacarpophalangeal joint (Fig. 17-2). In contrast, the design of many dynamic splints immobilizes the wrist and metacarpophalangeal joints in static positions when correcting interphalangeal joint contractures.

Casting may also provide the positioning necessary to rebalance externally what has become imbalanced internally by a selective muscle loss. When the intrinsic muscles of the hand are lost in the presence of healthy extrinsic muscles, such as happens after ulnar or median nerve paralysis, an imbalance of the extensor mechanism (overpull of the proximal phalanx by the extensor digitorum communis into extension and absent translational forces of the intrinsics on the dorsal hood) prevents the fingers from being fully extended at the interphalangeal joints (Fig. 17-3, *A*). In addition, the metacarpophalangeal joints have lost their primary flexor, and these joints flex only after flexion of the interphalangeal joints by the flexor digitorum superficialis and profundus.

Casting of the interphalangeal joints into extension allows the fingers to be brought into full extension by the extensor digitorum communis and into flexion at the metacarpophalangeal joints by the flexor digitorum superficialis and profundus (Fig. 17-3, *B*). Thus the casting allows for an external rebalancing of the fingers and can be used temporarily before and after intrinsic replacement surgery in lieu of ''dynamic'' splinting.

The hyperextension in the intrinsic minus hand that is usually present at the metacarpophalangeal joint (often progressing to a deformity if allowed to remain) does not usually continue after the casts are applied, because primary flexion to the metacarpophalangeal joint has been restored. The plaster casts are contraindicated if the patient continues to hyperextend at the metacarpophalangeal joints with the casts on, but this is not usually a problem. Postsurgically, because of the power of the extensor digitorum communis to give the fingers extension at the metacarpophalangeal joints, a patient must be guarded against early full extension and any hyperextension at the metacarpophalangeal joint for at least 6 weeks. Since the patient must be guarded in this fashion regardless of the casts, the casts can be used in lieu of dynamic splinting. A dorsal block not allowing the metacarpophalangeal joints to fully extend is usually used in this case in conjunction with the finger casts for the first few weeks (Fig. 17-3, *C*).

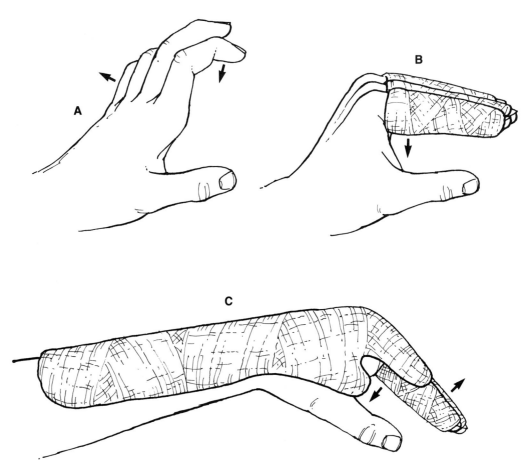

Fig. 17-3. Correction of finger extrinsic muscle imbalance caused by loss of intrinsic musculature. **A,** Without casting, the fingers primarily extend at the metacarpophalangeal joint, and primarily flex at the distal interphalangeal joint and interphalangeal joints. **B,** Preoperative casting transfers flexion of the superficialis and profundus to the metacarpophalangeal joint restoring primary flexion. **C,** Postoperative casting and metacarpophalangeal block helps augment desired action of the intrinsic transfers at the metacarpophalangeal joint.

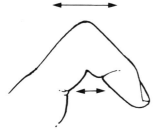

Fig. 17-4. Palmar skin becomes shortened in long-standing joint contractures. These often require skin grafting before other surgery unless remodeled by plaster cylinder casting.

SOFT TISSUE REMODELING

The traditional definition of static splint and the traditional use of plaster casting for support and immobilization make it hard to understand the intent of using plaster in the remodeling of soft tissue. To understand the technique, one has to discard the previous conception that the plaster is only forming a mold around the part. One also has to abandon the conception that force while the plaster is setting is what is required to reposition the joint and soft tissue into correction. Instead, one must begin to appreciate the dynamic and remodeling properties of soft tissue and realize that a change is occurring in the soft tissue itself. Soft tissue is alive and possesses viscoelastic properties that allow it to contract and be stretched within a certain range. It is also responsive to influences that can stimulate it to change its basic resting length.

Soft tissue is constantly undergoing remodeling. Even in the absence of injury and scar, there is a constant replacement of tissue as cells age and are replaced with new cells. This process is accelerated after injury as the tissue fights to renew itself and continues at an accelerated rate long after the visible signs of healing are completed. The rate of repair, although greatest immediately after injury, may continue at an accelerated rate for a year or longer. The remodeling/replacement process does not stop even after a year, but continues as long as the tissue is alive.

It is this remodeling process that is taken advantage of in plaster casting to increase range of motion. Soft tissue tends to increase or ''grow'' where it is being asked to grow; it tends to accommodate what is asked by the firmer structures of the body that give the soft tissue support. Occasionally the design or ordering of the growth is upset by the damage of some parts, changing the signals to the tissue. A joint that has not been extended for a while undergoes changes in its viscoelastic properties, which makes it harder for the joint to extend or be extended. Eventually, if not corrected, the joint develops a fixed contracture. What has happened is that soft tissue, such as skin and ligaments, has been reabsorbed to accommodate the reduced requirements. This is seen in joint flexion contractures, which without casting require skin grafts to have enough skin length to extend the finger after tendon transfer (Fig. 17-4).

The regrowth of soft tissue may be harmful as well as beneficial. If regrowth did not occur there would be no healing after injury, and the body would not survive. But scar is the regrowth of tissue that sometimes binds many structures together in an effort to heal. Since many of these structures must be mobile in planes of movement, the challenge is to either keep the soft tissue planes of movement free as a wound heals, or to regain these planes of movement as soon as possible after the wound has healed.

Scar tissue, in addition to binding some structures together is less compliant than other soft tissue and renders it less elastic. It has a natural tendency to contract during healing, greatly adding to the possibilities of contracture. If it is constantly stressed with intermittent forces, it may become hypertrophic and contract even more. Scar, however, is also undergoing a constant remodeling process, like other soft tissue, if it is held near the end of its elastic limit, it tends to regrow and relax in this position, allowing it to be lengthened just a little further. Thus the gentle positioning of contracted soft tissue at the end of its elastic limit by the use of plaster casting has a real advantage over "dynamic splinting", which supplies intermittent positioning of the contracted soft tissue. This may account for the success of the cylinder casting method over elastic traction splinting for longstanding contractures of the interphalangeal joints. Obviously, exercise in between casting is necessary to maintain active range of motion. The casts are changed for exercise at least every other day, or a minimum of twice a week. Depending on individual requirements, patients may be instructed to remove their casts for 10 to 15 minutes of exercise as often as every 3 to 4 hours.

Force

Skin and other soft tissues have elastic properties. They can be elongated when tension (a force) is applied and will contract when tension is released. They also have viscous properties. Each tissue has its own viscoelastic index. The skin is relatively elastic when compared with tissue such as a tendon, which is relatively inelastic. Each tissue has a limit to its ability to elongate. These are referred to as elastic limits (Fig. 17-5).

There is a point beyond which the tissue will elongate no more—the end of its elastic limit. Applied force that exceeds the tissue's elastic limit deforms and tears the tissue. When tissues and cells are torn, protein is released from the cells, which in turn forms more scar. Scar formation, then does not only reduce the elasticity of the tissue, but tends to make the tissue shorten even more.

Therefore plaster casting is a gentle positioning of the contracted tissue near the end of its elastic limit. No force greater than that which would be used to extend the tissue is applied. Measurements of the force required vary between 100 and 300 gm, which is minute compared with the force often used to manipulate a stiff contracted joint, which has been measured as high as 800 to 1000 gm. Rubber band tension required to improve a contracted joint by dynamic traction by comparison is as high as 450 gm applied at 2 to 3 cm from the axis of the joint.

Dr. Paul Brand, realizing these concepts early in his work, conceived the idea of

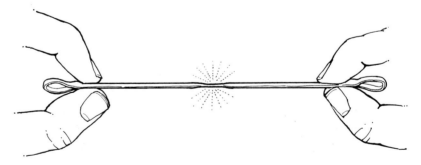

Fig. 17-5. Skin and other soft tissue have viscoelastic properties and will elongate and contract to a predetermined limit. Force beyond this limit deforms the tissue and tears some cells just as it would a rubber band.

casting for the remodeling of soft tissue and has used this technique throughout his work. He refers to the concept as the "inevitability of gradualness." The tissue is simply held near the end of its elastic limit until it relaxes or grows into this position and elongates a little further. The process is continued in this fashion, resetting the resting length and the ends of the tissue's elastic limits until maximum correction is achieved. The technique has been used successfully in a variety of patients with different causes of soft tissue contractures.

ADVANTAGES OF PLASTER

The remodeling of soft tissue may be accomplished by other types of splints and positioning devices, but plaster has unique characteristics which make it an optimal material for this method.

Plaster has the ability to conform precisely to a joint angle and skin surface, sometimes even retaining papillary ridges. This means it can be relied on to actually maintain the joint and skin at a chosen position near the ends of their elastic limit. Other material, such as thermoplastics, does not conform as effectively. Since only 1 or 2 degrees of change is expected with each cast change, a material that allows some play or does not secure the soft tissue may not achieve the same result. Thermoplastic splints are often used as holding or retainer splints after joint correction has been achieved, but they do not work as effectively as the plaster for corrective splints.

Unless the person doing the casting inadvertently exerts finger pressure on the cast during fabrication, the plaster distributes forces on the cast throughout the length of the cast. For example, in casting the proximal interphalangeal joint of the finger, the pressure is distributed over the length of the finger, not at three specific points, such as with joint jacks and other corrective devices. This is particularly important when one considers the delicate balance of the finger extension mechanism and how dangerous it is to apply a force anywhere close to the dorsum of the proximal interphalangeal joint. Yet this is specifically where a major portion of the pressure must be to correct a stiff joint by elastic or spring traction. Boutonniere deformities, and joint subluxations in particular, are often irritated by the force necessary to achieve correction by splints other than plaster casting.

The plaster allows skin underneath to breathe somewhat and therefore, in contrast to other materials such as plastic, does not macerate the skin if applied directly. The plaster is particularly helpful in allowing wounds to be held in an immobilized position and has even been observed to speed wound healing. This has led to a technique of casting for wound healing. One factor in this may be the plaster's ability to wick exudate away from a wound.

The most damaging force to skin is not direct pressure but sheer, or translational, forces. Because the plaster conforms so precisely, sheer force from movement of the finger under the cast is reduced.

In comparison with other materials and techniques, the plaster is relatively inexpensive, readily available, less cumbersome, easily set with water (sterile if desired), and not as likely to lose its corrective positioning.

DISADVANTAGES OF PLASTER
Wet plaster

Plaster of Paris casts should not become wet. If a cast becomes damp, it does not always lose its correction, but the dampness presents a problem. If the cast softens and changes position, pressures can be increased at specific sites, such as the dorsum of a proximal interphalangeal joint. To prevent the plaster from becoming wet, patients may wash around it or place a plastic cover over it. In some cases the cast may be made removable for washing. A wet cast needs to be changed.

Swelling under the cast

Swelling is never increased by plaster casting and is most often decreased because the cast keeps the joint or part quiet for periods of rest. The patient is always instructed to remove the cast if it appears too tight, but this is not usually necessary. The reason for this is that the casting is most often used in nonacute situations. But even when casting is used in the first few postoperative days, such as following a collateral ligament release, to gain a few degrees more extension, swelling is not usually a problem. Swelling from joint dislocations tends to decrease under the cast due to restriction of mechanical irritation. Even swelling from infections tends to decrease under the cast due to the restriction of mechanical irritation. This has enabled casting to be used for wound healing. Still, any situation that may induce swelling should be watched carefully. More important, the circulation of the finger or part is checked after cast application to make sure the vascular supply is not compromised. Excessive force during casting may compromise circulation to tissues that have become contracted. Blood vessels also become shortened in contracted tissue and may shut down if a contracted joint is extended too fast, thus preventing remodeling to occur. It is not surprising to find that blood vessels also elongate with the other soft tissue if time to remodel is allowed.

Patient far from therapy

Two of the biggest deterrents to the use of cylinder casting for remodeling of soft tissue are the time it takes to change progressive casts and patients who cannot return frequently. Although it is always preferable for the therapist to change the cast, the casting is such a relatively safe and noninvasive way of remodeling the joint that it can occasionally be done by another family member who has been carefully instructed in the technique. In a few cases, patients have even casted themselves. If the patient understands the objectives of the techniques and that too much force is harmful, he is not so apt to apply excessive force. If something goes wrong, he can always soak the cast and remove it, which is what he should do if there are problems with a therapist-applied cast. The casting may always be reapplied at a later date.

INDICATIONS FOR USE

As with any type of splinting, casting for range of motion increase is not generally used with patients responding well to exercise and gentle range of motion. It is used where there is a need to increase the range of motion by positioning tissues near the ends of their elastic limit. New injuries are often responsive to simple exercise, and although joint range of motion may be restricted by tissue swelling, new injuries have not had the time to develop tissue contractures from the remodeling process. The casting, in general, is most helpful for older injuries where some remodeling has taken place. In cases of fixed contracture it is often the only form of treatment other than surgical correction that will achieve satisfactory correction.

Serial casting both widens the possibility of surgical corrections and improves the chances of successful results. For example, in a fixed contracture that has undergone palmar skin shortening, surgical correction probably requires a skin graft as well as a collateral ligament release, in addition to correction of the original cause of the contracture. These cannot very well be done together, and the additional scar formed from a skin graft in a first-stage procedure may only lessen the chances of a successful repair. If the joint is remodeled with cylinder casting, the skin graft and collateral ligament releases are made unnecessary, and surgery can correct other problems, such as an intrinsic muscle loss.

The casting method is often successful with contractures other than those due to bony restrictions, but there are some joint contractures better left alone. If for any reason a joint would be unstable or painful if range of motion were increased, one would not want to use the method unless for a specific objective. Casting does not improve irregular joint surfaces damaged by factors such as fractures; these may remodel themselves through movement over time. It is not applicable to arthritic joints, in instances where the eroded joint surfaces may cause irritation and pain if more movement is obtained.

Fabrication of proximal interphalangeal cylinder casts

Materials
Quick-setting plaster
Paper towel
Water (sterile if desired)
Bandage scissors
Curved scissors
Wire cutters (for removal)
Lanolin (optional)

Procedure
1. Cut plaster gauze into strips 2.5 cm wide and 18 cm long.
2. Wet plaster gauze and dry excess on a paper towel.
3. Fold edge 0.5 cm for the first 2.5 cm to make a smooth edge for the cast (Fig. 17-6, *A*).
4. Begin wrapping the finger, placing the smooth edge under the palmar metacarpophalangeal crease (interphalangeal crease in distal interphalangeal joint casting) (Fig. 17-6, *B*).
5. Wrap in a figure-of-eight fashion to the tip of the finger, leaving only the fingertip exposed.
6. Prepare a second strip, as in step 3. Place the edge of the tip of the finger and wrap in a figure-of-eight fashion in the opposite direction. Trim length not needed (Fig. 17-6, *C*). The cast may be made with only one strip, but wrapping from proximal to distal, then distal to proximal, allows the last length of material to be available where most needed—usually for additional strength under the

palmar surface of the proximal interphalangeal joint. The cast should not be thick but should be about two layers at every point. A figure-of-eight wrap provides the best strength for the thin plaster cast; circular wraps can have weak points.

7. Once the finger is wrapped, the person casting should not hold the finger being casted firmly but, with continuous finger movement smoothing the cast, should support the finger until the plaster becomes warm and sets firmly. The plaster makes a firm cast in a few minutes. It does not reach maximum strength until completely dry in several hours, so the patient is instructed to be gentle with it until then (Fig. 17-6, *D*).

8. The cast is changed every other day, or at least once a week, and the finger exercised for a short period. If the cast is left off for long periods the tissue is not held continuously at the ends of its elastic limits, and progress is compromised. The cast is removed with wire cutters (with elongated tips) or curved scissors, or soaked off the finger.

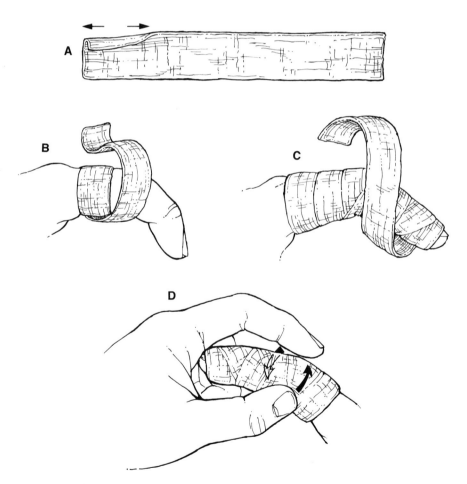

Fig. 17-6. Technique for proximal interphalangeal cylinder casts.

Padding

Plaster is used in the remodeling of soft tissue specifically because the plaster makes a firm mold around the finger and secures the skin preventing damaging sheer forces. Padding under plaster shifts and repositions as the hand is used, allowing soft tissue being corrected to return slightly toward the direction of contracture (Fig. 17-7). The plaster casting technique originally described by Brand does not use padding. The use of padding changes the technique and may not achieve the same results. Casting has been used clinically for years without the use of padding, and it is not considered necessary for the prevention of pressure. The cast itself distributes pressure if done correctly. If padding is used, it should at least be kept to a minimum. A small piece of cotton fluff seems to work the best. The fluff tends to expand and relieve the cast slightly at the desired site. This may help over the dorsum of an interphalangeal joint and at places where the cast makes an edge (Fig. 17-8).

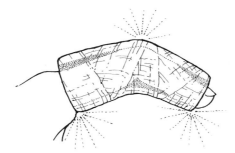

Fig. 17-7. Padding under the cast can shift slightly or compact, allowing pressure to be concentrated at specific points.

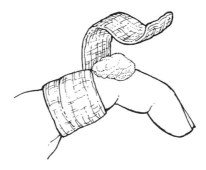

Fig. 17-8. When padding is used, a small piece of cotton fluff may be placed over the dorsum of an interphalangeal joint or where the cast makes an edge against the finger. As explained in this chapter, padding is not required except in cases of specific need.

REMOVABLE CASTS

For the cast to be easily removable for exercise it must be loosened slightly along its length and removed once just after it has become firm and then replaced. For maximum correction of the joint in the shortest time, the cast should not be removable. However, sometimes it is inadvisable to immobilize the finger until the next cast change, such as when adhesions are present along a flexor tendon in the finger. In this situation a removable cast is permitted.

Lanolin or other oil is not always necessary but helps to prepare a finger for a removable cast. A small spot of lanolin placed inside the cast assists replacement on the finger.

If the finger is too severely flexed for the cast to be easily removed, the cast should be relieved to avoid shear stress at the dorsum of the proximal interphalangeal joint on replacement. A cast may be made removable in one of two ways: a small cut can be made in the proximal dorsum of the cast (Fig. 17-9, *A*), or a U can be cut in the cast and the top removed (Fig. 17-9, *B*). The cast may be cut with curved scissors to remove the proximal portion. It should be noted that the cast is more secure without the cuts, and correction is achieved faster if the casts do not have to be removed. When replaced on the finger, the cast may be secured with skin tape.

The casting should never compromise blood supply to the skin or part. An opening left at the tip of the fingers as a precaution in cylinder casts allows recognition of problems. Occasionally, to allow for adequate circulation, a finger must be recasted with less tension.

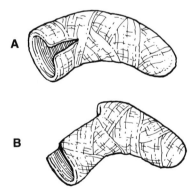

Fig. 17-9. Cutting to relieve a cast for removable casting. **A,** A small cut can be made in the proximal dorsum of the cast. **B,** A window can be cut in the cast and the top removed.

OTHER JOINTS AND TENDONS

Even though casting for increase of range of motion is most frequently used for finger joint contractures, the casting technique has broad application to other joints and problems requiring tissue remodeling. The concept of casting was first used by Brand in the correction of clubfeet in children. It has been used successfully with wrist, thumb web space, and elbow contractures, to name a few. The second most common use is for musculotendinous contractures (either flexion or extension contractures). So often the positioning necessary to reduce or eliminate tension on a repaired tendon while it is healing causes an adhesive restriction in the excursion of the tendon. In other cases, tendon length may have been lost as a part of the injury, or a tendon repair-transfer was made a little tight. Casting may be used to statically position tendons restricted by an excursion problem at their greatest limit of extension or flexion. Exercise in between casting has often been successful in improving tendon excursion problems. Brand does not endorse any theory that the casting can change the length of the tendon, but he

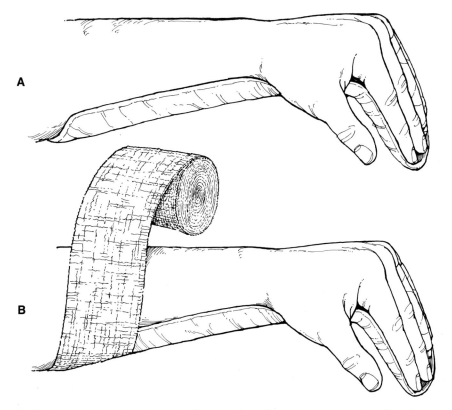

Fig. 17-10. Removable casting for extrinsic musculotendinous contractures. A minimal amount of padding is used, and a circular plaster bandage is wrapped around a plaster slab.

believes the scar and other soft tissue restricting the tendon may be remodeled and that muscle fibers may be lengthened. There is evidence that the muscle can increase its number of sarcomeres while contractures are successfully reduced, and that the muscle loses sarcomeres when it becomes contracted.

The technique of casting other parts and areas is based on the same principles as casting for finger interphalangeal joint contractures. A minimal amount of padding or no padding is used, and point pressure is avoided. For forearm casts, including the fingers and wrist, casting is best accomplished in two stages: (1) a slab thickness that fits palmarly (Fig. 17-10, *A*) and (2) a thin circular wrap of plaster that secures the slab and distributes pressure along the length of the cast (Fig. 17-10, *B*).

The forearm and hand are first wrapped with a very light cotton Webril-like dressing, and the palmar slab (six layers of plaster), which has been cut to approximate the length and shape of the fingers and forearm, is placed on the hand while it is held gently in its maximum position of correction. Once this sets, a plaster roll is then wrapped around the hand and forearm to secure the slab. Only a thin roll is needed—one or two layers. The plaster may then be smoothed along its length and around the fingers (plaster bandage will dimple in finger creases) to secure them in position.

Less padding is necessary in the staged cast because the thin layer of plaster conforms well to the curvatures of the fingers and joints, minimizing shear stress. Most of the pressure sores that occur with other forms of casting are from point pressure under the cast, causing ischemia, and from shear stress where the cast moves and rubs against the tissue. Without padding, the cast is more secure. If plaster is directly applied to the dorsum of the fingers, it sticks to the tissue, holding it more securely in position. Because of the thin layer the patient or therapist can easily cut the cast with scissors if there seems to be a problem.

The cast may be removed without the use of a cast cutter. A cast cutter (circular saw) *should not be used* on the thin plaster because it has little or no padding.

CASTING IN TWO DIRECTIONS

Some joint contractures of the hand require casting in two directions. In proximal interphalangeal joint contractures, regaining extension of the fingers is usually more difficult than regaining flexion. The finger flexor muscles through location and positioning have a mechanical advantage over the extensors. Often during casting to increase joint extension, flexion range of motion may be increased by exercise in between casting. This is true particularly in joints that have been recently subluxed, where stiffness is often present during both flexion and extension of the involved joint. When gains in flexion are not satisfactory, the casting may be alternated for periods of both flexion and extension. Approximately every 2 days the casting direction may be alternated. Some of the benefits of casting in one direction might initially be lost when this is done. However, the casting does effect a change in the tissue, and progress can be seen when the casting is continued for a week or more.

TWO-STAGE CASTING

Boutonniere and swan neck deformities require two-stage casting because of the joint forces they produce in opposite directions. Casting with one stage usually is not successful and may actually be harmful because cast pressures are concentrated where they could cause damage.

Boutonniere deformity

Casting is done first for the distal interphalangeal joint with the proximal interphalangeal joint in full flexion (Fig. 17-11, *A,B*). This reduces the tension on the lateral bands. At the first casting flexion of the distal interphalangeal joint may seem impossible. But as cast changes are made, improvement in flexion of this joint can be demonstrated. Once the plaster has set firmly around the distal interphalangeal joint, the proximal interphalangeal joint can be extended and a second cast made (Fig. 17-11, *C*), beginning at the metacarpophalangeal crease. Casting of both joints at the same time is impossible because the very short lever arm of the distal phalanx makes it difficult to control this joint and the proximal interphalangeal joint in the opposite direction. By casting the distal interphalangeal joint into flexion first, one has a longer and more powerful lever arm to extend the proximal interphalangeal joint. Although the force to extend the proximal interphalangeal joint is only that at the end of its elastic limit, one is able to accomplish this more effectively once the distal interphalangeal joint is casted. Gradually, the lateral bands causing the deformity relax, and casting in opposite directions becomes easier.

In this deformity, migration of the lateral bands has occurred so that they have become flexors of the proximal interphalangeal joint and extensors of the distal interphalangeal joint. Casting does not usually correct the underlying problem, only the joint stiffness, and the patient requires surgical correction. The joint stiffness returns quickly if casting is discontinued and surgery is not performed. If the deformity is recognized early and casting in the described fashion is done, occasionally the migration of the lateral bands may be arrested. This is probably due to an incomplete division of the

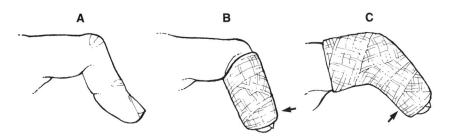

Fig. 17-11. A, Two stage casting of a boutonniere deformity. **B,** With proximal interphalangeal joint fully flexed, cast distal interphalangeal joint into flexion. **C,** Once cast is firm, cast proximal interphalangeal joint into extension.

dorsal hood supporting the lateral bands. If the finger is not casted for a while after injury, active flexion of the proximal interphalangeal joint increases tension on the dorsal hood and the migration of the lateral bands. The finger then quickly develops fixed joint contractures (Fig. 17-11).

Two to 3 weeks after surgical correction of the underlying problem a cylinder cast of only the proximal interphalangeal joint may be made, leaving the distal interphalangeal joint free to maintain extension of the joint. Restriction of the proximal interphalangeal joint maintains this joint in extension and allows early *protected gliding* of the dorsal hood repair as the distal joint moves. The cast may be removed for gentle controlled flexion of the proximal interphalangeal joint. Forced flexion is avoided for several weeks until the surgical repair has matured and the deformity is less likely to recur.

Swan neck deformity

The swan neck deformity is similar to the boutonniere deformity in that it quickly becomes a fixed contracture and usually requires surgical correction of the underlying problem to prevent contractures from recurring. Rupture of the lateral bands at their attachment on the distal interphalangeal joint or the palmar plate at the proximal interphalangeal joint can cause the deformity. If recognized and casted or splinted early, deformity might be arrested or prevented.

The distal interphalangeal joint is first casted into extension, beginning with a plaster wrap at the proximal interphalangeal joint (Fig. 17-12, *A*). With other forms of splinting

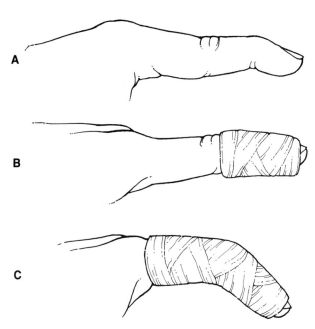

Fig. 17-12. A, Two stage casting of a swan neck deformity. **B,** Cast distal interphalangeal joint into extension. **C,** Once cast is firm, cast proximal interphalangeal joint into flexion.

the distal phalanx is such a short lever arm, it is sometimes impossible to extend this joint after a swan neck injury without causing more injury. The dispersion of the pressure of the cast over the length of the distal end of the finger helps prevent localized pressure to the dorsum of the distal interphalangeal joint, where injury often occurs.

Once the distal joint is casted, the lever arm is increased, and when the cast is firm the finger can be gently flexed at the proximal interphalangeal joint and casted with a second cast, beginning at the metacarpophalangeal joint (Fig. 17-12, *B*).

CASTING AND ELASTIC TRACTION SPLINTING

Casting for tissue remodeling is not meant to replace elastic traction splinting as an adjunct to therapy, but to extend the possibilities for therapy correction. In general, "dynamic" splinting works better on acute injuries where soft tissue remodeling has not yet taken place, than on long standing injuries where treatment of contracture is a part of the correction.

There are times when casting as a technique can be combined with "dynamic" splinting to reduce the amount of splinting necessary and to allow for correction of multiple problems at the same time. An example is correcting stiff interphalangeal joints into extension and metacarpophalangeal joints into flexion. If casting is done to correct interphalangeal joint problems, these casts, by stabilizing the interphalangeal joints, transfer power of the finger flexors proximal to the metacarpophalangeal joint. If this is not enough to accomplish increases in flexion range of motion at the metacarpophalangeal joint, an elastic traction splint can be used with the casts to augment the flexion. Since the casts stabilize the interphalangeal joints, they provide a longer lever arm for traction to be distributed over the length of the fingers. In this way more tension of the rubber bands can be used to provide more flexion at the metacarpophalangeal joints, while the possibilities of tissue injury and circulation compromise from the elastic traction are minimized (Fig. 17-13).

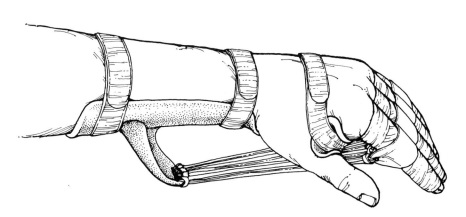

Fig. 17-13. Casting of the interphalangeal joints in extension allows rubber band traction to the metacarpophalangeal joint at a position of mechanical advantage. Possibilities of tissue injury are minimized by the cast displacement of pressure on the dorsum of the fingers.

The traction cuff then produces more tension at a better mechanical advantage because the tension of the rubber band can be farther away from the joint axis, for example, over the dorsum of the proximal interphalangeal joint, where it could not be if the fingers were casted. Other combinations of cylinder casting and elastic traction splinting are, of course, possible.

SUMMARY

Casting for soft tissue remodeling as conceived originally by Brand is an effective tool. It may be utilized in a variety of clinical situations where joint and soft tissue increases in range of motion are desired. The technique is often misunderstood and does not require force other than that required to gently position soft tissue near the ends of its elastic limit, allowing for a regrowth and remodeling of the tissue. Although used mostly at the interphalangeal joints of the fingers, the principles can and have been used for other structures and parts of the body. The unique properties of plaster make it an ideal choice for the remodeling of tissue. Very little if any padding is used in the processes to avoid shifting of padding and increases of joint pressure, and to ensure positioning of tissues near the ends of their elastic limits.

CHAPTER 18

Negative and positive molds

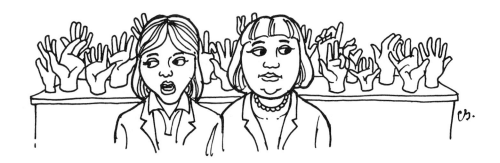

"DO YOU HAVE THE FEELING THAT WE ARE NOT ALONE?"

A negative mold provides the external frame or shell for a positive reproduction of the hand in plaster, dental acrylic, or similar material. The negative mold is prepared directly on the patient's hand. After removal, it is filled with a liquid material that, through an endogenous heat process, dries and hardens. When this material is completely solid, the negative mold is peeled away, leaving a positive duplication of the hand. This positive mold may then be used in the fabrication of splints and in the education of persons involved in wearing or making hand splints. The intent of this chapter is to acquaint the reader with the basic purposes of negative and positive molds and to briefly describe the construction process of these molds with two differing materials: plaster and dental acrylic.

Because early splint materials were often too caustic or too hot to be placed directly on a patient's skin, positive molds were indispensable in providing inert replicas on which splints could be fitted without harm to the patient. When necessary, the construction of negative and positive molds added considerably to fabrication time. Since they produced rigid duplications of normally mobile structures, the splints shaped to the molds frequently required further refinement to accommodate active hands, again adding to the total fabrication time. With the advent of low-temperature plastics that allow

467

warm splint materials to be fitted directly to the patient, the need to produce positive molds for splint fabrication has almost disappeared. Technological advances in materials have allowed more efficient splint fabrication, thereby making it unnecessary to use a negative/positive mold system on every patient requiring a hand splint. There are, however, specific instances when their production is indicated.

The use of positive molds can be invaluable in teaching patients, students, and other professionals (Fig. 18-1). For example, studying a splint without the corresponding

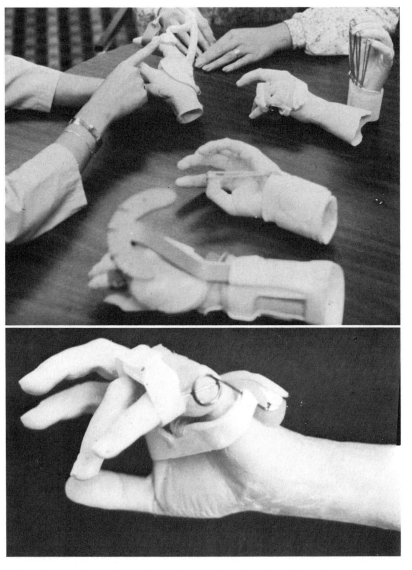

Fig. 18-1. Positive molds used as visual aids may be of considerable assistance in the education of patients or students.

anatomic landmarks can confuse and mislead even the most experienced clinician, to say nothing of its effect on an apprehensive patient who has never encountered such a device. When the splint is placed on a positive mold of a hand, however, familiar points of reference are readily apparent, allowing the patient or student to direct full attention to the instructions or explanation being given, instead of groping for spatial orientation. Serial positive molds may also provide a permanent three-dimensional record of postural changes in the hand as a result of therapeutic or surgical intervention or through a pathologic process occurring over a period of time (Fig. 18-2). In addition to providing permanent records of the changes in deformity in a given hand, these serial molds may be of considerable assistance in general patient counseling and teaching. There are also specific occasions when a positive mold may be helpful because of unusual patient circumstances, either environmental or medical. For instance, patients who will need periodic splint replacement but do not have ready access to the hand clinic may have additional splints fabricated by having permanent positive molds available at the clinic.

Although medical circumstances necessitating construction of positive molds are rare, they can and do occur. Overly anxious, hypersensitive, or hyperactive individuals comprise the majority of problem patients in this area, often requiring some means of anesthesia for the fabrication of the negative mold. A final situation requiring the preparation of negative/positive molds is when high-temperature plastics, caustic materials, or metal must be used for splint construction. The use of a positive mold during the construction and fitting processes of these types of splints frees the patient from involvement in tedious hours of splint fabrication.

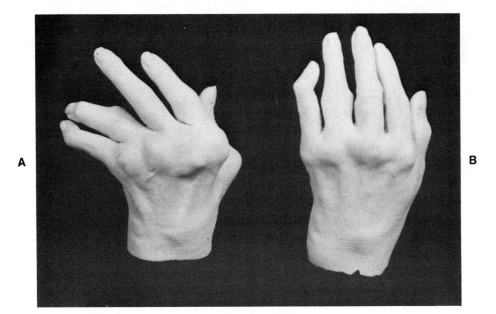

Fig. 18-2. Molds may provide a permanent record of postural changes in the hand, as does this set of preoperative (**A**) and postoperative (**B**) molds.

As previously mentioned, two methods of constructing molds are described in this chapter. Although the fundamental concepts are identical, the use of different materials produces positive molds with heterogeneous physical properties. The choice of material depends on the ultimate use intended for the positive mold. Although both techniques require similar construction times, plaster is considerably less expensive but produces a more fragile, less detailed finished product. This is sufficient for splint fabrication but lacks the durability needed for teaching models that will be handled and used daily. The more expensive dental acrylic molds are durable, and, if made correctly, reproduce the minute surface detail of the original hand (Fig. 18-3). It is important to note that the chemical reaction producing the endogenous heat process for curing the dental acrylic is toxic to the respiratory system. It is therefore imperative to work in a well-ventilated room.

To employ time efficiently and reduce the amount of clutter, all materials and equipment for the preparation of hand molds should be organized before initiating work. The patient and work area, including the floor, should have protective coverings. If the patient is unable to independently maintain the hand posture required, an assistant should be present to help.

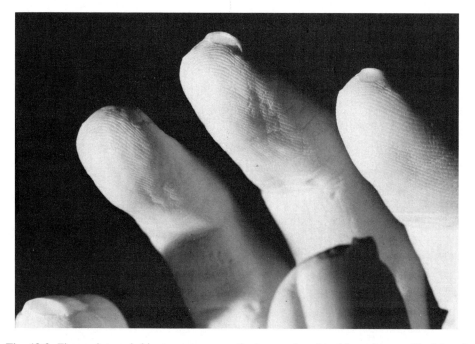

Fig. 18-3. Fingerprints and skin creases are exactingly reproduced in this positive mold of dental acrylic.

PLASTER MOLDS
General considerations

Plaster cures through endogenous heat created by a catalytic reaction between water and crystalized gypsum. The strength of plaster is proportionate to the ratio of plaster of Paris and water. Its curing time may, to some extent, be regulated by adjusting the water temperature. An increased temperature externally augments the catalytic heat response and decreases the curing time. Plaster-impregnated bandage is available in a range of approximate setting times and should be selected according to the specific task and the expertise of the clinician. When applied, wet layers of plaster bandage should be worked until the plaster layers are integrated and smooth. Adjustments during the 20- to 30-minute curing time necessary for most plaster bandage molds should be kept to a minimum because disruption of the plaster molecules at this stage may cause weakness in the mold.

Liquid plaster should be mixed to the consistency of heavy cream. Whipping motions that could induce air bubbles into the mixture should be avoided. The molds into which liquid plaster is poured should be rotated and gently tapped to release air bubbles trapped by the contours of the mold.

Fabrication of a negative plaster mold

Materials
Apron, smock
Newspaper, plastic sheeting
Pan of warm water
Bandage scissors
Petroleum jelly
Paper towels
Three rolls of fast-curing 2-inch plaster bandage

Procedure
1. Cover patient and work area with protective garments or materials.
2. Precut plaster bandage strips according to length of intended mold and size of the hand and forearm. Following are measurements for a forearm and hand mold on an adult patient:
    a. Twelve to fifteen 14-inch lengths (includes 2-inch distal overlap) for forearm/hand
    b. Several ½-inch widths 8 inches long for reinforcement of thumb, first web space, and fingers
    c. One 18- to 24-inch length for final spiraling wrap
3. Evenly coat patient's arm and hand with petroleum jelly, taking care to cover dorsal hair (Fig. 18-4).
4. Position fingers, wrist, and thumb.
5. Roll strips, and as needed dip into water, gently wringing to remove excess water.

6. Apply wet strips longitudinally to forearm and hand, alternating dorsally and palmarly. The 2-inch additional length of each strip is brought around fingertips and run in a proximal direction to provide overlapping of strip ends. Work around forearm with overlapping strips until two or three layers have been worked together (Fig. 18-5).

7. Use narrower bandage strips when working on thumb and reinforcing first web space and fingers (Fig. 18-6).

8. Spiral the final strip around the extremity to provide circumferential stability.

9. Allow plaster to set approximately 10 to 15 minutes.

10. Loosen negative mold by having patient pronate and supinate forearm.

11. Cut mold with bandage scissors to allow extraction of hand. Cut should be in the shape of an elongated Y following radial aspect of forearm and first and second metacarpals (Fig. 18-7).

12. Remove negative mold by pulling gently in a distal direction.

13. Close the radial cut and externally reinforce weak areas of negative mold with additional strips (Fig. 18-8).

Text continued on p. 477.

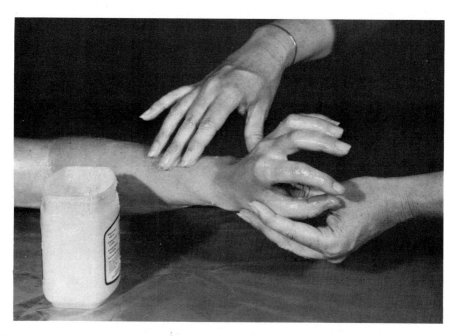

Fig. 18-4. Hair should be thoroughly covered with petroleum jelly to prevent adherence to the inner surfaces of the negative mold.

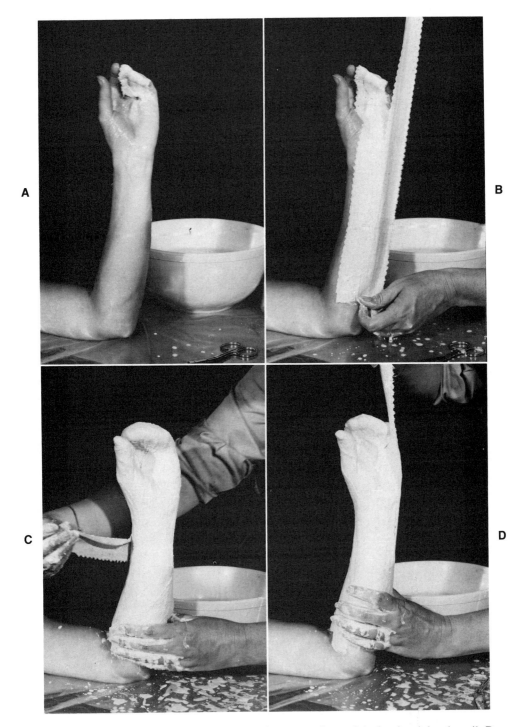

Fig. 18-5. A to **C,** Plaster strips are applied to alternate surfaces of the hand and thumb until, **D,** a thickness of three layers is reached.

A

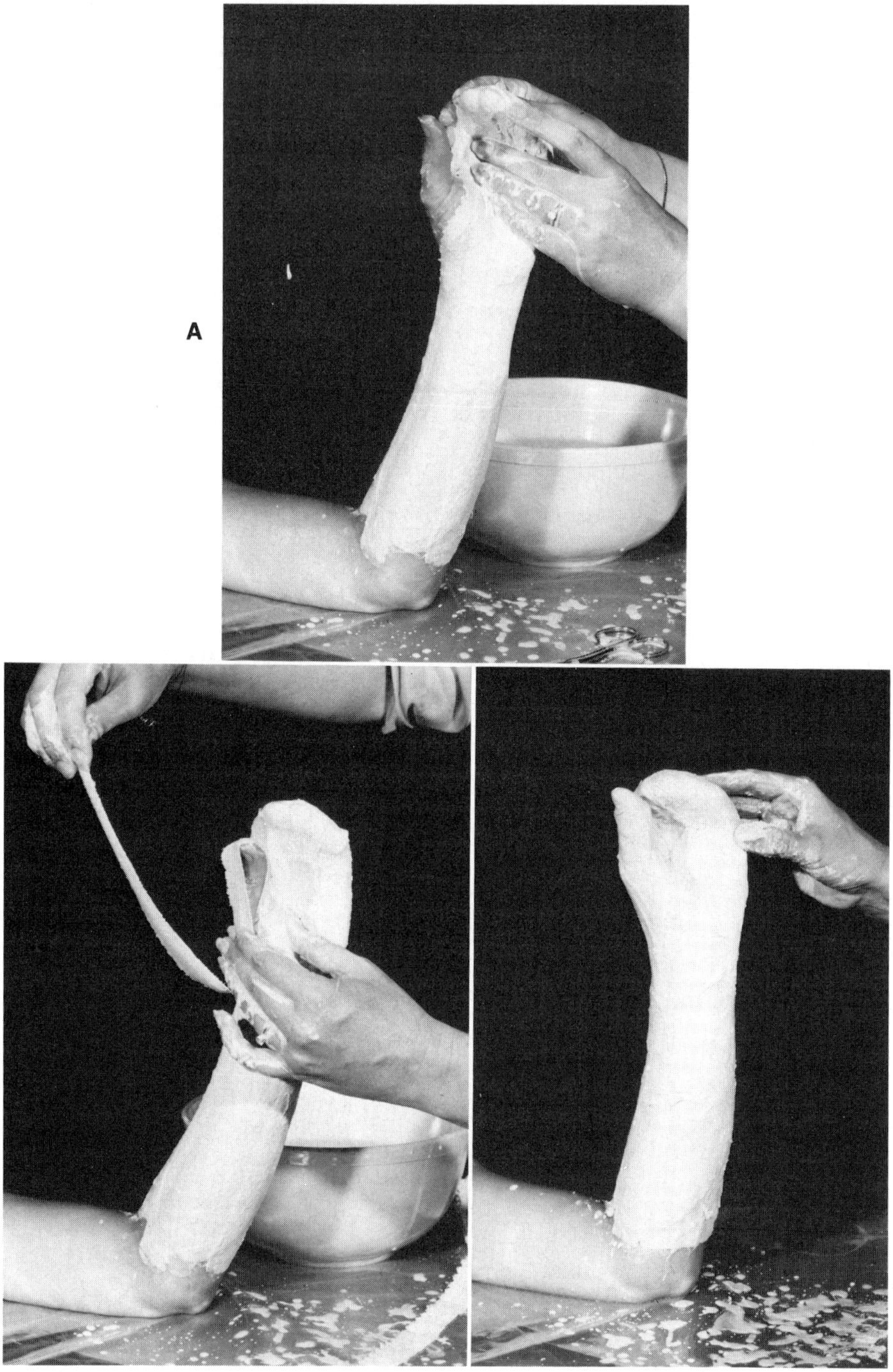

B

C

Fig. 18-6. Because of the potential for collapse at the time of removal, care should be taken to reinforce the thumb, first web space, and fingers.

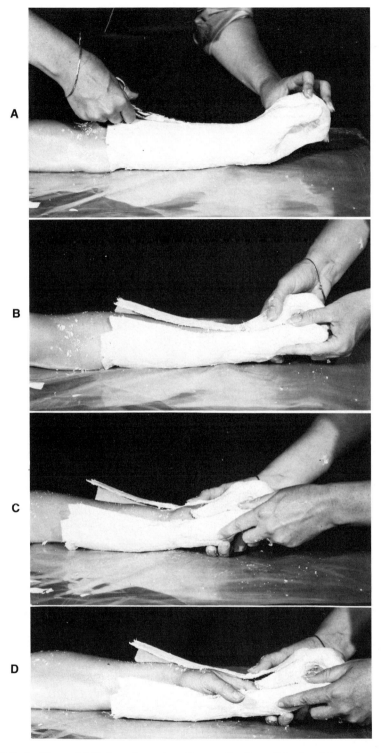

Fig. 18-7. A, The radial Y-shaped opening allows extraction of the hand from the plaster negative. Because of pressure from the scissors on underlying tissue, the course of the cut should run slightly dorsal to the prominences of the head of the radius and first metacarpal and slightly palmar to the lateral aspect of the second metacarpal. **B** to **E,** Once the cut is complete, the negative mold is removed from the hand by gently pulling distally. *Continued.*

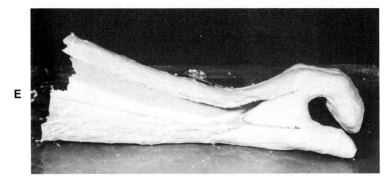

Fig. 18-7, cont'd. For legend see p. 475.

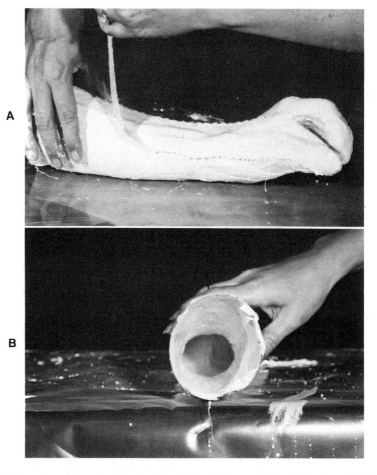

Fig. 18-8. A, The radial cut is closed with additional layers of plastic bandage. **B,** Visual examination of the internal surfaces of the mold by holding it to a light source will reveal weak areas in the layers of plaster.

Fabrication of a positive plaster mold

Materials
Apron, smock
Newspapers, plastic sheeting
Plaster of Paris
Two basins
Water
Separator (1 part kerosene, 1 part liquid soap)
Pencil
Dowel rod or pipe (optional)

Procedure
1. Cover work area with protective material.
2. Hold negative mold over basin, and pour approximately 1 cup of separator into mold. Coat all internal surfaces by rotating mold. Pour remaining separator in mold back into original container.
3. Mix plaster and water to consistency of heavy cream. The amount depends on size of negative mold.
4. Pour small amount of wet plaster into negative mold, rotating and shaking mold to allow plaster to flow into the more distal crevices.

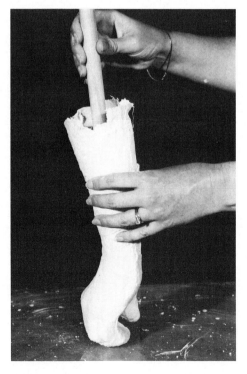

Fig. 18-9. A dowel rod incorporated into the positive mold at the time of pouring allows the finished mold to be secured in a vise.

5. Fill mold with plaster, and continue to rotate and shake mold gently to dislodge air bubbles.

6. If a dowel rod is to be included in the positive mold (Fig. 18-9), it should be inserted into the wet plaster and held until plaster is solid enough to support it.

7. When plaster maintains an impression, inscribe patient's initials and date to facilitate mold identification.

8. When plaster is completely solid and cool to the touch, gently peel negative mold away from positive mold. During this process, special care must be taken when working on thumb and isolated fingers since they break easily.

9. Finish the positive mold by lightly smoothing surface irregularities with fine sandpaper.

SILICONE RUBBER AND DENTAL ACRYLIC MOLDS
General considerations

It is important to be aware that, because of noxious fumes produced by catalytic reaction, the fabrication of molds from silicone rubber or dental acrylic must be carried out in a well-ventilated area. In contrast to the rigid plaster bandage negative mold, a silicone rubber negative mold is slightly flexible, allowing for easier removal of the patient's hand from the mold. Both silicone rubber and the dental acrylic require the addition of a separate catalyst to create the endogenous heat necessary for the conversion from a liquid to solid state. As with the plaster technique, care should be taken to minimize production of air bubbles in the liquid materials during the mixing and pouring stages. This may be done by avoiding whipping motions and by rotating and tapping the filled negative mold. The curing process may be accelerated by increasing the ratio of catalyst to base material. Care should be taken to prevent a setting time that is too rapid. This will result in sufficient time to apply the material or to pour it into the mold. Because the positive and negative materials are not homogeneous, the application of a separator to the internal surfaces of the negative mold is not necessary.

Fabrication of a silicone rubber negative mold

Materials
Apron, smock
Newspapers, plastic sheeting
Dow Corning 310 RTV silicone rubber
Dow Corning RTV Catalyst no. 1 or no. 4
Petroleum jelly
Paper towels
Wax paper
9-inch paper cups
Tongue depressors

Procedure

1. Protect patient and work area with appropriate coverings.
2. Place sheets of wax paper over immediate work area.
3. Coat hand and arm lightly with petroleum jelly. Too much jelly will decrease the final amount of surface detail. Be certain to adequately cover hair.
4. Pour catalyst into 9-inch cup, rotating to evenly coat inner surfaces. Pour excess back into bottle.
5. Fill cup to 2 inches from top with silicone rubber, and mix thoroughly with tongue depressor.
6. Position patient's thumb, fingers, and wrist.
7. Pour mixture slowly over patient's forearm and hand as patient gradually pronates and supinates extremity. Scrape excess material from wax paper and reapply to hand. Cover all areas of hand and forearm with substance (Fig. 18-10).
8. Maintain this posture of the covered extremity until curing process is completed (approximately 15 to 30 minutes).
9. Begin hand removal process by having patient pronate and supinate forearm and hand.
10. If negative mold includes forearm, it may be necessary to make small cut in negative mold at radial wrist level to allow hand to be pulled out of mold, depending on individual hand size and configuration.
11. Remove mold by gently pulling in distal direction (Fig. 18-11).
12. Externally repair any cuts or tears in negative mold with tape or silicone rubber.

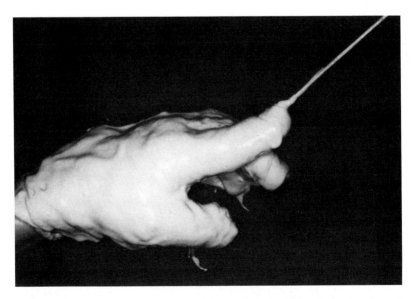

Fig. 18-10. To ensure adequate coverage, careful attention should be directed to the web spaces and adjacent finger surfaces.

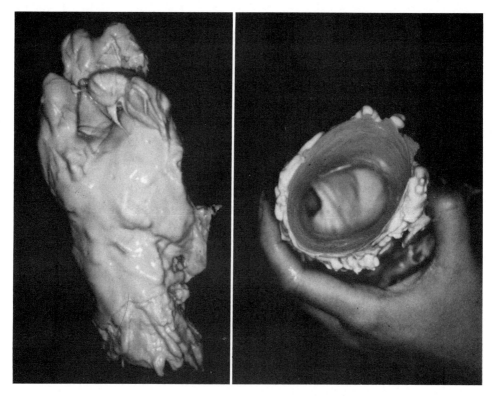

Fig. 18-11. The patient may assist in removal of the negative mold by gently pronating and supinating the hand and wiggling the fingers.

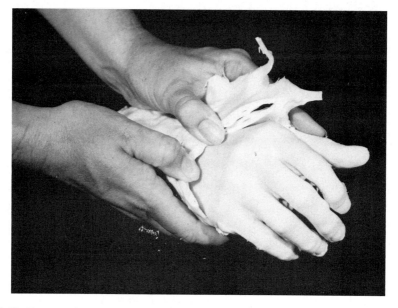

Fig. 18-12. Because the materials are heterogeneous, the negative mold is easily peeled away from the positive without the need for an intervening separator substance.

Fabrication of a dental acrylic positive mold

Materials
Apron, smock
Newspapers, plastic sheeting
Syborn Kerr Formatray powder
Dow Corning Catalyst M (stannous octoate)
9-inch paper cups
Tongue depressor

Procedure
1. Protect work area with appropriate covering.
2. Pour dental acrylic powder into cup to 4- to 5-inch level.
3. Add catalyst and mix. Material should be consistency of heavy cream.
4. Pour into negative mold, gently shaking and rotating mold to free bubbles trapped by mold contours.
5. Mix second batch of dental acrylic, if needed, and pour in similar manner.
6. Allow acrylic to fully cure (material becomes very warm and then cools).
7. Peel silicone rubber negative mold away from positive mold (Fig. 18-12).
8. Finish by sanding or filing surface irregularities from positive mold.

SUMMARY

Although negative/positive molds are not used as they formerly were, a definite place remains for the technique in certain clinical situations. In addition, accurate hand reproductions created by these methods may be of considerable value in teaching clinicians and educating patients, as well as providing a permanent record of a particular hand or changes in its deformity.

Appendices

APPENDIX A

Mathematic equations for Chapter 5

Fig. 5-12: $F \times FA = R \times RA$
$F \times 3 = 0.9 \times 2.5$
$F \times 3 = 2.25$
$F = 0.75$

$F \times 5 = 0.9 \times 2.5$
$F \times 5 = 2.25$
$F = 0.45$

$F \times 7 = 0.9 \times 2.5$
$F \times 7 = 2.25$
$F = 0.32$

Scale: 1 cm = 0.5 pound

Fig. 5-13: $F \times FA = R \times RA$
$F \times 1.5 = 4(0.5) \times 5$
$F1.5 = 10$
$F = 6.67$

$F \times 3.75 = 4(0.5) \times 5$
$F3.75 = 10$
$F = 2.67$

$F \times 5.75 = 4(0.5) \times 5$
$F5.75 = 10$
$F = 1.74$

Scale: 1 cm = 1 pound

Fig. 5-15: $\text{Sine} = \dfrac{\text{Opposite side}}{\text{Hypotenuse}} = \dfrac{O}{H}$ $\quad$ $\text{Cosine} = \dfrac{\text{Adjacent side}}{\text{Hypotenuse}} = \dfrac{A}{H}$

	Sine	Cosine
30°	$0.5 = \dfrac{O}{8}$	$0.866 = \dfrac{A}{8}$
	$4.0 = O$	$6.928 = A$
45°	$0.707 = \dfrac{O}{8}$	$0.707 = \dfrac{A}{8}$
	$5.656 = O$	$5.656 = A$
60°	$0.866 = \dfrac{O}{8}$	$0.5 = \dfrac{A}{8}$
	$6.928 = O$	$4.0 = A$
90°	$1 = \dfrac{O}{8}$	$0.0 = \dfrac{A}{8}$
	$8 = O$	$0.0 = A$
120°	*See* 60°	
135°	*See* 45°	
150°	*See* 30°	

Fig. 5-19:   Sine $= \dfrac{\text{Opposite side}}{\text{Hypotenuse}} = \dfrac{O}{H}$ Cosine $= \dfrac{\text{Adjacent side}}{\text{Hypotenuse}} = \dfrac{A}{H}$

30° $0.3420 = \dfrac{O}{4}$ $0.9848 = \dfrac{A}{4}$

$1.37 = O$ $3.9392 = A$

45° $0.4226 = \dfrac{O}{4}$ $0.9063 = \dfrac{A}{4}$

$1.69 = O$ $3.63 = A$

60° $0.5446 = \dfrac{O}{4}$ $0.8387 = \dfrac{A}{4}$

$2.18 = O$ $3.35 = A$

Fig. 5-20:   Torque $=$ Force $\times$ length
$T = 8 \times 1$
$T = 8$ inch-ounces

$T = 8 \times 2.25$
$T = 18$ inch-ounces

Fig. 5-26, A: $F \times FA = R \times RA$
$F \times 9 = 0.9 \times 3$
$F9 = 2.7$
$F = 0.3$
$0.3 + 0.9 = 1.2$

Fig. 5-26, B: $F \times 3.5 = 0.9 \times 3$
$F3.5 = 2.7$
$F = 0.77$
$0.77 + 0.9 = 1.67$

Fig. 5-26, C: 6.67 from Fig. 5-13
$2 + 6.67 = 8.67$

Fig. 5-26, D: 1.74 from Fig. 5-13
$2 + 1.74 = 3.74$

Scale: 1 cm $=$ 1 pound

Materials and equipment

SPLINTING MATERIALS

A. No external heat
  1. Plaster of Paris
    a. Chemical compound: Manufactured from a solid crystalline material known as gypsum or calcium sulfate. The gypsum is pulverized to break up the crystals and then subjected to intense heat to drive off the water of crystallization. The resulting powder is plaster of Paris.

    $$2\ CaSO_4 \cdot 2\ H_2O \rightarrow (CaSO_4)_2 \cdot H_2O + 3\ H_2O$$

    b. Advantages: $2\ [CaSO_4 \cdot 2\ (H_2O)] \xrightarrow[500°\ F]{\triangle} (CaSO_4)_2 \cdot H_2O + 3(H_2O)$
      (1) Quick to work with
      (2) Gives rigid immobilization
      (3) Inexpensive
    c. Disadvantages
      (1) Does not hold up over time
      (2) Cannot become wet
    d. Working temperature is 70°-75° F (21°-24° C) water
    e. Other features
      (1) Setting time is 5-8 minutes for fast-setting plaster and 2-4 minutes for extra fast-setting plaster. It may take 20-30 minutes for the plaster to dry completely.
      (2) Material is porous and creamy and has serrated edges in bandage form.
    f. Clinical problems: No known allergic reactions. Should, however, protect skin from excessive perspiration since skin rash could develop.
    g. Precautions: Overwrapping the freshly applied cast, placing it on a pillow or mattress, covering it with a blanket, or insulating the cast from free access to the air causes a sharp rise in the temperature of the material. Conversely, the most effective way to reduce the temperature of a cast is to increase circulation of air by such means as blowing air over the cast with a circulating fan.

B. Low-temperature thermoplastics
  1. Ezeform
     a. Chemical Composition: plastic polymer
     b. Advantages
        (1) Easy to handle.
        (2) Provides excellent strength and rigidity.
        (3) Not susceptible to aging.
        (4) Edges trim and roll easily.
        (5) Does not stretch excessively.
        (6) Does not leave fingerprints on material.
     c. Disadvantage: Does not drape and contour precisely.
     d. Heating
        (1) Working temperature is 170° F (75° C)
        (2) Hot water is recommended for softening. Material can also be heated in a hot air oven. A heat gun can be used for spot heating.
        (3) Cools in 4-6 minutes.
     e. Other features:
        (1) Can be purchased in smooth or perforated sheets ⅛ inch thick.
        (2) Color is white.
        (3) Can be washed with mild soap and cool water.
        (4) Material is self-bonding without solvent.
        (5) Scraps are not recyclable.
     f. Suggested use: Can be used for larger orthoses as well as some smaller splints.
     g. Clinical problems: No known allergic reaction; however, it may be desirable to provide the patient with a stockinette liner to protect the skin from excess perspiration.
     h. Precautions: Patient should be instructed to keep splint away from excessive heat and should not leave the splint in a hot car.
  2. Polyform
     a. Chemical composition: Plastic polymer
     b. Advantages
        (1) Molds easily.
        (2) Contours and drapes precisely to the hand.
        (3) Provides excellent strength and rigidity.
        (4) Does not shrink.
        (5) Edges can be smoothed or rolled easily.
        (6) Not susceptible to aging and will not discolor.
     c. Disadvantages
        (1) Care must be taken to avoid leaving fingerprints on the material.
        (2) If overheated, this material will become very soft and stretch excessively.
     d. Heating
        (1) Working temperature of 160° F (70° C).

(2) Hot water is suggested for heating the material. A heat gun can be used for spot heating.

(3) Cools in 3-5 minutes.

e. Other features

(1) Can be purchased in smooth or perforated sheets ⅛ inch thick.

(2) Color is white.

(3) Can be cleaned with cool water and soap.

(4) Can be bonded with Kay-Splint cement.

f. Suggested uses: Works well for smaller orthoses and when exact contouring is desired, such as in an ulnar nerve palsy splint.

g. Clinical problems: No known allergic reactions. However, it may be desirable to provide the patient with a stockinette liner to protect the skin from excessive perspiration.

h. Precautions: Patient should be instructed to keep splint away from excessive heat and should not leave the splint in a hot car.

3. Polyflex II

a. Chemical composition: Plastic polymer and rubber

b. Advantages

(1) Molds easily.

(2) Contours and drapes moderately well to the hand.

(3) Provides excellent strength and rigidity.

(4) Not susceptible to aging and will not discolor.

(5) Edges can be smoothed and rolled easily.

c. Disadvantages

(1) Care must be taken to avoid leaving fingerprints on the material.

(2) May stretch excessively if overheated.

d. Heating

(1) Working temperature of 160° F (70° C) is recommended for softening.

(2) Hot water is suggested for heating material. Heat gun can be used for spot heating.

(3) Cools in 3-5 minutes.

e. Other features

(1) Can be purchased in smooth or perforated sheets ⅛ inch thick.

(2) Color is white.

(3) Can be washed with mild soap and cool water.

(4) Can be bonded with solvent.

(5) Scraps are recyclable.

f. Suggested uses: Can be used for larger orthoses such as elbow splints or fracture braces as well as smaller splints.

g. Clinical problems: No known allergic reaction; however, it may be desirable to provide the patient with a stockinette liner to protect the skin from perspiration.

h. Precautions: Patient should be instructed to keep splint away from excessive heat and should not leave the splint in a hot car.

4. Orthoform
   a. Chemical composition: Transpolyisoprene
   b. Advantages
      (1) Easy to handle.
      (2) Provides good strength and durability.
      (3) Edges are easily smoothed and rolled.
      (4) Can be used for a large variety of splint designs.
      (5) Bonds well to itself without adhesive.
      (6) Does not appear to be affected by exposure to light and air.
   c. Disadvantage: Does not drape and contour as precisely as the plastic polymer materials.
   d. Heating
      (1) Working temperature is 160°-180° F (70°-80° C).
      (2) Can be heated in hot water or with a heat gun.
      (3) Cools in 8-10 minutes.
   e. Other features: Can be purchased in white or flesh color.
   f. Suggested uses: May be used for a wide variety of splints. A versatile material.
   g. Clinical problems: Skin rash may develop from excess perspiration. Stockinette liner may be required.
   h. Precautions
      (1) Material has some shrinkage when cooling. As splint is molding, gently stretch out edges of splint.
      (2) Patient should be instructed to keep splint away from excessive heat and should not leave splint in a hot car.
5. Hexcelite
   a. Chemical composition: Polymers, filler, and pigment impregnated onto cotton netting.
   b. Advantages
      (1) Good ventilation
      (2) Lightweight
      (3) Rigidity can be controlled to some degree by the number of layers of material used.
   c. Disadvantages
      (1) Because of open weave, the splint may not be as strong as that made from other thermal plastics.
      (2) If overheated, holes may stretch.
   d. Heating
      (1) Hot water is recommended for softening.
      (2) Water temperature of 160°-180° F (60°-80° C) is suggested.
   e. Other features
      (1) Can be purchased in rolled bandage or flat sheets.
      (2) Self-adhesive.

f. Suggested uses

(1) Good for small finger splints.

(2) Good when splint needs to be lightweight and when only light support is necessary.

g. Clinical problems: None known. A liner of stockinette is suggested.

h. Precautions: Watch that all rough edges left when cutting the open weave are smooth. Moleskin on edges may be necessary. May cause pressure from open weave design.

6. Orthoplast

a. Chemical composition: Transpolyisoprene.

b. Advantages

(1) Easy to handle.

(2) Provides good strength and durability.

(3) Edges are easily smoothed and rolled.

(4) Can be used for large variety of splint designs.

(5) Bonds well to itself without adhesive.

c. Disadvantages

(1) Does not drape and contour as precisely as the plastic polymer materials.

(2) Material is susceptible to yellowing if left out in the air and light. Therefore store in original box.

(3) Material may lose its adhesive properties if left out in the air and light or if the material becomes soiled. In some cases this may be reversed by cleaning the surfaces with nonflammable spot remover.

d. Heating

(1) Working temperature is 160°-180° F (70°-80° C).

(2) Can be heated in hot water or with a heat gun.

(3) Cools in 8-10 minutes.

e. Other features: Can be purchased in smooth or perforated sheets.

f. Suggested uses: May be used for a wide variety of splints. A versatile material.

g. Clinical problems: Skin rash may develop from excess perspiration. Stockinette liner may be required.

h. Precautions

(1) Material has some shrinkage when cooling. As splint is molding, gently stretch out edges of splint.

(2) Patient should be instructed to keep splint away from excessive heat and should not leave splint in hot car.

7. Aquaplast (original sticky)

a. Chemical composition: Poly(epsilon)caprolactone. This is a thermoplastic crystalline polyester. No surface coating.

b. Advantages

(1) Forms a precise mold of the hand, since it clings to the skin as it hardens.

(2) Transparency while soft allows for observation of the extremity while

splint is being molded. Potential pressure areas can be located and modifications made.

(3) Not affected by overheating.

(4) Material resists fingerprints

c. Disadvantage: Edges do not smooth and roll as easily as some of the other splinting materials.

d. Heating:

(1) Working temperature of 160°-180° F (70°-80° C) is recommended for softening.

(2) Hot water is suggested for heating. Dry heat tends to make the material excessively sticky.

e. Other features

(1) Available in ⅛-inch and ¹⁄₁₆-inch thicknesses of either smooth or perforated sheets.

(2) Self-bonding.

(3) Will adhere to synthetic casting materials.

(4) Can be cleaned with soap and cool water.

f. Suggested uses: Versatile material. Good for a variety of splints. Start with smaller splints until experience is gained in using the material.

g. Clinical problems: Occasional skin rash usually caused by perspiration. It may be desirable to provide the patient with a stockinette liner.

h. Precautions

(1) Apply petroleum jelly or hand lotion to heated material if applying to fragile skin or to skin with sutures still remaining to prevent material from sticking to skin.

(2) When working with the sticky material, it is easier to work if the therapist's fingers are wet with cold water.

(3) Aquaplast shrinks 2% while cooling and may become too tight unless splint is deliberately spread. It is recommended that this be done as the partially hardened splint is removed from the patient's extremity.

8. Aquaplast T (nonstick)

a. Chemical composition: Polycaprolactone with surface coating.

b. Advantages:

(1) Forms and contours well with nonstick surface.

(2) Transparency while soft allows for observation of the extremity while splint is being molded.

(3) Not affected by overheating.

(4) Material resists fingerprints.

(5) Has elastic memory.

c. Disadvantages:

(1) Edges do not smooth and roll as easily as some of the other splinting materials. Save edge finishing for final step (due to elastic memory edges go square during splint revision).

(2) Material will form weak bond to itself with deliberate pressure. It is suggested that the nonstick surface be abraded or a splinting solvent be used for a rigid bond.

d. Heating:

(1) Working temperature of 160°-180° is suggested.

(2) May be heated in hot water, with a heat gun, or in an oven. Hot water, however, seems preferable.

e. Other features:

(1) Available in ⅛″, ⅟₁₆″, and ³⁄₁₆″ thicknesses of either solid or perforated sheets.

(2) Can be cleaned with soap and cool water.

f. Suggested uses: Versatile material. Can be used for most hand splints. Start with smaller splints until experience is gained.

g. Clinical problems: Same as Aquaplast.

h. Precautions: Material shrinks 2% while cooling and may become too tight unless splint is deliberately spread. It is recommended that this be done as the partially hardened splint is removed from the patient's extremity.

9. Manorthos

a. Chemical composition: Polycaprolactone, other polymers, and pigment; like Aquaplast.

b. Advantages:

(1) Pliability can be adjusted from firm to soft by adjusting the water temperature

(2) Handles easily

(3) Self-bonding

(4) Edges can be smoothed or rolled easily

(5) Resists fingerprints.

c. Heating: Same as for Aquaplast.

d. Other features: Available in smooth or perforated sheets ⅛ inch thick.

e. Suggested uses: Good for hand and wrist splints. Since one can control the pliability, it can also be used for larger splints such as elbow splints.

f. Clinical problems: Same as for Aquaplast.

g. Precautions: Material shrinks 2% while cooling and may become too tight unless splint is deliberately spread. It is recommended that this be done as the partially hardened splint is removed from the patient's extremity.

10. Green Stripe Aquaplast

a. Chemical composition: Polycaprolactone, with or without a surface coating.

b. Advantages

(1) Not affected by overheating.

(2) Material resistant to fingerprints.

c. Disadvantage: Less pliable material with less conforming capabilities.

d. Heating: Same as for Aquaplast.

e. Other features

(1) Available in sticky and nonsticky surfaces.

(2) Available in ⅛-inch and ⅟₁₆-inch thicknesses of smooth or perforated sheets.

f. Suggested uses: Good for larger splints where exact detail and conformity are not necessary.

g. Clinical problems: Same as for Aquaplast.

h. Precautions: Material shrinks 2% while cooling and may become too tight unless splint is deliberately spread. It is recommended that this be done as the partially hardened splint is removed from the patient's extremity.

11. Burns Quality Aquaplast: (Blue stripe)

a. Chemical composition: Polycaprolactone, with a surface coating.

b. Advantages

(1) This material is extra pliable and will provide a firm, equal pressure necessary for burn patients or in other situations where hypertrophic scarring may be a problem.

(2) When soft, the material will flow and drape for maximum conformity.

c. Heating

(1) Working temperature of 160°-180° F (70°-80° C).

(2) Hot water is recommended for softening.

d. Other features

(1) Available in ⅛-inch thickness in smooth and perforated sheets.

(2) Can be cleaned with soap and cool water.

(3) Material is nonsticky but can be specially ordered with sticky surface.

(4) Recommend cutting out pattern while *translucent* (not transparent). When material is softened until transparent, remove from hot water on frypan guard to prevent stretching.

e. Suggested uses: Good when exact contouring is needed in splints for scar control or intricately molded hand splints.

f. Clinical problems: Same as for Aquaplast.

g. Precautions: Material shrinks 2% while cooling and may become too tight unless splint is deliberately spread. It is recommended that this be done as the partially hardened splint is removed from the patient's extremity.

12. Kay-Splint Series 3

a. Chemical composition: Plastic polymer.

b. Advantages

(1) Easy to handle.

(2) Provides excellent strength and rigidity.

(3) Not susceptible to aging.

(4) Edges trim and roll easily.

(5) Does not stretch excessively.

(6) Does not leave fingerprints on material.

c. Disadvantage

(1) Does not drape and contour as precisely as other materials.

    d. Heating
      (1) Working temperature is 170° F (78° C).
      (2) Hot water is recommended for softening the material. This material may also be heated in a hot air oven. A heat gun can be used for spot heating.
      (3) Cools in 3-5 minutes.
    e. Other features
      (1) Can be purchased in smooth or perforated sheets ⅛ inch thick.
      (2) Color is beige.
      (3) Can be washed with mild soap and cool water.
      (4) Material is self-bonding without solvent.
      (5) Scraps are not recyclable.
    f. Suggested uses: Can be used for larger orthoses as well as some smaller splints.
    g. Clinical problems: No known allergic reaction; however, it may be desirable to provide the patient with a stockinette liner to protect the skin from excess perspiration.
    h. Precautions: Patient should be instructed to keep splint away from excessive heat and should not leave the splint in a hot car.
13. Kay-Splint Isoprene
    a. Chemical composition: Plastic polymer and rubber.
    b. Advantages
      (1) Molds easily.
      (2) Contours and drapes moderately well to the hand.
      (3) Provides excellent strength and rigidity.
      (4) Not susceptible to aging and will not discolor.
      (5) Edges can be smoothed and rolled easily.
    c. Disadvantages
      (1) Care must be taken to avoid leaving fingerprints on the material.
      (2) May stretch excessively if overheated.
    d. Heating
      (1) Working temperature of 150°-160° F (66°-72° C) is suggested for softening.
      (2) Hot water is recommended for heating the material. A heat gun can be used for spot heating but will not provide uniform softening over a larger area.
      (3) Cools in 2-3 minutes.
    e. Other features
      (1) Can be purchased in smooth or perforated sheets ⅛ inch thick.
      (2) Color is beige.
      (3) Can be washed with mild soap and cool water.
      (4) Can be bonded using solvent.
      (5) Scraps are recyclable.

f. Suggested uses: Can be used for larger orthoses such as elbow splints or fracture braces as well as smaller splints.

g. Clinical problems: No known allergic reaction, however, it is desirable to provide the patient with a stockinette liner to protect the skin from perspiration.

h. Precautions: Patient should be instructed to keep splints away from excessive heat and should not leave the splint in a hot car.

14. Kay-Splint I

a. Chemical composition: Plastic polymer.

b. Advantages

(1) Molds easily.

(2) Contours and drapes precisely to the hand.

(3) Provides excellent strength and rigidity.

(4) Does not shrink.

(5) Edges can be smoothed or rolled easily.

(6) Not susceptible to aging and will not discolor.

c. Disadvantages

(1) Care must be taken to avoid leaving fingerprints on the material.

(2) If overheated, this material will become very soft and stretch excessively.

d. Heating:

(1) Temperature of 150°-160° F (66°-72° C) is recommended for softening.

(2) Hot water is suggested for heating material. A heat gun can be useful for spot heating but will not provide uniform softening over a larger area.

(3) Cools in 2-3 minutes.

e. Other features:

(1) Can be purchased in smooth or perforated sheets ⅛ inch thick.

(2) Color is beige.

(3) Can be cleaned with cool water and soap.

(4) Can be bonded with Kay-Splint cement.

f. Suggested uses: Works well for smaller orthoses and when exact contouring is desired, such as in an ulnar nerve palsy splint.

g. Clinical problems: No known allergic reactions. However, it is desirable to provide the patient with a stockinette liner to protect the skin from excess perspiration.

h. Precautions: Patient should be instructed to keep splint away from excessive heat and should not leave the splint in a hot car.

15. JU 1000 Splinting Compound

a. Chemical composition: plastic polymer

b. Advantages

(1) Molds easily to body contours.

(2) Bonds well when heated.

(3) Edges seal and finish well.

  c. Disadvantages

    (1) Care must be taken to avoid leaving fingerprints on material.

    (2) Will stretch if overheated.

  d. Heating

    (1) Working temperature of 160°-170° F (70°-80° C) is recommended for softening.

    (2) Cools in 3-4 minutes.

  e. Other features

    (1) Color is beige.

    (2) Not susceptible to aging.

  f. Suggested uses: A versatile material. Can be used for a variety of splinting applications.

  g. Clinical problems: None known. Skin rash may develop from excess perspiration. Stockinette liner may be required.

  h. Precautions: Keep splint away from excessive heat. Do not leave splint in a hot car.

16. MR 2000 Splinting Compound

  a. Chemical composition: plastic polymer

  b. Advantages

    (1) Material drapes well.

    (2) Will bond well with solvent.

    (3) Edges can be rolled to finish edges.

  c. Disadvantages

    (1) Care should be taken to avoid fingerprints on material.

    (2) May stretch if overheated.

  d. Heating

    (1) Working temperature 160°-170° F (70°-80° C) is recommended for softening.

    (2) Cools in 3-4 minutes.

  e. Other features

    (1) Color of material is white.

    (2) Not susceptible to aging.

    (3) Material has memory retention.

  f. Suggested uses: Can be used for a variety of splint designs.

  g. Clinical problems: None known. Skin rash may develop from excess perspiration. Stockinette liner may be required.

  h. Precautions: Keep splint away from excessive heat. Do not leave splint in a hot car.

17. RS 3000 Splinting Compound

  a. Chemical composition: plastic polymer

  b. Advantages

    (1) Pliable and easily molded.

  (2) Material self-adherent.

  (3) Edges are easily smoothed.

  (4) Fingerprints can be smoothed out.

 c. Disadvantage: Does not drape and conform as closely as some other materials.

 d. Heating

  (1) Working temperature of 160°-170° F (70°-80° C) is recommended for softening.

  (2) Cools in 3-4 minutes.

 e. Other features

  (1) Color of material is off-white.

  (2) Not susceptible to aging.

 f. Suggested uses: A versatile material. Well suited for hand and wrist splinting.

 g. Clinical problems: None known. Skin rash may develop from excess perspiration. Stockinette liner may be required.

 h. Precautions: Keep splint away from excessive heat. Do not leave splint in a hot car.

18. Summary

	Polycaprolactone	Other polymers	Transpolyisoprene	Other elastomers	Pigments	Fillers	Surface coating	Conformability*
Ezeform	X			X	X	X	X	L
Polyform	X	X			X	X	X	M
Polyflex II	X	X			X	X	X	H
Orthoplast			X		X	X		L
Orthoform			X		X	X	X	L
Hexcelite		X			X	X		L
Manorthos	X	X			X		X	M
Green Stripe AQ	X						X	L
Burns Quality AQ	X						X	H
Aquaplast T	X						X	M
Aquaplast Sticky	X							H
Kay Splint Series 3	X			X	X	X	X	L
Kay Splint Isoprene	X	X			X	X	X	H
Kay Splint I	X	X			X	X	X	M
JU 1000	X	X			X	X	X	M
MR 2000	X	X			X	X	X	M
RS 3000	X	X			X	X	X	L

*Conformability: *L*, low, resists stretching and fingerprints, conforms to gross contours well; *M*, general purpose; *H*, stretches easily and conforms closely to soft tissue.

C. High-temperature thermoplastics
   1. Vinyl
      a. Chemical composition: Polyvinyl chloride
      b. Advantages
        (1) Slightly elastic when hot.
        (2) Can be cut with a band saw with edges finished by sanding.
        (3) Has high-impact strength.
      c. Disadvantages
        (1) Material cannot be formed directly on the patient's skin without protective stockinette.
        (2) Does not contour as well as many of the low-temperature materials.
        (3) Does not bond to self.
      d. Heating
        (1) Working temperature 200°-225° F (93°-107° C).
        (2) May be heated in an oven or hot water. May be spot heated with heat gun.
      e. Other features
        (1) Vinyl is a smooth, transparent, blue-tinted sheet.
        (2) In hot water the material becomes cloudy.
      f. Suggested use: May be used for splints requiring strength and durability.
      g. Clinical problem: Occasional skin rash may occur. Stockinette liner may be required.
      h. Precautions: With wear or excessive force, material may fracture at narrow parts of splint.
   2. Kydex
      a. Chemical composition: Copolymer of polyvinyl chloride and acrylic.
      b. Advantage
        (1) Due to its strength, 3/16 inch of Kydex is suitable for outriggers.
      c. Disadvantages
        (1) Material cannot be formed on the skin because of the high working temperature and should be fitted on a mold or over a stockinette.
        (2) If overheated, it will form bubbles and discolor.
      d. Heating: Working temperature is 350° F (177° C). Requires dry heat oven or heat gun.
      e. Other features
        (1) Sheets of Kydex are smooth on one side and textured on the other.
        (2) The material can be cut with a band saw and finished with a file and sandpaper.
        (3) Kydex is thermoplastic and is rigid.
      f. Suggested uses: Bar design splints, outriggers.
      g. Clinical problem: Occasional skin rash may occur. Stockinette liner may be required.
      h. Precautions: When fitted on positive mold, splint may require further adjustments to accommodate hand mobility.

3. W-Clear
   a. Chemical composition: W-clear is a transparent polyester-based orthotic material (copolyester of polyethylene terephthalate).
   b. Advantages
      (1) Provides strong immobilization.
      (2) Completely transparent when hard.
      (3) Gamma ray or gas sterilizable.
   c. Disadvantages
      (1) Material must be shaped or molded over a plaster positive mold.
   d. Heating
      (1) Material softens at 175°-375° F.
      (2) Ideal temperature is approximately 325° F.
      (3) May be vacuum formed or shaped by hand wearing cotton gloves.
      (4) May be reshaped repeatedly with a heat gun.
   e. Other features: Material comes in ⅛-inch and ¹⁄₁₆-inch thicknesses.
   f. Suggested uses: Face masks, hand splints, lower extremity orthoses, burn splints.
   g. Clinical problems: None known. Skin rash may develop from excess perspiration. Stockinette liner may be required.
   h. Precautions: When fitted on positive mold, splint may require further adjustments to accommodate hand mobility.

EQUIPMENT AND SOURCES*

Equipment	Source
Supplies	
Ace bandage	Local pharmacy or surgical supply house (e.g., Abbey Medical)
Acetone (solvent for ethyl cyanoacrylate glue)	Local pharmacy or surgical supply house
Cabinets (storage)	Local hardware store
Chair with adjustable seat height for patient	Local pharmacy or surgical supply house
D rings	Splinting equipment supply house
Dressings (e.g., sterile Kling or 4- × 4-inch surgical pads)	Local pharmacy or surgical supply house
Ethyl cyanoacrylate (Permabond)	Local pharmacy surgical supply house, or drug store
Finger cuffs	Splinting equipment supply house
Fingernail clips (no. 2 dress hooks and eyes)	Local fabric store
Goniometer	Splinting equipment supply house, or local pharmacy or surgical supply house
Patterns (e.g., paper towels or surgical gloves)	

Equipment	Source
Pen (not water soluble)	
Petroleum jelly (Vaseline)	Local pharmacy or surgical supply house
Piano wire	Local music company
Rivets (rapid, pop)	Splinting equipment supply house
Rubber bands	Splinting equipment supply house
Stockinette	Local pharmacy or surgical supply house
Surgical gloves	Local pharmacy or surgical supply house
Tape (adhesive, Micropore)	Local pharmacy or surgical supply house
Velcro (1-inch hook, plain and adhesive backed; 2-, 1-, and ¾-inch loop)	Splinting equipment supply house, local pharmacy or surgical supply house

Tools

Equipment	Source
Band saw	Local hardware store
Electric drill and bits	Local hardware store
Files	Local hardware store
Goggles (safety)	Local hardware store
Hammer	Local hardware store
Heat gun and spot heater	Splinting equipment supply house
Hydrocollator	Splinting equipment supply house
Jig to construct springs	Local welding shop
Pan (jumbo electric frying— one for dry heat and one for wet heat)	Splinting equipment supply house
Pliers (needlenose)	Local hardware store
Punch (drive and rotary)	Local Tandy Leather Co. or hardware store
Ruler	Local hardware store
Sander (electric)	Local hardware store
Sandpaper	Local hardware store
Scissors	Local fabric store
Screwdrivers (Phillips and regular)	Local hardware store
Sewing machine	Local fabric store
Sink	
Vise	Local hardware store
Wire cutters	Local hardware store
Wrench (adjustable)	Local hardware store

Forms

Administration
Range of motion
Volume
Strength
Sensibility and pain
ADL/Homemaking
Orthotics/Prosthetics
Combined hand evaluation

Administration

PRESCRIPTION FORM FOR EVALUATION AND TREATMENT

Patient Name	Date
Diagnosis	

Date of Onset/Injury	Type of Surgery (if any)	Date of Surgery

Treatment and Modalities Requested:

Precautions/Comments:

Physician's Signature

Courtesy Cynthia Philips, M.A., O.T.R., A.S.H.T.

SPLINTING AND HAND THERAPY REFERRAL

Name: _____

Address: _____

Phone number: _____

Diagnosis:

Referral for extremity: ☐ Right ☐ Left

    ☐ Evaluation and report
    ☐ Evaluation and treatment
       ☐ Range of motion
       ☐ Strengthening
       ☐ Dexterity
       ☐ Sensory reeducation
       ☐ Desensitization
       ☐ Activities of daily living
       ☐ Work/home evaluation
       ☐ Joint protection (arthritic program)
       ☐ Upper extremity prosthetic training
       ☐ Upper extremity Jobst garment measurement and fitting
       ☐ Transcutaneous stimulation
       ☐ Upper extremity Jobst pump
       ☐ Other (specify): _____
    ☐ Splint fabrication:

Check joints desired to be incorporated in splint*:

Immobilize (specify position of joint in degrees)		Mobilize
	Elbow	
	Ext	
	Flex	
	Wrist	
	Ext	
	Flex	
	UD	
	RD	

SPLINTING AND HAND THERAPY REFERRAL—cont'd

Immobilize (specify position of joint in degrees)						Mobilize				
					TH	TH				
					CMC					
					Ext					
					Flex					
					Abd					
Ind	Long	Ring	Sm	Th		Th	Ind	Long	Ring	Sm
					MP					
					Ext					
					Flex					
					RD					
					UD					
					PIP (IP)					
					Ext					
					Flex					
					DIP					
					Ext					
					Flex					

*Ext, Extension; *Flex*, flexion; *RD*, radial deviation; *UD*, ulnar deviation; *MP*, metacarpophalangeal; *PIP*, proximal interphalangeal; *DIP*, distal interphalangeal; *ABD*, abduction; *Th*, thumb; *Ind*, index; *Sm*, small.

Describe the function you would like the splint or splints to provide:

The correct fabrication of the splint is important. Therefore, please call for any specific instructions (phone number _____).

NEW PATIENT FORM

Last Name   First Name

Home Address _____
    Number   Street

_____
City   State   ZIP Code

Work Telephone Number _____ _____

Home Telephone Number _____ _____

Age _____ Birthdate _____
                        Month   Date   Year

Employer: _____

Doctor's Name

Number   Street

City

State   ZIP Code

Telephone: _____

Employer's Address: _____
                Number   Street   City   State   ZIP Code

Occupation: _____ Were you injured at work? Yes _____ No _____

Injured Hand: Right _____ Left _____   Are you working now: Yes _____ No _____

Were you injured in an accident? Yes _____ No _____ Date _____

Did you have surgery? Yes _____ No _____ Date _____

Referred by: Doctor _____ Rehabilitation Nurse _____ Insurance Co. _____

FOR OFFICE USE ONLY

Compensation _____ Private _____ Date Policy Explained: _____

Insurance Co.: _____ Telephone No.: _____

Address: _____
    Number   Street   Street   City   ZIP Code

CLAIM NO.: _____

Bills should be sent to the attention of: _____

Rehabilitation Nurse: _____

Eval. Date:

Time:

Therapist:

GH/
2/15/82

Courtesy A. Gloria Hershman, O.T.R., F.A.O.T.A., A.S.H.T.

DAILY PATIENT LOG

DATE:_____ a.m.
p.m.

		N A M E										

E	VOLUME											
V	TEMPERATURE											
A	RANGE OF MOTION											
L	MUSCLE TEST											
U	SENSIBILITY											
A	COORDINATION											
T	ADL/HOMEMAKING											
I	EMPLOYMENT											
O	PROSTHETIC											
N	SPLINT											
	JOBST MEASUREMENT											
	EMG											
	NCV											
	OTHER											
	INITIAL											
	PROGRESS											
	FINAL											
T	PASSIVE EXERCISE											
R	ACTIVE EXERCISE											
E	RESISTIVE EXERCISE											
A	FUNCTIONAL ACTIVITY											
T	EARLY MOBILIZATION											
M	JOINT MOBILIZATION											
E	DESENSITIZATION											
N	SENSORY REEDUCATION											
T	DEBRIDEMENT											
	JOINT PROTECTION											
	HOME PROGRAM											
	OTHER											
M	BIOFEEDBACK											
O	ELEC STIMULATION											
D	TNS											
A	WHIRLPOOL											
L	HOT PACKS											
I	PARAFFIN											
T	FLUIDOTHERAPY											
I	INTERMIT PRESSURE											
E	OTHER											
S												
S	IMMOBILIZATION											
P	MOBILIZATION											
L	SIMPLE											
I	COMPOUND											
N	COMPLEX											
T	EQUIPMENT											
S	OTHER											

Therapist: _____

		Upper Extremity Assessment Battery
NAME	DATE OF SERVICE	
THERAPIST	LOCATION	**HAND THERAPY ROUTING SLIP**
DIAGNOSIS		

CODE		DESCRIPTION	CODE		DESCRIPTION
9770		ADL EVALUATION	29126		DYNAMIC ARM/HAND SPLINT
97720		STRENGTH/CO-ORD EVALUATION	291301		JOINT JACK
95832		MUSCLE TEST HAND	291302		FINGER GUTTER
95852		ROM TEST HAND	291303		ALUMNA FOAM SPLINT
95999		SENSORY EVALUATION	291304		STAX SPLINT
			29131		LMB-DYNAMIC FINGER SPLINT
97110		THERAPEUTIC EXERCISE - 30'	29260		ELBOW/WRIST STRAP
97112		NEUROMUSCULAR RE-ED - 30'	29280		TENNIS ELBOW STRAP
97114		FUNCTIONAL ACTIVITIES - 30'	292801		HAND/FINGER STRAP
97124		RETRO/FRICTION MASSAGE	977991		REPAIR/REVISION SPLINT
97145		PHYSICAL MED-ADD'L 15'			
97540		ADL TRAINING - 30'	29799		COMPRESSION DRESSING
97541		ADL TRAINING - ADD'L 15'	990701		ACE BANDAGE
97500		ORTHOTIC TRAINING - 30'	990702		DERMAL PADS
97501		ORTHOTIC TRAINING-ADD'L 15'	990703		ELASTOMER MOLD/UNIT
97520		PROSTHETIC TRAINING - 30'	990704		PROSTHETIC FOAM MOLD/UNIT
97521		PROSTHETIC TRNG - ADD'L 15'	990705		COBAN
97740		KINETIC ACTIVITIES - 30'	990706		TUBIGRIP/UNIT
97741		KINETIC ACT - ADD'L 15'	990707		THERAPY PUTTY - 2 OZ./UNIT
97139		HOME PROGRAM	990708		HAND HELPER EXERCISE AID
971391		(SPECIFY)	990709		SWANSON GRIP X
97799		JOBST MEASUREMENT/FITTING	9907010		THERABAND/UNIT
97010		HOT/COLD PACKS	9907011		SPONGE EXERCISER
97016		VASOPNEUMATIC DEVICE	9907012		COMPRESSION GLOVE
97018		PARAFFIN BATH	9907013		ISOTONER GLOVE
97022		WHIRLPOOL	9907014		FLEXION GLOVE
97118		ELECTRICAL STIMULATION	9907015		EXERCISE STABILIZER
97126		CONTRAST BATH	9907016		SENSORY STICKS/UNIT
97039		TENS	9907017		DYNAGRIP
90900		BIOFEEDBACK TRAINING	9907018		T FOAM SHEET/UNIT
90906		THERMAL FEEDBACK TRAINING	9907019		(SPECIFY)
970391		(SPECIFY)			
			97003		OFFICE VISIT 45'
29105		LONG ARM SPLINT			
29125		STATIC SHORT ARM/HAND SP.			**DAILY TOTAL - $** _____

Courtesy Joan E. Sullivan, M.A.O.T., O.T.R., A.S.H.T.

STATEMENT

PATIENT

CHARGES OR
PAYMENTS MADE
AFTER LAST DATE
SHOWN WILL APPEAR
ON YOUR NEXT
STATEMENT

BALANCE
FORWARD

TH. IN	DATE	DETAIL	CHARGES	PAYMENTS	BALANCE

SAFEGUARD

PLEASE PAY LAST AMOUNT IN BALANCE COLUMN →

TAXPAYER IDENTIFICATION NUMBER

EVS—Evaluation Session
CTS—Clinic Treatment Session
HPE—Home Program and Exercises
WTS—Work Tolerance Session
EVT—Evaluation Time
CTT—Clinic Treatment Time
SHS—Simple Hand Splint
    Fabrication and Materials
CHS—Complex Hand Splint
    Fabrication and Materials

SPF—Splint Fitting
SPA—Splint Adjustment
SPL—Splint
WS—Wire Splint
BA—Bandaging
FH—Finger Hooks
SPG—Splint Glue
JF—Jobst Fitting
JC—Jobst Check
TH—Theraplast

ISG—Stretch Glove/Isotoner
PNF—P.N.F.
NC—Nivea Cream/Lanolin
FLG—Flexion Glove
HHE—Hand Helper Exerciser
MS—Medical Supply
ES—Electric Stim
TENS—Trams Nerve Stim
BIO—Biofeedback

Courtesy A. Gloria Hershman, O.T.R., F.A.O.T.A., A.S.H.T.

VENDOR BILLS TO BE PAID

VENDOR NAME	AMOUNT	P	DATE PAID	CHECK #	INITIALS

TOTAL$ _____

Courtesy A. Gloria Hershman, O.T.R., F.A.O.T.A., A.S.H.T.

Range of motion

RANGE OF MOTION
HAND

DATE:	THUMB	CHANGE +/−	INDEX	CHANGE +/−	LONG	CHANGE +/−	RING	CHANGE +/−	SMALL	CHANGE +/−
MP	( )	( )	( )	( )	( )	( )	( )	( )	( )	( )
PIP	IP ( )	( )	( )	( )	( )	( )	( )	( )	( )	( )
DIP	CMC ( )	( )	( )	( )	( )	( )	( )	( )	( )	( )
TAM (TPM)	( )	( )	( )	( )	( )	( )	( )	( )	( )	( )

DATE:	THUMB	CHANGE +/−	INDEX	CHANGE +/−	LONG	CHANGE +/−	RING	CHANGE +/−	SMALL	CHANGE +/−
MP	( )	( )	( )	( )	( )	( )	( )	( )	( )	( )
PIP	IP ( )	( )	( )	( )	( )	( )	( )	( )	( )	( )
DIP	CMC ( )	( )	( )	( )	( )	( )	( )	( )	( )	( )
TAM (TPM)	( )	( )	( )	( )	( )	( )	( )	( )	( )	( )

DATE:	THUMB	CHANGE +/−	INDEX	CHANGE +/−	LONG	CHANGE +/−	RING	CHANGE +/−	SMALL	CHANGE +/−
MP	( )	( )	( )	( )	( )	( )	( )	( )	( )	( )
PIP	IP ( )	( )	( )	( )	( )	( )	( )	( )	( )	( )
DIP	CMC ( )	( )	( )	( )	( )	( )	( )	( )	( )	( )
TAM (TPM)	( )	( )	( )	( )	( )	( )	( )	( )	( )	( )

KEY:

Active: extension/flexion
Passive: (extension/flexion)
Thumb CMC: adduction/abduction
Change: record in red

Name: _____
Number: _____
Hand: _____

RANGE OF MOTION
WRIST, FOREARM, ELBOW, SHOULDER

		DATE:			DATE:			DATE:		
			CHANGE +/−			CHANGE +/−			CHANGE +/−	
W R I S T	EXTENSION	(	) (	)	(	) (	)	(	) (	)
	FLEXION	(	) (	)	(	) (	)	(	) (	)
	RADIAL DEVIATION	(	) (	)	(	) (	)	(	) (	)
	ULNAR DEVIATION	(	) (	)	(	) (	)	(	) (	)
F O R E A R M **E L B O W**	SUPINATION	(	) (	)	(	) (	)	(	) (	)
	PRONATION	(	) (	)	(	) (	)	(	) (	)
	EXTENSION	(	) (	)	(	) (	)	(	) (	)
	FLEXION	(	) (	)	(	) (	)	(	) (	)
S H O U L D E R	EXTENSION	(	) (	)	(	) (	)	(	) (	)
	FLEXION	(	) (	)	(	) (	)	(	) (	)
	ABDUCTION	(	) (	)	(	) (	)	(	) (	)
	INTERNAL ROTATION	(	) (	)	(	) (	)	(	) (	)
	EXTERNAL ROTATION	(	) (	)	(	) (	)	(	) (	)

KEY:
    Active: #0
    Passive: (#0   )
    Change: Record in red

Name: _____

Number: _____

Extremity: _____

SUMMARY SHEET
TOTAL ACTIVE MOTION / TOTAL PASSIVE MOTION

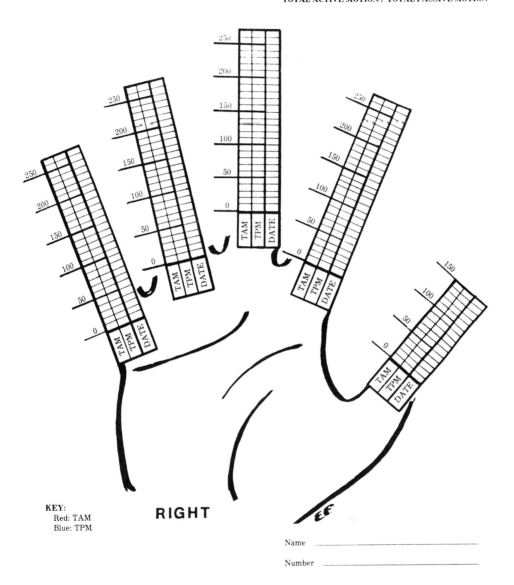

KEY:
Red: TAM
Blue: TPM

RIGHT

Name _____

Number _____

EXAMPLE OF COMPLETED ROM FORM

DATE: 8-17-84	THUMB	CHANGE +/−		INDEX	CHANGE +/−		LONG	CHANGE +/−		RING	CHANGE +/−		SMALL	CHANGE +/−	
MP	( )	(	)	30/70 (0/90)	+ 10 (	)	10/30 ( )	(	)	( )	(	)	( )	(	)
PIP	IP ( )	(	)	45/60 (0/90)	+ 15 (	)	30/45 ( )	(	)	( )	(	)	( )	(	)
DIP	CMC ( )	(	)	10/80 (0/90)	+ 5 (	)	0/75 ( )	(	)	( )	(	)	( )	(	)
TAM (TPM)	( )	(	)	125 (270)	(	)	110 ( )	(	)	( )	(	)	( )	(	)

*Total motion provides a single numerical value for composite digital motion: summation of digit flexion (30 + 45 + 75 = 150); summation of digit-extension deficits (10 + 30 + 0 = 40); flexion sum minus extension deficit sum (150 - 40 = 110); total active motion of digit = 110 degrees. (Long Finger)

Volume

VOLUME

VOLUMETER MEASUREMENTS:

Date _____ Date _____ Date _____ Date _____ Date _____ Date _____

800 ml						
700 ml						
600 ml						
500 ml						
400 ml						
300 ml						
200 ml						

NORMAL VOLUME (opposite hand): _____ ml.

CIRCUMFERENCE / DIAMETER c:

Biceps* _____ _____ _____ _____ _____ _____

Forearm* _____ _____ _____ _____ _____ _____

DPC _____ _____ _____ _____ _____ _____

Digit (_____) _____ _____ _____ _____ _____ _____

NORMAL MEASUREMENT (opposite hand):

Biceps _____ Forearm _____ DPC _____ Digit _____

c Circle method used.

* 10 cm. above/below the medial
   epicondyle of the humerus

Name: _____

Number: _____

Hand: _____

Strength

JAYMAR DYNAMOMETER # _____

	1st	2nd	3rd	4th	5th
150					
140					
130					
120					
110					
100					
90					
80					
70					
60					
50					
40					
30					
20					
10					
0					

A V E R A G E P O U N D S

TRIALS:　　　　　　HANDLE POSITION

NORMAL

Date _____ (———)

	1st	2nd	3rd	4th	5th
(1)	_____	_____	_____	_____	_____
(2)	_____ *	_____ *	_____ *	_____ *	_____
(3)	_____	_____	_____	_____	_____
Average:	_____	_____	_____	_____	_____

Date _____ (· · · · ·)

	1st	2nd	3rd	4th	5th
(1)	_____	_____	_____	_____	_____
(2)	_____ *	_____ *	_____ *	_____ *	_____
(3)	_____	_____	_____	_____	_____
Average:	_____	_____	_____	_____	_____

Date _____ (· · · · ·)

	1st	2nd	3rd	4th	5th
(1)	_____	_____	_____	_____	_____
(2)	_____ *	_____ *	_____ *	_____ *	_____
(3)	_____	_____	_____	_____	_____
Average:	_____	_____	_____	_____	_____

Date _____ (xxxxx)

	1st	2nd	3rd	4th	5th
(1)	_____	_____	_____	_____	_____
(2)	_____ *	_____ *	_____ *	_____ *	_____
(3)	_____	_____	_____	_____	_____
Average:	_____	_____	_____	_____	_____

* 5 Minute rest period.

Name _____

Number _____

Hand _____

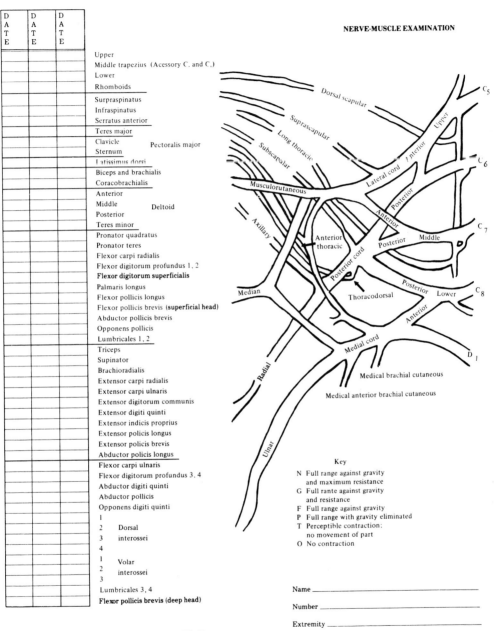

NERVE-MUSCLE EXAMINATION

	DATE	DATE	DATE
Upper			
Middle trapezius (Acessory C. and C.)			
Lower			
Rhomboids			
Surpraspinatus			
Infraspinatus			
Serratus anterior			
Teres major			
Clavicle — Pectoralis major			
Sternum			
Latissimus dorsi			
Biceps and brachialis			
Coracobrachialis			
Anterior			
Middle — Deltoid			
Posterior			
Teres minor			
Pronator quadratus			
Pronator teres			
Flexor carpi radialis			
Flexor digitorum profundus 1, 2			
Flexor digitorum superficialis			
Palmaris longus			
Flexor pollicis longus			
Flexor pollicis brevis **(superficial head)**			
Abductor pollicis brevis			
Opponens pollicis			
Lumbricales 1, 2			
Triceps			
Supinator			
Brachioradialis			
Extensor carpi radialis			
Extensor carpi ulnaris			
Extensor digitorum communis			
Extensor digiti quinti			
Extensor indicis proprius			
Extensor policis longus			
Extensor policis brevis			
Abductor policis longus			
Flexor carpi ulnaris			
Flexor digitorum profundus 3, 4			
Abductor digiti quinti			
Abductor pollicis			
Opponens digiti quinti			
1			
2 — Dorsal			
3 — interossei			
4			
1			
2 — Volar			
3 — interossei			
Lumbricales 3, 4			
Flexor pollicis brevis (deep head)			

Key
N Full range against gravity
and maximum resistance
G Full rante against gravity
and resistance
F Full range against gravity
P Full range with gravity eliminated
T Perceptible contraction;
no movement of part
O No contraction

Name _____

Number _____

Extremity _____

Adapted from form by Lorraine F. Lake, Ph.D.

Sensibility and pain

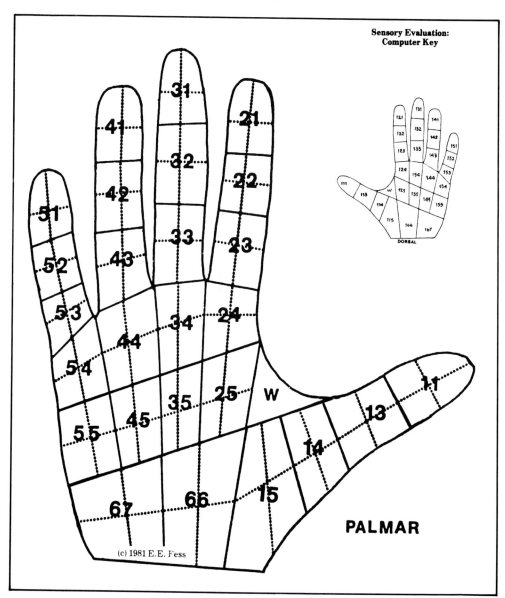

Sensory Evaluation:
Computer Key

PALMAR

(c) 1981 E.E. Fess

Longitudinal:
10s = Thumb ray
20s = Index ray
30s = Long ray
40s = Ring ray
50s = Small ray
60s = Carpus*

Transverse:
1s = Distal phalanx
2s = Middle phalanx
3s = Proximal phalanx
4s = Distal palm
5s = Mid palm
6/7s = Proximal palm*

Anterior/Posterior
10s = Volar
100s = Dorsal

Subdivisions:
D = Distal
P = Proximal
R = Radial
U = Ulnar

*Modification suggested by J. Bell, 1982.

**SENSORY EVALUATION:
TINEL'S SIGN & TROPHIC CHANGES**

Tinel's Sign	Ninhydrin/Wrinkle

Date _____

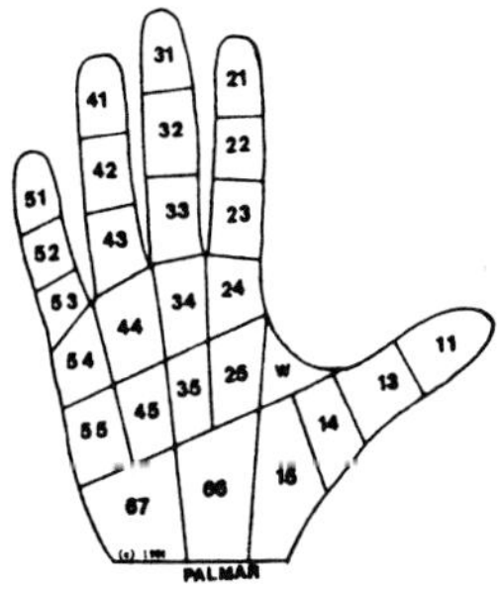

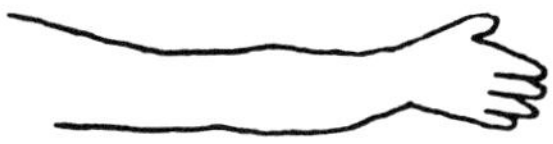

Date _____

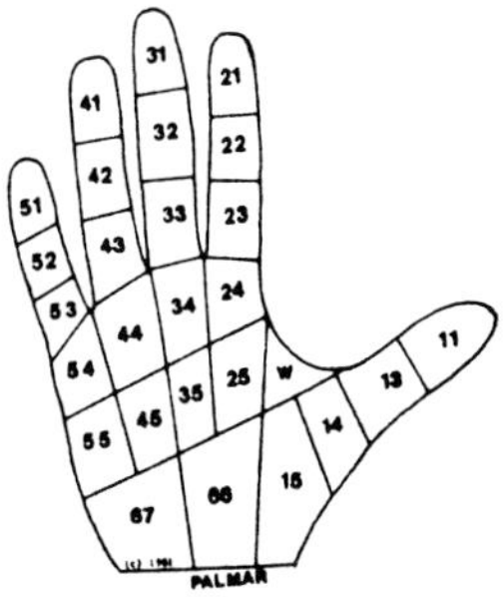

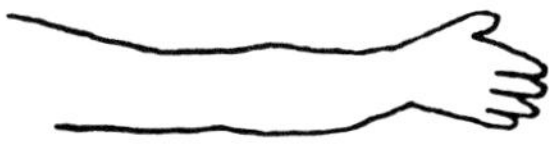

Date _____

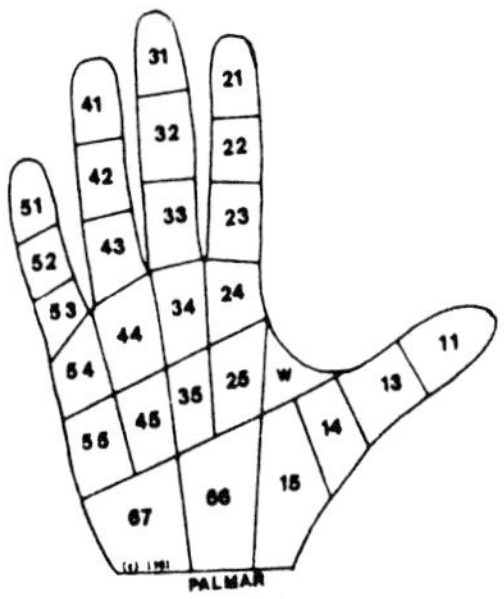

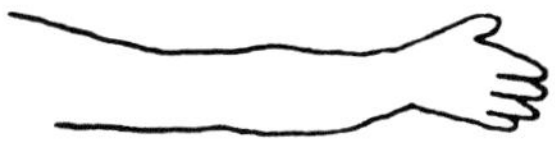

KEY:

☒ Tinel's

⬚ Ninhydrin

▨ Wrinkle

Name _____

Number _____

Hand _____

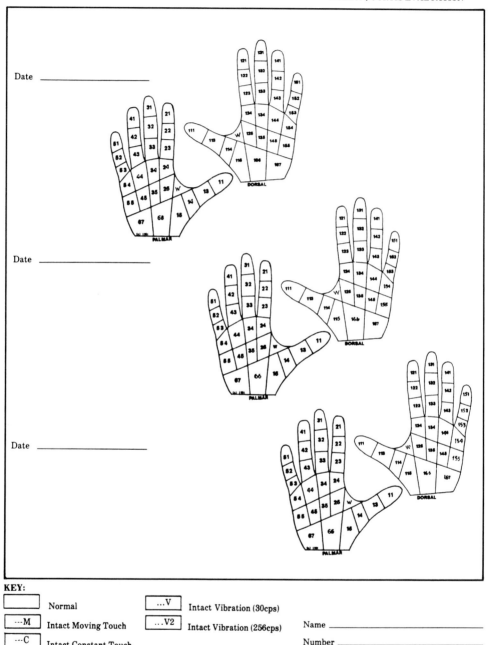

Date _____

Date _____

Date _____

KEY:

	Normal
---M	Intact Moving Touch
---C	Intact Constant Touch

...V	Intact Vibration (30cps)
...V2	Intact Vibration (256cps)

Name _____

Number _____

Hand _____

SENSORY EVALUATION:
SEMMES-WEINSTEIN CALIBRATED MONOFILAMENTS

PALMAR/DORSAL   (circle):

Date:	Thumb U—1—R	Index U—2—R	Long U—3—R	Ring U—4—R	Small U—5—R
_1					
_2					
_3					
_4					
_5					
_6/_7	////	_6_		_6_	

PALMAR/DORSAL   (circle):

Date:	Thumb U—1—R	Index U—2—R	Long U—3—R	Ring U—4—R	Small U—5—R
_1					
_2					
_3					
_4					
_5					
_6/_7	////	_6_		_6_	

PALMAR/DORSAL   (circle):

Date:	Thumb U—1—R	Index U—2—R	Long U—3—R	Ring U—4—R	Small U—5—R
_1					
_2					
_3					
_4					
_5					
_6/_7	////	_6_		_6_	

KEY:*

		Filament	Pressure
	Normal	1.65 - 2.83	1.45 - 4.86
Blue	Dimished light touch	3.22 - 3.61	11.1 - 17.7
Purple	Diminished protective sensation	3.84 - 4.31	19.3 - 33.1
Red	Loss of protective sensation	4.56 - 6.65	47.3 - 439.0
Red-lined	Untestable	6.65	439.0

*Levine, S., Pearsall, G., & Ruderman, R.: J Hand Surg., 3:211, 1978.   (gm/mm2)

Name _____

Number _____

Hand _____

SENSORY EVALUATION:
2 POINT DISCRIMINATION

PALMAR/DORSAL   (circle):

Date:	Thumb 1 U — R	Index 2 U — R	Long 3 U — R	Ring 4 U — R	Small 5 U — R
_1					
_2					
_3					
_4					
_5					
_6/_7	////////	_6_		_6_	

PALMAR/DORSAL   (circle):

Date:	Thumb 1 U — R	Index 2 U — R	Long 3 U — R	Ring 4 U — R	Small 5 U — R
_1					
_2					
_3					
_4					
_5					
_6/_7	////////	_6_		_6_	

PALMAR/DORSAL   (circle):

Date:	Thumb 1 U — R	Index 2 U — R	Long 3 U — R	Ring 4 U — R	Small 5 U — R
_1					
_2					
_3					
_4					
_5					
_6/_7	////////	_6_		_6_	

KEY:*

	Normal	Less than 6mm
Blue	Fair	6 - 10mm
Purple	Poor	11 - 15mm
Orange	Protective	One point perceived
Orange-lined	Anesthetic	No point perceived

***ASSH:** *The hand - examination and diagnosis,* Aurora, Colorado 1978.

Name _____

Number _____

Hand _____

SENSORY EVALUATION:
MOVING 2 POINT DISCRIMINATION & RIDGE TEST

Moving Two Point Discrimination

PALMAR/DORSAL (circle):

Date:	Thumb U—1—R	Index U—2—R	Long U—3—R	Ring U—4—R	Small U—5—R
1					
2					
3					
4					
5				6	
6/ 7		6			

PALMAR/DORSAL (circle):

Date:	Thumb U—1—R	Index U—2—R	Long U—3—R	Ring U—4—R	Small U—5—R
1					
2					
3					
4					
5				6	
6/ 7		6			

PALMAR/DORSAL (circle):

Date:	Thumb U—1—R	Index U—2—R	Long U—3—R	Ring U—4—R	Small U—5—R
1					
2					
3					
4					
5				6	
6/ 7		6			

(mm)

Ridge Test

PALMAR/DORSAL (circle):

Date:	Thumb U—1—R	Index U—2—R	Long U—3—R	Ring U—4—R	Small U—5—R
1					
2					
3					
4					
5				6	
6/ 7		6			

PALMAR/DORSAL (circle):

Date:	Thumb U—1—R	Index U—2—R	Long U—3—R	Ring U—4—R	Small U—5—R
1					
2					
3					
4					
5				6	
6/ 7		6			

PALMAR/DORSAL (circle):

Date:	Thumb U—1—R	Index U—2—R	Long U—3—R	Ring U—4—R	Small U—5—R
1					
2					
3					
4					
5				6	
6/ 7		6			

(cm)

Name _____
Number _____
Hand _____

Proprioception & Hypersensitivity

Date _____

Date _____

Date _____

KEY:

| ✓ | Intact proprioception |

| * | Hypersensitivity |

Moberg Picking Up Test:

Date:							
	R	L	R	L	R	L	(seconds)
Without Blindfold	/		/		/		
With Blindfold							
Identification	/		/		/		

Patient's Subjective Estimate of Sensation:

"If this is a $1.00," (touch normal area)
"how much would this be in comparison? (touch symptomatic area)*

$.10   .20   .30   .40   .50   .60   .70   .80   .90   (circle and date)

Pain: *G. Blatt, M.D., 9/82*

Date:			
With Motion			
Without Motion			
Stops Activity			

Name _____

Number _____

Hand _____

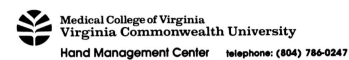

Medical College of Virginia
Virginia Commonwealth University

Hand Management Center   telephone: **(804) 786-0247**

PAIN EVALUATION

Name _____   Date _____

Right Arm

INTENSITY

UNPLEASANTNESS

DORSAL   PALMAR

Courtesy Karen Hull Prendergast, M.A., R.P.T.

ADL/Homemaking

ADL EVALUATION

Rating guide
✔ = Normal performance
0 = Impossible
+ = Adequate with mechanical aid
– = Awkward or slow
N = Not indicated for testing

Activity	Date	Comments
Feeding		
Eating with fingers		
Eating with spoon		
Eating with fork		
Cut with knife		
Cut with fork		
Drink from cup		
Drink from glass		
Drink from straw		
Drink from pitcher		
Butter bread		
Serve from one dish to another		
Dressing		
Put on-remove		
Gloves		
Overcoat		
Overshoes		
Trousers or shirt		
Shirt or blouse		
Slip over garment		
Shoes		
Hose		
Bra		
Girdle		
Underpants		
Catheter bag		
Eyeglasses		
Clothes from hanger		
Tie bow or tie		
Manipulate		
Shoelaces		
Buttons		
Zippers		
Hygiene		
Turn on faucet		
Turn off faucet		
Brush teeth		
Wash extremities (sponge bath)		
Wash face		
Comb, brush hair		
Flush toilet		
Adjust clothing		
Use urinal		
Shave or apply cosmetics		
Shampoo, set hair		
Use handkerchief		
Clean eyeglasses		
Care for fingernails		
Care for toenails		

Activity	Date	Comments
Communication, utilities		
Operate light switch:		
Toggle		
Wall plug		
Hanging cord		
Table lamp		
Plug in cord		
Wrap, unwrap package		
Use telephone		
Write		
Use typewriter		
Hold newspaper, book		
Turn pages		
Handle money, use purse		
Handle own mail		
Sharpen pencil		
Use scissors		
Turn radio, television		
Wind watch or clock		
Open and close:		
Pull drawers		
Spring lock		
Padlock		
Latched cupboard door		
Slide bolt latch		
Trunk and suitcase latches		
Blinds, window shade		
Sash window		
Roll-out window		
Gate hook		
Door		
Car door		
Play/work		
Put object in pocket		
Remove object from pocket		
Light cigarette—match		
Light cigarette— lighter		
Use safety pin		
Use needle and thread		
Shuffle cards		
Pick up object:		
From floor		
From table		
Heavy object		
Small object		
High object		
Additional remarks:		

Name
Number
Hand

HOMEMAKING EVALUATION

Rating guide:

- ✓ = Normal performance
- O = Impossible
- + = Adequate with mechanical aid
- ± = Normal, but awkward or slow
- N = Not indicated for testing

Activity	Date	Comments
Cleaning		
Pick up objects from floor		
Wipe up spills		
Make bed (daily)		
Use dust mop		
Dust high surfaces		
Mop floor		
Sweep with broom		
Use dust pan, broom		
Use vacuum cleaner		
Carry light cleaning tools		
Clean bathtub		
Meal preparation		
Carry pan of water		
Turn on water		
Turn on stove		
Pour hot water		
Open packaged goods		
Carry pan from sink to stove		
Use can opener		
Handle milk bottle		
Dispose of garbage		
Remove things from refrigerator		
Bend to low cupboards		
Reach to high cupboards		
Peel vegetables		
Cut up food		
Handle sharp tools safely		
Break an egg		
Stir against resistance		
Use egg beater		
Measure flour		
Remove batter to pan		
Open oven door		
Put pan in and out of oven		
Roll dough		
Store to serving dishes		
Unscrew jar top		

Activity	Date	Comments
Meal service		
Set table		
Carry hot food to table		
Clear table		
Scrape and stack dishes		
Wash dishes		
Wipe silver		
Wash pots and pans		
Wipe up stove and work areas		
Wring dish cloth		
Carry glasses		
Laundry		
Wash lingerie		
Wring out, squeeze		
Hang to dry		
Sprinkle clothes		
Iron blouse or slip		
Fold ironed clothes		
Use washer and dryer		
Sewing		
Thread needle, make knot		
Sew on buttons		
Mend rip		
Darn socks		
Use sewing machine		
Crochet		
Knit		
Embroider		
Cut with shears		
Heavy household activities		
Household laundry, washing		
Hanging clothes		
Clean range, refrigerator		
Wax floors		
Marketing		
Turn mattresses		
Wash windows		
Put up curtains		
Clean rugs		

Name _____

Number _____

Hand _____

Orthotics/Prosthetics

SPLINT CHECKOUT FORM

	Yes	No	Comments
DESIGN			
Does the splint meet general design concepts, including adaptation for:			
1. Individual patient factors			
2. Total utilization time			
3. Simplicity			
4. Optimum function			
5. Optimum sensation			
6. Efficient construction and fit			
7. Ease of application and removal			
8. Exercise regimen			
Does the splint meet specific design concepts, including adaptation for:			
9. Influencing key joints			
10. Attaining purpose			
a. Augment passive motion			
b. Substitute for active motion			
11. Types of forces used			
12. Surface of application			
13. Anatomic variables			
14. Material properties			
MECHANICS			
Does the splint meet specific mechanical concepts, including adaptation for:			
1. Reduction of pressure			
2. Increased mechanical advantage (Ratio of FA to RA)			
3. Optimum rotational force (90°)			
4. Torque			
5. Variance of passive mobility of successive joints			
6. Optimum utilization of parallel forces			
7. Material strength			
8. Elimination of friction			

SPLINT CHECKOUT FORM—cont'd

	Yes	No	Comments
CONSTRUCTION			
Has the splint been fabricated appropriately to provide:			
1. Good cosmesis			
2. Rounded corners			
3. Smooth edges and surfaces			
4. Stable joints			
5. Finished rivets			
6. Ventilation			
7. Secure padding			
8. Secure straps			
FIT			
Has the splint been fitted appropriately to adapt to:			
1. Bony prominences			
2. Dual obliquity			
3. Ligamentous stress			
4. Arches			
5. Joint axis alignment			
6. Skin creases			
7. Kinematic changes			
8. Kinetic concepts			
DYNAMIC ASSIST(S)			
Does each dynamic assist meet appropriate requisites for:			
1. Magnitude of force application			
2. Physical properties correlated with patient needs			
3. Physical properties correlated with splint design			
4. Mechanical concepts			
a. 90° rotational force			
b. Torque			
c. Pressure			
5. Fit			
a. Ligamentous stress			
b. Kinematic changes			
c. Kinetic changes			
6. Maintenance of force magnitude			

SPLINT INSTRUCTIONS

Patient _____ Date _____

A _____ splint has been made for you. The purpose of the splint is to

_____

_____.

You are to wear the splint _____.

Other instructions for you to follow are: _____

_____

_____

_____

_____.

Precautions:

1. Note any areas of redness, pressure, or rash on your skin or any pain or numbness. If any of these problems develop *notify therapist* to have necessary adjustments made.
2. Keep splint away from heat such as a stove or heating unit. Do not leave your splint in the car in the hot weather. The heat will soften the splint and change its shape.
3. The splint may be cleaned with mild soap and cool water. The inside of the splint may be cleaned with rubbing alcohol. The pieces of stockinette given to you with your splint should be worn under the splint and should be kept clean.

If you have any further questions or if any problems develop with the splint contact your therapist.

Therapist: _____

Phone: _____

Courtesy Cynthia Philips, M.A., O.T.R.

INSTRUCTIONS FOR
PROPER CARE AND WEARING OF SPLINTS

Your splint was constructed for you; if you have any questions concerning its proper application, fit, or wearing schedule, please contact the hand rehabilitation center.

Please read the following instructions for proper care and wearing of your splint.

Precautions

1. Contact the hand rehabilitation center if your splint causes:
   a. Excessive swelling or stiffness
   b. Severe pain
   c. Pressure area (an irritated skin area resembling the beginning of a blister).
   d. A skin rash on areas in direct contact with the splint.
2. Splints should not be used while operating machinery unless you have specific permission from your physician.
3. Your splint will lose its shape if exposed to heat sources such as radiator, stove, or being left on a car seat during the summer.

Adjustments in rubber band tension

1. A light steady pull (approximately 8 ounces) on your fingers is better than a strong pull.
2. If rubber bands become stretched, replace them with new ones.

Cleaning your splint

1. Your splint may be cleaned with soap and lukewarm (never hot) water when perspiration and dirt collect inside. To thoroughly clean straps, it may be necessary to scrub them with a small brush.
2. For ink or spots that are difficult to remove, use a cleanser with chlorine.
3. If your sutures have been removed and your wound closed and you have no pins protruding from your skin, you may use talcum powder or cornstarch on your hand and arm to help absorb excess moisture.

Wear

☐ Night and rest periods only.
☐ Daytime: for _____ minutes/hours at a time, _____ times a day.
☐ Remove splint every _____, and do active and/or passive range-of-motion exercises.
☐ _____

_____

_____

_____

**UPPER EXTREMITY AMPUTEE
PROSTHESIS CHECKOUT**

Amputee type: R _____ L _____ BE _____ AE _____ SD _____ WD _____ ED _____ Other _____

	Test	Performance	Standard
I	Conformance to prescription		Conform to written prescription
II	Workmanship and appearance		
III	Control system efficiency	Hook Hand	
	1. Force applied at terminal device	_____ lb _____ lb	B/E should be 70% or greater.
	2. Force applied at harness	_____ lb _____ lb	A/E should be 50% or greater.
	3. Efficiency = $\dfrac{\text{Force at T.D.}}{\text{Force at harness}}$	_____ % _____ %	
IV	Compression fit and comfort		Socket compression should cause no pain or discomfort.
V	Tension stability	_____ in displacement	50 lb (or ⅓ body weight) axial pull should not displace socket more than 1 in. Harness should not fail.
VI	Terminal device—opening and closing	Hook Hand	Full opening and closing should be obtained with forearm at 90°.
	1. Mechanical range	_____ in _____ in	
	2. Active range (forearm at 90°)	_____ in _____ in	B/E 70% (A/E 50%) opening at mouth and waist.
	3. Active range (waist)	_____ in _____ in	
	4. Active range (mouth)	_____ in _____ in	

Date: _____   Patient: _____

Additional below-elbow specifications

VII	Amount of forearm	Prosthesis off _____ Prosthesis on _____	Should be within 10° of range with prosthesis off, except for very short stumps
VIII	Amount of forearm rotation	Prosthesis off _____ Prosthesis on _____	Total rotation with prosthesis should be half that with prosthesis off (Practical only for long B/E and W/D)
IX	Placement of artificial elbow		Should be not more than below normal elbow on adult
X	Range of glenohumeral motion with prosthesis on	Abduction Flexion Extension Rotation	90° 90° 30° Prosthesis on Variable
XI	Glenohumeral flexion required to flex forearm fully	_____ °	Should not exceed 45°
	Prosthetic elbow—mechanical range	_____ °	To 135°
	Prosthetic elbow—active range	_____ °	To 135°
XII	Force required to initiate forearm flexion from a position of 90° flexed	_____ lb	Should not exceed the force necessary to open terminal device or 10 lb
XIII	Socket rotation stability		Resist force of 3 lb 12 in from elbow center Applied laterally and medially

Prosthesis passed _____   Prosthesis rejected _____

Returned for following reasons: _____

_____

_____   Patient _____

From Prosthetic-Orthotic Department at Northwestern University, Chicago.

Combined hand evaluation

HAND EVALUATION

Patient Name		Occupation	
Date of Evaluation	Dominant Hand ☐ Left ☐ Right		Affected Hand ☐ Left ☐ Right
Diagnosis			

RANGE OF MOTION					
		Right		**Left**	
		Active	Passive	Active	Passive
Wrist	Elbow Ex/Flex				
	Forearm Pron/Sup				
	Dorsiflex/Palmar Flex				
	Radial Dev./Ulnar Dev.				
Thumb	Radial/Palmar Abd.				
	MP Ext/Flex./IP Ext/Flex				
	Opp. to Tip of 5th Finger				
	Opp. to 5th MP Crease				
Index	MCP Ext/Flex				
	PIP Ext/Flex				
	DIP Ext./Flex				
	Flex to Palmar Crease				
Middle	MCP Ext/Flex				
	PIP Ext/Flex				
	DIP Ext/Flex				
	Flexion to Palmar Crease				
Ring	MCP Ext/Flex				
	PIP Ext/Flex				
	DIP Ext/Flex				
	Flexion to Palmar Crease				
Little	MCP Ext/Flex				
	PIP Ext/Flex				
	Dip Ext/Flex				
	Flexion to Palmar Crease				

7092 5/86

Courtesy Cynthia Philips, M.A. O.T.R.

Hand Evaluation (cont.)

Grip Strength:		Pinch Strength: Lateral		Pulp:		3-Jaw Pinch (3-Point)	
R:	L:	R:	Lat. L:	R:	L:	R:	L:
Circumference Around Forearm		Hand Spread-Tip of Thumb to 5th Finger		Circumferential Measurement - Around MCP Joints			
R:	L:	R:	L:	R:	L:		
Circ. Measurement - Around Wrist		Volumeter Measurement					
R:	L:	R:	L:				

Treatment Goals:

Circumferential Measure: Around PIP Joint	
R	L
I:	I:
M:	M:
R:	R:
L:	L:

Plan:

Comments:

Signature of Therapist

Splint room organization

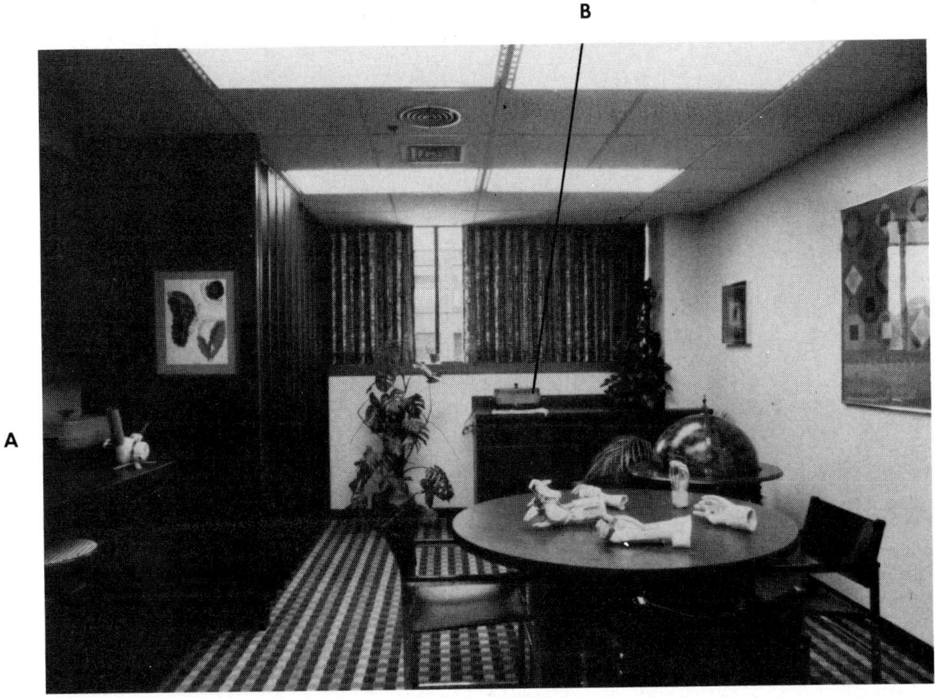

B

A

Fig. D-1. This room was designed to serve two purposes. With the folding doors closed and equipment in cabinets, it is used as a small conference room. During patient office hours, it is quickly converted to an efficient splinting area large enough to accommodate two therapists and four or five patients at a time. A "dry" **(A)** and a "wet" **(B)** skillet allow low-temperature splinting materials to be preheated and held at the malleable stage until needed.

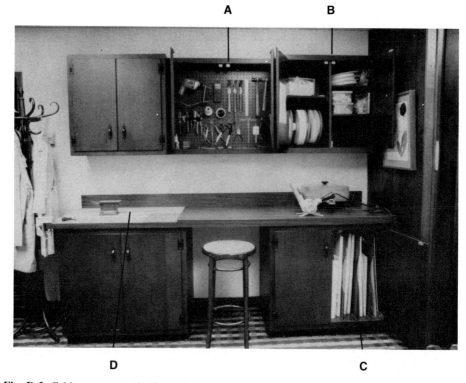

Fig. D-2. Cabinets are specifically designed for storage of **(A)** tools, **(B)** Velcro, and **(C)** plastics. The finished cabinet top **(D)** slides off to expose a workbench suitable for working with equipment such as hand tools and vises.

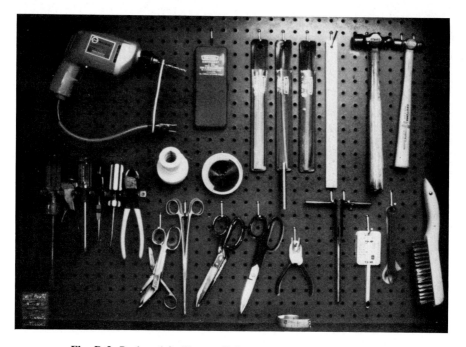

Fig. D-3. Pegboard facilitates efficient storage of small hand tools.

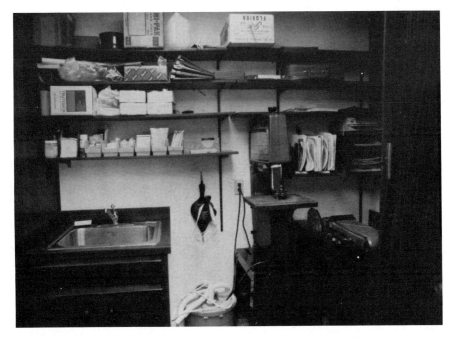

Fig. D-4. Heavy power equipment, a sink, and additional storage shelves are hidden behind the folding door, which may be opened at either end. The sander and band saw are attached to a portable vacuum system to reduce shavings and dust in the area.

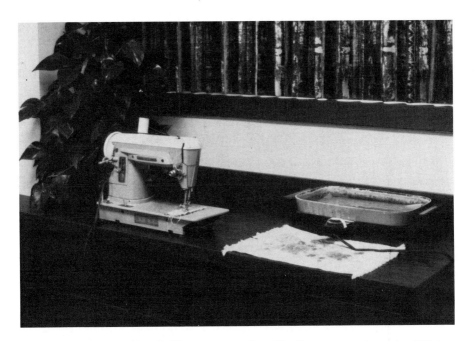

Fig. D-5. A sewing maching facilitates construction of splint components made of Velcro or cloth. A drying towel is placed next to the wet-heat skillet.

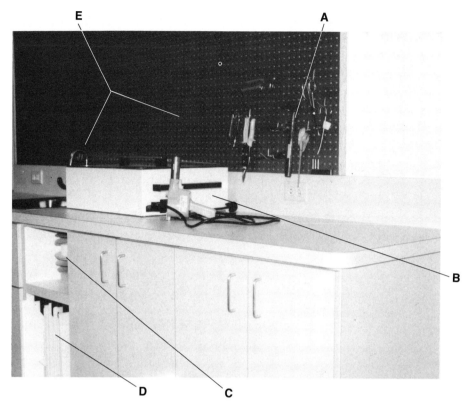

Fig. D-6. Another example of splint room organization: **(A)** Tools, **(B)** heating equipment, **(C)** Velcro, **(D)** plastics, and **(E)** space for display of splint samples.

American Society for Surgery of the Hand clinical assessment recommendations*

A. Sensibility

Apply two-point discrimination with a blunt instrument in a longitudinal axis of the digit. Do not blanch the skin.

Ratings:

1. Normal, less than 6 mm
2. Fair, 6 to 10 mm
3. Poor, 11 to 15 mm
4. Protective, one point perceived
5. Anesthetic, no point perceived

B. Strength

1. Grip: Use a grip dynamometer with the handle preferably in second position. Alteration from this would be recorded as such. Make three successive determinations, record, and calculate percentage relative to pretreatment value as well as to value from contralateral hand.

2. Pinch: Use a standard, commercially available pinch meter. Key pinch is the thumb tip to the radial aspect of the middle phalanx of the index finger and is the most universal and preferred value. Record three successive efforts, and calculate percentage relative to pretreatment as well as to contralateral hand values. (Tip pinch value will be slightly less than key pinch.)

3. Reverse key pinch: Index tip to ulnar tip of thumb. Recordings are the same as those for key pinch.

---

*From The American Society for Surgery of the Hand: The hand examination and diagnosis, ed. 2, © 1983, Churchill Livingstone, New York.

MP, Metacarpophalangeal.

PIP, Proximal interphalangeal.

DIP, Distal interphalangeal.

C. Motion

1. Total passive motion (TPM): Sum of angles formed by MP, PIP, and DIP joints in maximum passive flexion minus the sum of angles of deficit from complete extension at each of these three joints: (MP + PIP + DIP) − (MP + PIP + DIP) = Total flexion − Total extensor lag = TPM.

2. Total active motion (TAM): Sum of angles formed by MP, PIP, and DIP joints in maximum active flexion, that is, fist position, minus total extension deficit at the MP, PIP, and DIP joints with active finger extension. Significant hyperextension at any joint, particularly the PIP and DIP joints, is recorded as a deficit in extension and is included in the total extension deficit. Hyperextension must be considered an abnormal value in swan neck (PIP) and boutonniere deformities (DIP). Comparison of pretreatment and posttreatment TAM values will be significant; however, comparison as a percentage of normal value is invalid. TAM is a term applied to one finger and is:

   a. Sum of active MP flexion plus active PIP flexion plus active DIP flexion
   b. Minus sum of incomplete active extension if any is present (Figs. E-1 to E-3)

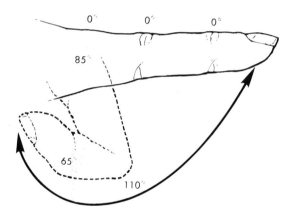

Fig. E-1. Normal range of motion.

	Active	Flexion	Extension lack
MP		85°	0°
PIP		110°	0°
DIP		65°	0°
TOTALS		260°	0°

$$\text{TAM} = 260° - 0° = 260°$$

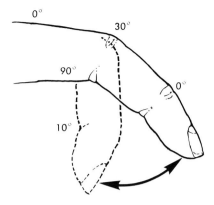

Fig. E-2. Stiff metacarpophalangeal and limited proximal interphalangeal joint extension.

Active	Flexion	Extension lack
MP	0°	0°
PIP	90°	30°
DIP	10°	0°
TOTALS	100°	30°

$$\text{TAM} = 100° - 30° = 70°$$

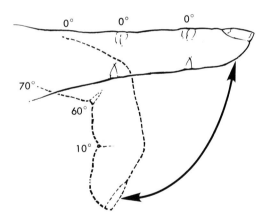

Fig. E-3. Limited metacarpophalangeal and proximal interphalangeal joint flexion with good extension.

Active	Flexion	Extension lack
MP	70°	0°
PIP	60°	0°
DIP	10°	0°
TOTALS	140°	0°

$$\text{TAM} = 140° - 0° = 140°$$

D. Vascular status

Patients who have vascular repair are evaluated in the following manner:

1. Examination for tissue survival.
2. Objective evidence of patent vessels by Allen test and/or ultrasonic pulse detector.
3. Revascularized part examination in resting and postexercise state by one of several methods:
   a. Presence of capillary filling
   b. Physiologic testing such as ultrasonic pulse detector
      When possible, comparison with evaluation before and after 3-minute tourniquet ischemia.
4. Evaluation regarding cold tolerance of the part.

   Ratings:
   a. Failure, no survival
   b. Poor, tissue survival
   c. Fair, objective evidence of patent vessels
   d. Good, function not limited by circulation
   e. Excellent, no cold intolerance

Bibliography

SPLINTING AND ORTHOTICS

American Academy of Orthopaedic Surgeons: Atlas of orthotics: biomechanical principles and application, St. Louis, 1975, The C.V. Mosby Co.

American Occupational Therapy Association, Practice Division: Hand, Rockville, Md, 1984, The Society.

Anderson, M. In Sollers, R., editor: Upper limb orthotics, Springfield, Ill., 1965, Charles C Thomas, Publisher.

Anderson, M.N.: Upper extremities orthotics, Springfield, Ill., 1965, Charles C Thomas, Publisher.

Ansell, B.M., Williams, J.G., Cheshire, L., Lawton, S., and Haines, R.E.: Farnham Park modular splint system, Rheumatol. Phys. Med. **11**:334-336, 1972.

Araicoj, J.L., and Ortiz, J.M.: An internal wire splint for adduction contracture of the thumb, Plast. Reconstr. Surg. **48**:339-342, 1971.

Bacon, G., and Olszewski, E.: Sequential advancing flexion retention attachment, Am.J. Occup. Ther. **32**:577, 1978.

Barr, N.: The hand: principles and techniques and simple splint making in rehabilitation, London, 1975, Butterworths.

Bean, C., Semelis-Last, E., and Rothenberg, S: The functional hand: a guide to splinting, Cambridge, Mass., 1982, Mt. Auburn Hospital.

Beasley, R.W.: The addition of dynamic splinting to hand casts, Plast. Reconstr. Surg. **44**:507, 1969.

Bennett, R.L.: Wrist and hand slip-on splints. In Arthritis and physical medicine, New Haven, 1960, Elizabeth Licht Publishers.

Bergfeld, J.A., Weiker, C.G., Andrish, J.T., and Hall, R.: Soft playing splint for protection of significant hand and wrist injuries in sports, Am. J. Sports Med. **10**(5):293-296, 1982.

Betts, G.A.: An adjustable plastazote splint for the hand or arm. Nurs. Times **66**:1556-1557, 1970.

Bielawski, T., and Bear-Lehman, J.: Brief or new: a gauntlet work splint, Am. J. Occup. Ther. **40**(3), 1986.

Boyes, J.H.: Bunnell's surgery of the hand, ed. 5, Philadelphia, 1970, J.B. Lippincott Co.

Bradley, K.: Basic splinting manual, Unpublished handout, Indianapolis, 1968, Indiana University Medical Center, Occupational Therapy Program.

Bradley, K., Fess, E., and Keal, J.: Basic splinting manual, Unpublished handout, Indianapolis, 1972, Indiana University Medical Center, Occupational Therapy Program.

Buckner, F.: A dynamic finger splint, Am. J. Occup. Ther. **27**:477, 1973.

Buckner, G.: A dynamic finger splint, Am. J. Occup. Ther. **27**:39, 1973.

Bunch, W., and Keagy, R.: Principles of orthotic treatment, St. Louis, 1976, The C.V. Mosby Co.

Caldwell, H.: Progressive splinting manual utilizing the master template method, New Brunswick, N.J., 1970, Johnson & Johnson.

Callahan, A.D., and McEntee, P.: Splinting proximal interphalangeal joint flexion contractures: a new design, Am. J. Occup. Ther. **40**:6, 1986.

Callahan, A.D., and Yasaki, K.: Step-by-step construction of a cock-up splint, Philadelphia, 1980, Hand Rehabilitation Foundation.

Cannon, N.M., et al.: Manual of hand splinting, New York, 1985, Churchill Livingstone.

Capener, N.: Lively splints, Physiotherapy **53**:371-374, 1967.

Colditz, J.C.: Anatomic and kinesiologic considerations for dynamic splint design, Proceedings American Society of Hand Therapists, J. Hand Surg. **6**:299, 1981.

Colditz, J.C.: Dynamic splinting of the stiff hand. In

Hunter, J.M., et al., editors: Rehabilitation of the hand, ed. 2, St. Louis, 1984, The C.V. Mosby Co.

Colditz, J.C.: Low profile dynamic splinting of the injured hand, Am. J. Occup. Ther. **37**:182, 1983.

Colditz, J.C.: Spring wire splinting of the proximal interphalangeal joint. In Hunter, et al., editors: Rehabilitation of the hand, ed. 2, St. Louis, 1984, The C.V. Mosby Co.

Devore, G.L.: Low cost hand splinting, Hand Rehabilitation Center, Chapel Hill, N.C., 1968 University of North Carolina.

Dillner, S., et al.: Technical and clinical function testing of hand orthoses in Sweden, Int. J. Rehab. Res. **2**(1):47-60, 1979.

Engen, T.J.: Development of upper extremity orthotics. Part I: Research and development of powered and non-powered systems, Am. J. Orthot. Prosthet. **24**(1):12-29, 1970.

Engen, T.J.: Development of upper extremity orthotics. Part II: Patient applications and functional, Am. J. Orthot. Prosthet. **24**(2):1-31, 1970.

English, C.B., Rehm, R.A., and Petzoldt, R.L.: Blocking splints to assist finger exercise, Am. J. Occup. Ther. **36**(4):259-262, 1982.

Eyler, R.: Treatment of flexion contractures in occupational therapy, Am. J. Occup. Ther. **19**:86, 1965.

Fess, E.E.: Principles and methods of splinting for mobilization of joints. In Hunter, J.M., et al., editors: Rehabilitation of the hand, ed. 2, St. Louis, 1984, The C.V. Mosby Co.

Fess, E.E.: Rubber band traction: physical properties, splint design and identification of force magnitude, Proceedings American Society of Hand Therapists, J. Hand Surg. **9A**:610, 1984.

Fess, E.E.: Splinting for mobilization of the thumb. In Hunter, et al., editors: Rehabilitation of the Hand, ed. 2, St. Louis, 1984, The C.V. Mosby Co.

Fess, E.E., Gettle K.S. and Strickland, J.W.: Hand splinting: principles and methods, St. Louis, 1981, The C.V. Mosby Co.

Gelberman, R.H., et al.: J. Bone Joint Surg. **65A**:70-80, 1983.

Greenburg, S., and Braun, R.: Therapeutic uses of the air bag splint for the injured hand, Am. J. Occup. Ther. **31**(5):318-319, 1977.

Griffin, J.M., and Lissner, G.: Tape splinting for mallet finger, Mo. Med. **69**:813, 1973.

Hall, A.J., and Stenner, R.W.: Manual of fracture bracing, New York, 1985, Churchill Livingstone.

Henwood, J.: Hinged working splint for the elbow, Br. J. Occup. Ther. **38**:265, 1975.

Heuricj, M., and Polansky, S.: An adaptation of the glove flexion mitt, Am. J. Occup. Ther. **32**:110, 1978.

Hollis, I.: Splint substitutes, Am. J. Occup. Ther. **21**:139-145, 1967.

Hooper, R.M., and North E.R.: Dynamic interphalangeal extension splint design, Am. J. Occup. Ther. **36**:257, 1982.

Jones, M.S. (revised by P. Jay): An approach to occupational therapy, ed. 3, London, 1977, Butterworths.

Joshi, B.B.: Simple and economical splints for the hand (using readily available materials). In Pulvertaft, R.G., editor: Operative surgery on the hand, London, 1977, Butterworths.

Kalisman, M., Chesher, S.P., and Lister, G.D.: Adjustable dynamic external splint for control of first web contracture, Plast. Reconstr. Surg. **71**(2):266-267, 1983.

Keil, J.: Basic hand splinting: a pattern designing approach, Boston, 1983, Little, Brown & Co.

Kester, N.C., and Lehneis, H.R.: A combined ADL-long opponens orthosis, Arch. Phys. Med. Rehabil. **50**:219-222, 1969.

Ketchum, L.D., Hibbard, A., and Hassanein, K.M.: Follow-up report on the electrically driven hand splint, J. Hand Surg. **4**:474, 1979.

Knapp, M.E.: Orthotics: bracing in upper extremity, Postgrad. Med. **43**:215-219, 1968.

Kolumban, S.L.: The use of dynamic and static splints in straightening contracted proximal interphalangeal joints in leprosy patients: a comparative study. Presented at the Forty-seventh Annual Conference of the American Physical Therapy Association, Washington, D.C., 1960.

Kolumban, S.L.: The role of static and dynamic splints, physiotherapy techniques and time in straightening contractures of the interphalangeal joints, Lepr. India 323-328, 1969.

Laskin, R.S.: Simple splint for finger injuries, Postgrad. Med. **4**:174-175, 1970.

Lehneis, H.R.: Upper limb orthotics, Am. J. Orthot. Prosthet. **31**(4):14-20, 1977.

Leung, P.C., and Hui, K.M.: The thumbweb expanding splint: dynamic splintage for traumatic web contracture, Hand **13**:311-317, 1981.

Licht, S.H., and Kamenetz, H.L., editors: Orthotics etcetera, New Haven, Conn., 1966, Elizabeth Licht, Publisher.

Malick, M.H.: Manual on dynamic hand splinting with thermoplastic materials, ed. 2, Pittsburgh, 1978, Harmarville Rehabilitation Center.

Malick, M.H.: Manual on Static Hand Splinting, ed. 3, Pittsburgh, 1979, Harmarville Rehabilitation Center.

Mayou, B., and Jefferiss, C.: A simple splint to elevate the hand, Hand **9**(1):94, 1977.

McDougall, D.: Modern concepts in hand orthotics, Hand **7**:58-62, 1975.

McFarland, S.R., Laenger, C.J.S.R., Francis, P.N., and Ziperman, H.H.: Fiber reinforced composites for orthotics, prosthetics, and mobility aids, Biomed. Sci. Instrum. **11**:151-156, 1975.

McKenzie, M.W.: The Ratchet handsplint, Am. J. Occup. Ther. **27**:477-479, 1973.

Michon, J., and Pillet, J.: The GEM dynamic hand splint, Hand **6**:295-296, 1974.

Mildenberger, L.A.: Magnetic splint for object retrieval, Am. J. Occup. Ther. **38**:195, 1984.

Millender, L.H., and Phillips, C.: Uses of the proximal interphalangeal joint gutter splint, Am. J. Occup. Ther. **27**:8, 1973.

Moberg, E.: Dressings, splints and post-operative care in hand surgery, Surg. Clin. North Am. **44**:941, 1964.

Moberg, E., et al.: Splinting in hand therapy, New York, 1984, Thieme-Stratton, Inc.

Modern concepts in hand orthotics, Hand **7**(1):58-62, 1975.

Mould, C.: Pilot project to gather information on splint-making, Occup. Ther. Nov. 1973, p. 539.

Nalebuff, E., and Millender, L.: Robert B. Brigham Hospital dynamic hand splint, Midland, Mich., Dow Corning Medical Products.

Niehuss, J.E.: An improved method to attach straps to plaster splints, Phys. Ther. **45**:1059, 1965.

Parks, B.J., Barrett, K.P., and Voss, K.: The use of hexcelite in splinting the thumb, Am. J. Occup. Ther. **37**:266, 1983.

Peacock, E., Jr.: Dynamic splinting for the prevention and correction of deformities, J. Bone Joint Surg. [Am.] **34**:789-796, 1952.

Phelps, P.E., and Weeks, P.M.: Management of the thumb-index web space contracture, Am. J. Occup. Ther. **30**:543-550,1976.

Redford, J.B., editor: Orthotics etcetera, ed. 3, Baltimore, 1986, Williams & Wilkins Co.

Reid, R.L.: Position of immobilization for the hand, Milit. Med. **143**(9):626-628, 1978.

Ries, D.A.: A new material for splinting in hand surgery, Mo. Med. **64**:843, 1967.

Seller, J.: A low-profile dorsal dynamic splint, Am. J. Occup. Ther. **34**:213, 1980.

Silverstein, F.: Occupational therapy and the hand splint, Am. J. Occup. Ther. Sept. 1953.

Simard, T.G., and Ladd, H.W.: Hand orthotic device influence on fine neuromuscular control, Arch. Phys. Med. Rehabil. **57**:258-263, 1976.

Solie, G.A.: Short opponens hand orthosis, Am. J. Occup. Ther. **32**:588, 1978.

Spieker, J.L., and Lethcoe, B.J.: Upper extremity bracing: a follow-up study, Am. J. Occup. Ther. **25**:398, 1971.

Stern, G.R.: Thumb abduction splint, Phsiotherapy **66**(10):352, 1980.

Strong, M.L.: A new method of extension-block splinting for the proximal interphalangeal joint: preliminary report, J. Hand Surg. **5**(6):606-607, 1980.

Sutcliffe, B., and Clark, C.: A polythene and plastazote hand-resting splint, Physiotherapy **58**:138-139, 1972.

Tenney, C.G., and Lisak, J. M.: Atlas of hand splinting, 1986, Little, Brown & Co.

Torres, J.: Little finger splint, Am. J. Occup. Ther. **29**:230, 1975.

Truong, X.T.: Fluidic power and control for hand orthosis and prosthesis, Arch. Phys. Med. Rehabil. **54**:91-96, 1973.

Upper extremity orthotics, Physical Therapy **58**(3)263-320.

Van Straten, O., and Mahler, D.: Four new hand splints, Br. J. Plast. Surg **34**(3):345-348, 1981.

Vigliotta, C.L.: Traction splint for maximum interphalangeal joint flexion, Am. J. Occup. Ther. **32**(3):175-178, 1978.

Ward, C.G.: Vacuum splintage of the hand, Hand **9**(1):71-75, 1977.

Yeakel, M.H.: Polypropylene hinges for hand splints, J. Bone Joint Surg. [Am.] **48**:955-956, 1966.

Zide, B.M., Bevin, A.G., and Hollis, L.I.: Examples of simply fabricated custom made splints for the hand, J. Hand Surg. **6**(1):35-39, 1981.

Ziegler, E.M.: Current concepts in orthotics: a diagnosis-related approach to splinting, 1984, Rolyan Medical Products.

AMPUTATION

Dworecka, F., Wisham, L.H., and Smith, R.: A new device for the restoration of partially amputated hands, Mt. Sinai J. Med. **38**:462-469, 1971.

Malick, M.H.: A preliminary prosthesis for the partially amputated hand, Am. J. Occup. Ther. **29**:479-482, 1975.

ANATOMY AND KINESIOLOGY

Barron, J.N.: Structure and function of the skin of the hand, Hand **2**(2):93, 1970.

Basmajian, J.V.: Practical functional anatomy. In Hunter, J.M., Schneider, L.H., Mackin, E. J., and Bell, J.A., editors: Rehabilitation of the hand, St. Louis, 1978, The C.V. Mosby Co.

Basmajian, J.V.: Muscles alive, ed. 4, Baltimore, 1979, Williams & Wilkins Co.

Boyes, J.H., editor: Bunnell's surgery of the hand, ed. 4, Philadelphia, 1964, J.B. Lippincott Co.

Boyes, J.H., editor: Bunnell's surgery of the hand, ed. 5, Philadelphia, 1970, J.B. Lippincott Co.

Brumstrom, S.: Clinical kinesiology, ed. 3, Philadelphia, 1972, F.A. Davis Co.

Chase, R.A.: Atlas of hand surgery, Philadelphia, 1973, W.B. Saunders Co.

Chase, R.A.: Atlas of hand surgery, vol. 2, Philadelphia, 1984, W.B. Saunders Co.

Curtis, R.: Opposition of the thumb, Orthop. Clin. North Am. **5**(2):305, 1974.

Doyle, J.R., and Blythe, W.: The finger flexor tendon sheath and pulleys: anatomy and reconstruction. In American Academy of Orthopaedic Surgeons: Symposium on Tendon Surgery in the Hand, St. Louis, 1975, The C.V. Mosby Co.

Flatt, A.: Care of the arthritic hand, ed. 4, St. Louis, 1983, The C.V. Mosby Co.

Grant, J.C.: Grant's atlas of anatomy, ed. 6, Baltimore, 1986, The Williams & Wilkins Co.

Gray, H.: Gray's anatomy of the human body, Am. ed. 13, edited by C.D. Clemente, Philadelphia, 1985, Lea & Febiger.

Haines, R.: The mechanism of rotation of the first carpometacarpal joint, J. Anat. **78**:44, 1944.

Hollinshead, H.W.: Anatomy for surgeons, vol. 4: The back and limbs, New York, 1982, Harper & Row, Publishers.

Johnson, M., and Cohen, M.: The hand atlas, Springfield, Ill., 1975, Charles C Thomas, Publisher.

Kamaura, N., et al.: Patterns of static prehension in normal hands, Am. J. Occup. Ther. **34**:437-445,1980.

Kaplan, E.B.: Functional and surgical anatomy of the hand, ed. 2, Philadelphia, 1965, J.B. Lippincott Co.

Kaplan, E.B.: Anatomy and kinesiology of the hand. In Flynn, J.E., editor: Hand surgeries, ed. 2, Baltimore, 1975, The Williams & Wilkins Co.

Lampe, E.W.: Surgical anatomy of the hand. In Clinical symposia, New York, 1969, Ciba Pharmaceutical Co., Division of Ciba-Geigy Corp.; illustrations by F.H. Netter.

Landsmeer, J.: Atlas of anatomy of the hand, Edinburgh, 1976, Churchill Livingstone.

Marble, H.C.: The hand, a manual and atlas for the general surgeon, Philadelphia, 1960, W.B. Saunders Co.

Milford, L.: Retaining ligaments of the digits of the hand, Philadelphia, 1968, W.B. Saunders Co.

Napier, J.R.: The form and function of the carpometacarpal joint of the thumb, J. Anat. **89**:362-369, 1955.

Napier, J.R.: The prehensile movements of the human hand, J. Bone Joint Surg. [Br.] **38**:902-913, 1956.

Netter, F.H.: Illustrations for Surgical anatomy of the hand. In Clinical symposia, New York, 1969, Ciba-Geigy Corp.

Rasch, P., and Burke, R.: Kinesiology and applied anatomy, ed. 6, Philadelphia, 1978, Lea & Febiger.

Seddon, H.: Surgical disorders of the peripheral nerves, Baltimore, 1972, The Williams & Wilkins Co.

Smith, R.: Intrinsic muscles of the fingers: Function, dysfunction, and surgical reconstruction, Am. Acad. Orthop. Surgeons Instructional Course Lectures, **24**, St. Louis, 1975, The C.V. Mosby Co., 1974, p. 200.

Smith, R.: Balance and kinetics of the fingers under normal and pathological conditions, Clin. Orthop. **104**:92-111, 1974.

Spinner, M.: Kaplan's functional and surgical anatomy of the hand, ed. 3, Philadelphia, 1984, J.B. Lippincott Co.

Taleisnik, J.: Wrist anatomy, function and injury. In American Academy of Orthopaedic surgeons: Instructional Lecture Course Series, vol. 27, St. Louis, 1978, The C.V. Mosby Co.

Taleisnik, J.: The wrist, New York, 1985, Churchill Livingstone.

Thomas, D.H., Long, C., and Landsmeer, J.M.F.: Biochemical considerations of lumbricalis behavior in the human finger, J. Biomechanics **1**:107-115, 1968.

Von Lanz, T., and Wachsmuth, W.: Praktische anatomie, 1959. In Boyes, J.H., editor: Bunnell's surgery of the hand, ed. 5, Philadelphia, 1970, J.B. Lippincott Co.

Weber, E.R.: Concepts governing the rotational shift of the intercalated segment of the carpus. Orthop. Clin. North Am. **15**(2):193-207, 1984.

Zancolli, E.: Structural and dynamic bases of hand surgery, Philadelphia, 1968, J.B. Lippincott Co.

ARTHRITIS

Alexander, G.J., Hortas, C., and Bacon, P.A.: Bed rest, activity and the inflammation of rheumatoid arthritis, Br. J. Rheumatol. **22**:134-140, 1983.

Belsky, M.R., et al.: Hand involvement in psoriatic arthritis, J. Hand Surg. **7**:203, 1982.

Bennett, R.L.: Orthotic devices to prevent deformities of the hand in rheumatoid arthritis, Arthr. Rheumat. **8**:1006-1018, Oct. 1965.

Bens, D.E., and Krewer, S.E.: The hand gym: an exercise apparatus for the patient with rheumatoid arthritis, Arch. Phys. Med. Rehab. **55**:477, 1974.

Besser, M.J.B.: The conservative treatment of the swan-neck deformity in the rheumatoid hand, Hand **10**:91-93, 1978.

Buchanan, C., et al.: Postoperative care for patients with Silastic finger joint implants (Swanson design), Dow Corning Wright, 1979.

Calabro J.: Rheumatoid arthritis: clinical symposia, vol. 23, Ciba Pharmaceutical Products, Summit, N.J., 1971.

Carr, K.: Hand splints for rheumatoid arthritis, Can. J. Occup. Ther. **35**:17-18, 1978.

Carthum, C.J., Clawson, D.K.,and Decker, J.L.: Functional assessment of the rheumatoid hand, Am.J. Occup. Ther. **23**:122, 1969.

Clawson, D.K., et al.: Functional assessment of the rheumatoid hand, Clin. Orthop. Rel. Res. **77**:203, 1971.

Convery, F.R., and Minteer, M.: The use of orthoses in the management of rheumatoid arthritis, Clin. Orthop. Rel. Res. **102**:118-125, 1974.

Convery, F.R., Conaty, J.P., and Nickel, V.L.: Dynamic splinting of the rheumatoid hand, Orthot. Prosthet. **21**:249-254, Dec. 1967.

Convery, F.R., Conaty, J.P., and Nickel, V.L.: Dynamic splinting of the rheumatoid hand, Orthot. Prosthet. **22**:41-45, March 1968.

Czap, L.: Orthotic management of the rheumatoid hand, South. Med. J. **59**:1115-1117, 1966.

Davis, R.F., Weiland, A.J., and Dowling, S.: Swanson implant of the wrist in rheumatoid arthritis, Clin. Orthop. Rel. Res. **166**:132, 1982.

DeVore, G.L.: Preoperative assessment and postoperative therapy and splinting in rheumatoid arthritis. In Hunter, et al., editors: Rehabilitation of the hand, ed. 2, St. Louis, 1984, The C.V. Mosby Co.

Ehrlich, G.E.: Splinting for arthritis, Med. Times **96**:485-489, May 1968.

English, C.B., and Nalebuff, E.A.: Understanding the arthritic hand, Am. J. Occup. Ther. **25**(7):352-359, 1971.

Eyring, E.J., and Murray, W.R.: The effect of joint position on the pressure of intra-articular effusion, J. Bone Joint Surg. **46A**(6):1235-1241, Sept. 1964.

Feinberg, J., and Brandt, K.D.: Use of resting splints by patients with rheumatoid arthritis, Am. J. Occup. Ther. **35**(3):173-178, 1981.

Feinberg, J.R., and Brandt, K.D.: Factors influencing compliance of night splinting by patients with rheumatoid arthritis (abstract), J. Hand Surg. **7**:308, 1982.

Fess, E.E., Gettle, K., and Strickland, J.: Hand splinting principles and methods, St. Louis, 1981, The C.V. Mosby Co.

Flatt, A.E.: Care of the arthritic hand, ed. 4, St. Louis, 1983, The C.V. Mosby Co.

Gault, S.J., and Spyker, M.J.: Beneficial effect of immobilization of joints in rheumatoid and related arthritides: a splint study using sequential analysis, Arthritis Rheum. **12**:34-44, 1969.

Goodman, M.J., et al.: Arthroplasty of rheumatoid wrist with silicone rubber: early evaluation, J. Hand Surg. **5**:114, 1980.

Granger, C.V., et al.: Laminated plaster-plastic bandage splints, Arch. Phys. Med. **46**:585-589, August, 1965.

Gruen, H.: A postoperative dynamic splint for the rhuematoid hand, Am. J. Occup. Ther. **24**:284, 1970.

Hasselkaus, B.R., Kshepakaran, K.K., and Safrit, M.J.: Handedness and hand joint changes in rheumatoid arthritis, Am. J. Occup. Ther. **35**(11):705-710, 1981.

Hunter, J.M., et al., editors: Rehabilitation of the hand, St. Louis, 1984, The C.V. Mosby Co.

Johnson, B.M., Flynn, M.J.G., and Beckenbaugh, R.D.: A dynamic splint for use after total wrist arthroplasty, Am. J. Occup. Ther. **35**:79-84, 1981.

Kelley, W.N., et al., editors: Textbook of rheumatology, Philadelphia, 1985, W.B. Saunders Co.

Leonard, J., Swanson, A.B., and Swanson, G.: Postoperative care for patients with silastic finger joint implants (Swanson design), ed. 3, 1984, Dow Corning Wright.

Lesiak, A., and Seyfried, A.: Splinting of the rheumatoid hand in an apparatus in cases of ulnar deviation in the metacarpophalangeal joints, Reumatologia **7**:247-253, 1969.

MacBain, K.P.: Assessment of function in the rheumatoid hand, Can. J. Occup. Ther. **37**:95, 1970.

Madden, J.W., DeVore, G., and Arem, A.: A rational post-operative management program for metacarpophalangeal joint implant arthroplasty, J. Hand Surg. **2**:358-366, 1977.

Mannerfelt, L., and Fredricksson, K.: The effect of commercial orthoses on rheumatically deformed hands, Stepelsen For Teknisk Utveckling, S.T.U. information section, STU report no. 47, 1976.

McCann, V.H., Philips, C.A. and Quigley, T.R.: Preoperative and postoperative management: the role of the allied health professionsals, Orthop. Clin. North Am. **6**(3):881-905, 1975.

McKnight, P. and Schomburg, F.: Air pressure splint on hand symptoms of patients with rheumatoid arthritis, Arch. Phys. Med. Rehab. **63**(11):560-564, 1982.

Melvin, J.L.: Rheumatic disease: occupational therapy and rehabilitation, ed. 2, Philadelphia, 1982, F.A. Davis Co.

Millender, C.H., et al.: Interpositional arthroplasty for rheumatoid carpometacarpal joint disease, J. Hand Surg. **3**:533, 1978.

Mills, J.A., et al.: Value of bed rest in patients with rheumatoid arthritis, N. Engl. J. Med. **284**:453-458, 1971.

Moon, M.H., Moon, B.A., and Black, W.A.: Compliancy in splint-wearing behaviour of patients with rheumatoid arthritis, N. Zealand Med. J. **83**:360-365, 1976.

Nalebuff, E.A.: Diagnosis, classification and management of rheumatoid thumb deformities, Bull. Hosp. Joint Dis. **29**:199, 1968.

Nalebuff, E.A.: The rheumatoid thumb, Clin. Rheum. Dis. **10**:3, 1984.

Nalebuff, E.A., and Millender, L.H.: Surgical treatment of the swan-neck deformity in rheumatoid arthritis, Orthop. Clin. North Am. **6**(3):733-752, 1975.

Nalebuff, E.A., and Millender, L.H.: Surgical treatment of the boutonniere deformity in rheumatoid arthritis, Orthop. Clin. North Am. **6**(3):753-763, 1975.

Nalebuff, E.A., and Philips, C.A.: The rheumatoid thumb. in Hunter, et al., editors: Rehabilitation of the hand, St. Louis, 1984, The C.V. Mosby Co.

Nicholas, J.J., et al.: Splinting in rheumatoid arthritis. I. Factors affecting patient compliance, Arch. Phys. Med. Rehab. **63**:92-96, 1982.

Nicolle, F.V., and Presswell, D.R.: A valuable splint for the rheumatoid hand, Hand **7**:67-69, 1975.

Oakes, T.W.: Ward, J.R., Gray, R.M., Klauber, M.R., and Moody, P.M.: Family expectations and arthritis patient compliance to a hand resting splint regimen, J. Chronic Dis. **22**:757-764, 1970.

Opitz, J., and Linscheid, R.: Hand function after metacarpophalangeal joint replacement in rheumatoid arthritis, Arch. Phys. Med. Rehab. **59**(4):160-165, 1978.

Overton, J., and Wolcott, L.E.: The role of splints in the prevention of deformity in the rheumatoid hand and wrist, Missouri Med. **63**:423-427, 1966.

Pahle, J.A., and Raunia, P.: The influence of wrist position on finger deviation in the rheumatoid hand, J. Bone Joint Surg. **51B**:664-676, 1969.

Partridge, R.E., and Duthie, J.J.: Controlled trial of the effects of complete immobilization of the joints in rheumatoid arthritis, Ann. Rheum. Dis. **22**:91-99, 1963.

Philips, C.A.: Hand therapy in the early stages of rheumatoid arthritis, In Hunter, et al., editors: Rehabilitation of the hand, St. Louis, 1978, The C.V. Mosby Co.

Porter, S.F., Dapper, M.J., and Foran, C.: Adult arthritis; hand splints, Am. J. Nurs. **83**(2):276-278, 1983.

Quest, I.M., and Corderly, J.: A functional ulnar deviation cuff for the rheumatoid deformity, Am. J. Occup. Ther. **25**:32-37, 1971.

Quintner, J.L.: Hand splints in "Prenyl" for rheumatoid arthritis. A preliminary report, Ann. Phys. Med. **9**:280-281, 1968.

Ratcliff A.H.C.: Deformities of the thumb in rheumatoid arthritis, J. Bone Joint Surg. **54B**:557, 1972.

Rhinelander, F.W.: The effectiveness of splinting and bracing on rheumatoid arthritis, Arthr. Rheum. **2**:270-277, 1959.

Rotstein, J.: Simple splinting, Philadelphia, 1965, W.B. Saunders Co.

Rotstein, J.: Use of splints in conservative management of acutely inflamed joints in rheumatoid arthritis, Arch. Phys. Med. **46**:198-199, 1965.

Shalit, J.E., and Decker, J.L.: Silicone foam resting splints for rheumatoid arthritis, Lancet **1**:142-144, 1965.

Smith, E.M., et al.: Role of the finger flexors in rheumatoid deformities of the metacarpophalangeal joints, Arth. Rheum. **7**:467-480, 1964.

Smith, R.J., and Kaplan, E.B.: Rheumatoid deformities at the metacarpophalangeal joints of the fingers, J. Bone Joint Surg. **49A**(1), Jan. 1967.

Souter, W.A.: Splintage in the rheumatoid hand, Hand **3**:144-151, 1971.

Spelbring, L.M.: Splinting the arthritic hand, Am. J. Occup. Ther. **20**:40-41, 1966.

Swanson, A.B.: Flexible implant resection arthroplasty in the hand and extremities, St. Louis, 1973, The C.V. Mosby Co.

Swanson, A.B., and Coleman, J.D.: Corrective bracing needs of the rheumatoid arthritic wrist, Am. J. Occup. Ther. **20**:38-40, 1966.

Swanson, A.B., and Swanson, G.D.: Pathogenesis and pathomechanics of rheumatoid deformities in the hand and wrist, Orthop. Clin. North Am. **4**:1939-1956, 1973.

Swanson, A.B., Swanson, G., and Leonard, J.: Postoperative rehabilitation program for flexible implant arthroplasty of the fingers. In Inglis, editor: AAOS symposium on total joint replacement of the upper extremity, St. Louis, 1982, The C.V. Mosby Co.

Swanson, A.B., Swanson, G., and Leonard J.: Postoperative rehabilitation programs in flexible implant arthroplasty of the digits. In Hunter, et al., editors: Rehabilitation of the hand, ed. 2, St. Louis, 1984, The C.V. Mosby Co.

Swanson, A.B., Swanson, G., and Leonard, J.: Upper limb joint replacement. In Nichel, editor: Orthopedic rehabilitation, ed. 2, St. Louis, 1984, The C.V. Mosby Co.

Swezey, R.L.: Dynamic factors in deformity of the rheumatoid arthritic hand, Bull. Rheum. Dis. **22**:649-656, 1971-72.

VanBrocklin, J.D.: Splinting the rheumatoid hand, Arch. Phys. Med. **47**:262-265, 1966.

Williams, J.G.: Splints for the rheumatoid hand, Br. Med. J. **1**:106, 1970.

Young, P.J.: Use of splintage in the rheumatoid hand after surgery, Physiotherapy, **66**:371-374, 1980.

Zoeckler, A.A., and Nicholas, J.J.: Prenyl hand splint for rheumatoid arthritis, Phys. Ther. **49**:377-379, 1969.

ASSESSMENT

Aoer, C.L., Olivett, B.L., and Johnson, C.L.: Grasp and pinch strength in children 5 to 12 years old, Am. J. Occup Ther. **38**:107, 1984.

American Academy of Orthopaedic Surgeons: Joint motion—method of measuring and recording, Chicago, 1956, The Academy.

American Academy of Orthopaedic Surgeons: Atlas of orthotics: biomechanical principles and application, St. Louis, 1975, The C.V. Mosby Co.

American Society for Surgery of the Hand: Examination and diagnosis, Aurora, Colo., 1978, The Society.

American Society for Surgery of the Hand: The hand—examination and diagnosis, ed. 2, New York, 1983, Churchill Livingstone.

American Society of Hand Therapists: Clinical assessment recommendations, Raleigh, 1981, The Society.

Baxter, P.L., and Ballard, M.: Evaluation of the hand by functional tests. In Hunter, et al., editors: Rehabilitation of the hand, ed. 2, St. Louis, 1984, The C.V. Mosby Co.

Baxter, P.L., and McEntee, P.M.: Physical capacity evaluation. In Hunter, et al., editors: Rehabilitation of the hand, ed. 2, St. Louis, 1984, The C.V. Mosby Co.

Beach, R.B., and Bell, J.A.: Torque/ROM curve: an objective method of passive joint ROM measurement (abstract), J. Hand Surg. 7:308, 1982.

Bechtol, C.D.: Grip test: use of a dynamometer with adjustable handle spacing, J. Bone Joint Surg. 36A:820, 1954.

Bell, E., Jurek, K., and Wilson, T.: Hand skill measurement: a gauge for treatment, Am. J. Occup. Ther. 30:80, 1976.

Bell, J.: Sensibility evaluation. In Hunter, J., Schneider, L., Mackin, E., and Bell, J., editors: Rehabilitation of the hand, St. Louis, 1978, The C.V. Mosby Co.

Bell, J.: Symposium: assessment of levels of cutaneous sensibility, United States Public Health Service Hospital, Carville, Louisiana, 1980.

Bell, J.A.: Simplified measurement graphs: a new approach (abstract), J. Hand Surg. 8:626, 1983.

Bell, J.A.: Light touch–deep pressure testing using Semmes-Weinstein monofilaments. In Hunter et al., editors: rehabilitation of the hand, ed. 2, St. Louis, 1984, The C.V. Mosby Co.

Bell, J.A.: Sensibility testing: state of the art. In Hunter, et al., editors: Rehabilitation of the hand, ed. 2, St. Louis, 1984, The C.V. Mosby Co.

Bell, J., and Buford, W.: The force/time relationship of clinically used sensory testing instruments, Paper presented at the thirty-seventh annual meeting of the American Society for Surgery of the Hand, New Orleans, 1982.

Bell-Krotoski, J., and Tomancik, L.: Repeatability of the Semmes-Weinstein monofilaments, Paper presented at the ninth annual meeting of the American Society of Hand Therapists, New Orleans, 1986.

Blesh, T.E.: Measurement in physical education, ed. 2, New York, 1974, The Ronald Press Co.

Bowers, L.E.: Investigation of the relationship of the hand size and lower arm girths to hand grip strength as measured by selected dynamometers, Research Quart. 32:308, 1961.

Brand, P.W.: Clinical mechanics of the hand, St. Louis, 1985, The C.V. Mosby Co.

Brand, P., and Wood, H.: Hand volumeter instruction sheet, U.S. Public Health Service Hospital, Carville, Louisiana.

Bright, D., and Wright, S.: Postoperative management in replantation. In American Academy of Orthopedic Surgeons: Symposium on microsurgery: practical use in orthopaedics, St. Louis, 1979, The C.V. Mosby Co.

Callahan, A.D.: Sensibility testing: clinical methods. In Hunter, et al., editors: Rehabilitation of the hand, ed. 2, St. Louis, 1984, The C.V. Mosby Co.

Carlson, J.D., and Trombly, C.A.: The effect of wrist immobilization on performance of the Jebsen Hand Function Test, Am. J. Occup. Ther. 37(3):167-175, 1983.

Collins, R.D.: Illustrated manual of neurologic diagnosis, Philadelphia, 1962, J.B. Lippincott Co.

Cotton, D.J., and Bonnell, L.: Investigation of the T-5 cable tensiometer grip attachment for measuring strength of college women, Research Quart. 40:848, 1969.

Crawford small parts dexterity test, The Psychological Corporation, New York, 1956.

Creelnan, G.: Report on hand volumeter—accuracy and sensitivity of measurements, Idyllwild, Calif., 1979, Engraving Experts, Medical Supply Division.

Cronbach, L.J.: In Thorndike, R.L., editor: Educational measurement, ed. 2, Washington, D.C., 1971, American Council on Education.

Currier, D.P.: Elements of research in physical therapy, ed. 2, Baltimore, 1984, The Williams & Wilkins Co.

Dellon, A.: The moving two-point discrimination test: clinical evaluation of the quickly-adapting fiber receptor system, J. Hand Surg. 3:474, 1978.

Dellon, A.L.: Evaluation of sensibility and reeducation of sensation in the hand, Baltimore, Md., 1981, The Williams & Wilkins Co.

Dellon, A., Curtis, R., and Edgerton, M.: Reeducation of sensation in the hand after nerve injury and repair, Plast. Reconstr. Surg. 53:297, 1974.

DeVore, G.L., and Hamilton, G.F.: Volume measuring of the severely injured hand, Am. J. Occup. Ther. 22:16, 1968.

DeVore, G.L., et al.: Development and validation of a self-report hand functioning checklist (abstract), J. Hand Surg. 9A:611, 1984.

DeVore, G.L., and Smith, H.: A new method for measuring motion of flexor tendon grafts, Am. J. Occup. Ther. 24:336, 1970.

Downie, N.M.: Fundamentals of measurement: techniques and practices, ed. 2, New York, 1967, Oxford University Press.

Dyck, P.J., O'Brien, P.C., Bushek, W., and others: Clinical vs quantitative evaluation of cutaneous sensation, Arch. Neurol. **33**:651, 1976.

Fess, E.E.: The effects of Jaymar dynamometer handle position and test protocol on normal grip strength. Proceedings of the American Society of Hand Therapists, J. Hand Surg. **7**:308, 1982.

Fess, E.E.: Documentation: Essential elements of an upper extremity assessment battery, In Hunter, J., et al., editors: Rehabilitation of the hand, ed. 2, St. Louis, 1984, The C.V. Mosby Co.

Fess, E.E.: The need for reliability and validity in hand assessment instruments, J. Hand Surg. Sept. 1986.

Gelberman, R.H., et al.: Sensibility testing in peripheral nerve compression syndrome: an experimental study in humans, J. Bone Joint Surg. **65A**:632-638, 1983.

Gloss, D.S., and Wardle, M.G.: Reliability and validity of AMA's guide to ratings of permanent impairment, JAMA **248**(18):2292, 1982.

Heyward, V., McKeown, B., and Lesseman, R.: Comparison of Stoelting hand grip dynamometer and linear voltage differential transformer for measuring grip strength, Research Quart. **46**:262, 1975.

Hines, M., and O'Connor, J.: A measure of finger dexterity, Personnel J. **4**:379, 1926.

Hoppenfeld, S.: Physical examination of the spine and extremities, New York, 1976, Appleton-Century-Crofts.

Jebsen, R., et al.: An objective and standardized test of hand function, Arch. Phys. Med. Rehabil. **50**:311, 1969.

Kellor, M., et al.: Hand strength and dexterity, Am. J. Occup. Ther. **25**:77-83, 1971.

Kendal, H., Kendal, F., and Wadsworth, G.: Muscle testing and function, Baltimore, 1971, The Williams & Wilkins Co.

Kirkpatrick, J.: Evaluation of grip loss: a factor of permanent partial disability in California, Industr. Med. Surg. **26**:285, 1957.

Kirkpatrick, J.E., Evaluation of grip loss: factor of permanent disability in California: summation and conclusions of sub-committee for study of grasping power committee on industrial health and rehabilitation of California Medical Association, Calif. Med. **85**:314-320, 1956.

LaMotte, R.: Symposium: assessment of levels of cutaneous sensibility, United States Public Health Service Hospital, Carville, Louisiana, 1980.

Levin, S., Pearsall, C., and Ruderman, R.: Von Frey's method of measuring pressure sensibility in the hand: an engineering analysis of the Weinstein-Semmes pressure aesthesiometer, J. Hand Surg. **3**:211, 1978.

Louis, D.S., et al.: An evaluation of normal values for and variations between stationary moving 2-point discrimination, J. Hand surg. **8**:617, 1983.

Mathiowetz, V., Rennells, M.S., and Donahoe, L.: Effect of elbow position on grip and key pinch strength, J. Hand Surg. **10A**:694-696, 1985.

Mathiowetz, V., et al.: Reliability and validity of grip and pinch strength evaluations, J. Hand Surg. **9A**:222, 1984.

Mauer, G.L, et al.: A statistical analysis of methods in current use for evaluating the results of flexor tendon surgery, J. Hand Surg. **9A**:610: 1984.

Minnesota rate of manipulation test, Layfayette Instrument Co., Layfayette, Ind, 1969.

Mitchell, E.: Symposium: assessment of levels of cutaneous sensibility, United States Public Health Service Hospital, Carville, Louisiana, 1980.

Moberg, E.: Objective methods of determining the functional value of sensibility in the hand, J. Bone Joint Surg. **40B**:454, 1958.

Moberg, E.: Criticism and study of methods of examining sensibility in the hand, Neurology **12**:8-19, 1962.

Murray, J.: The patient with the injured hand. Presidential address, American Society for Surgery of the Hand, J. Hand Surg. **7**:543, 1982.

Nemethi, C.E.: Evaluation of hand grip in industry, Indust. Med. Surg. **21**:65, 1952.

Onne, L.: Recovery of sensibility and sudomotor activity in the hand after severe injury, Acta Chir. Scand. [Suppl.]:300, 1962.

O'Rain, S.: New and simple test for nerve function in the hand, Br. Med. J. **3**:615, 1973.

Payton, O.D.: Research: the validation of clinical practice, Philadelphia, 1984, F.A. Davis Co.

Phelps, P., and Walker, E.: Comparison of the finger wrinkling test results to establish sensory tests in peripheral nerve injury. Am. J. Occup. Ther. **31**:565, 1977.

Polley, H., and Hunder, G.: Physical examination of the joints, Philadelphia, 1978, W.B. Saunders Co.

Poppen, N., et al.: Recovery of sensibility after suture of digital nerves, J. Hand Surg. **4**:212, 1979.

Porter, R.W.: New test for fingertip sensation, Br. Med. J. **2**:927-928, 1966.

Pryce, J.: The wrist position between neutral and ulnar deviation that facilitates maximum power grip strength. J. Biomech. **13**:505, 1980.

Renfrew, S.: Fingertip sensation: a routine neurological test, Lancet **1**:396, 1969.

Rizzo, F., Hamilton, B.B., and Keagy, R.D.: Orthotics research evaluation framework, Arch. Phys. Med. Rehabil. **56**:304-308, 1975.

Schmidt, R., and Toews, J.: Grip strength as measured by the jaymar dynamometer, Arch. Phys. Med. Rehabil. June, pp. 321-327, 1970.

Seddon, H.J.: Surgical disorders of the peripheral nerves, Baltimore, 1972, Williams & Wilkins Co.

Seddon, H.: Surgical disorders of the peripheral nerves, ed. 2, New York, 1975, Churchill Livingstone.

Semmes, J., et al.: Somato-sensory changes after penetrating brain wounds in man, Cambridge, Mass., 1960, Harvard University Press.

Smith, R.: Clinical examination. In Lamb, D., and Kuezynski, K., editors: The practice of hand surgery, Boston, 1981, Blackwell Scientific Publications, Inc.

Stanley, J.: In Thorndike, R.L., editor: Educational measurement, ed. 2, Washington, D.C., 1971, American Council on Education.

Sunderland, S.: Nerves and nerve injuries, ed. 2, New York, 1978. Churchill Livingstone.

Swinscow, T.D.V.: Statistics at square one, London, 1983, British Medical Association.

Szabo, R.M., et al.: Vibratory sensory testing in acute peripheral nerve compression, J. Hand Surg. **9A:**104-109, 1984.

Tevaoka, T.: Studies on the peculiarity of grip strength in relation to body position and age, Kobe J. Med. Sci. **25:**1-17, 1979.

Thorngren, K.C., and Werner, C.O.: Normal grip strength, Acta Orthopaed. Scand. **50:**255-259, 1979.

Tiffin, J., and Asher, E.: The Purdue pegboard: norms and studies of reliability and validity, J. Appel Psychol. **32:**234, 1948.

Waylett, J., Seibly, D.: A study to determine the average deviation accuracy of a commercially available volumeter. (Abstract) J. Hand Surg. **6:**300, 1981.

Weber, E.: Data cited by Sherrington, C.S.: In Shafer's textbook of physiology, Edinburgh, 1900, Young J. Pentland.

Werner, J.L., and Omer, G.E.: Evaluation cutaneous pressure sensation of the hand, Am. J. Occup. Ther. **24:**347, 1970.

Wolf, L., Klein, L., and Cauldwell-Klein, E.: Comparison of torque strength measurements on two evaluation devices, Paper presented at the ninth annual meeting of the American Society of Hand Therapists, New Orleans, 1986.

Yerxa, E.J., et al.: Development of a hand sensitivity test for the hypersensitive hand, Am. J. Occup. Ther. **37**(3):176-181, 1983.

BIOMECHANICS, PHYSICS

Bauman, J.H., and Brand, P.W.: Measurement of pressure between foot and shoe, The Lancet, pp. 629-632, 1963.

Bennett, L.: "Transferring Load to Flesh, Part II. Analysis of Compressive Stress," Bull. of Prosthetic Research, BPR 10-16, Veterans Administration, Washington, D.C., pp. 45-63, 1971.

Brand, P.: Clinical mechanics of the hand, St. Louis, 1985, The C.V. Mosby Co.

Brand, P.W.: *Repetitive Stress on Insensitive Feet*, A Monograph Published by United States Public Health Service Hospital, Carville, Louisiana, 1975.

Hampton, George H.: "Therapeutic Footwear for the Insensitive Foot," *J. Physical Therapy*, V. 52, No. 1, pp. 23-29, January, 1979.

Jensen, A., and Chenoweth, H: Statics and strengths of materials, New York, 1975, McGraw-Hill Book Co.

Levinson, I.: Introduction to mechanics, ed. 2, Englewood Cliffs, N.J., 1968, Prentice-Hall, Inc.

Markenscoff, X.: I.V. Yannas, on the Stress-Strain Relation for Skin. J. Biomechanics, Vol. 12, pp. 127-129, 1979.

Murphy, E.F.: "Transferring Load to Flesh, Part I. Concepts," Bull. of Prosthetics Research, BPR 10-16, Veterans Administration, Washington, D.C., pp. 38-44, 1971.

Sakata K., Parfitt, G., and Pinder, K.L.: Compressive Behavior of a Physiological Tissue, *Biorheology*, Vol. 9, pp. 173-184, 1972.

Thompson, D.E.: The pathomechanics of soft tissue damage. *The Diabetic Foot*, Mosby Co., ed. 3, In Levin, M.A. and O'Neal, L.W., editors: pp. 148-161, 1983.

Williams, M., and Lissner, H.: Biomechanics of human motions, Philadelphia, 1962, W.B. Saunders Co.

BURNS

Boswich, J.: Mangagement of fresh burns of the hand and deformities resulting from burn injuries, Clin. Plast. Surg. **1**(4):621, 1974.

Buchan, N.G.: Experience with thermoplastic splints in the post-burn hand, Br. J. Plast. Surg. **28:**8193-8197, 1975.

Evans, E.B.: Orthopaedic measures in the treatment of severe burns, J. Bone Joint Surg. **48A:**643, 1966.

Fishwick, G.M., and Tobin, D.G.: Splinting the burned hand with primary excision and early grafting, Am. J. Occup. Ther. **32**(3):182-183, 1978.

Habal, M.B.: The burned hand: a planned treatment program, J. Trauma, **18**(8):587-595, 1978.

Herman, H.: Compliance with splint wearing schedule on a burn unit (abstract), J. Hand Surg. **9A:**610, 1984.

Johnson, C.J., and Graham, W.P.: Use of thermoplastic splints in the treatment of burned hands, Plast. Reconstr. Surg. **44:**399-400, 1969.

Larson, D., et al.: Splints and traction. In Polk, H., and Stone, H., editors: Contemporary Bone Management, Boston 1971, Little Brown & Co.

LaVore, J.S., and Marshall, J.H.: Expedient splinting of the burned patient, Phys. Ther. **52:**1036-1042, 1972.

Malick, M.: Management of the severely burned patient, Br. J. Occup. Ther. **38**(4), 1975.

Malick, M.H., and Carr, J.A.: Flexible elastomer molds in burn scar control, Am. J. Occup. Ther. **43:**603-608, 1980.

Miles, W.K.: Remodeling of scar tissue in the burned patient. In Hunter, et al., editors: Rehabilitation of the Hand, ed. 2, St. Louis, 1984, The C.V. Mosby Co.

Newmeyer, W.L., and Kilgore, E.S., Jr.: Management of the burned hand, Phys. Ther. **57**(1);16-23, 1977.

Newton, N., and Bubenickova, M.: Rehabilitation of the autografted hand in children with burns, Phys. Ther. **57**(12):1383-1388, 1977.

Reardon, J.C.: Occupational therapy treatment of the patient with thermally injured upper extremity, Major Probl. Clin. Surg. **19:**127-147, 1976.

Robetaille, A., et al.: Correction of keloid and finger contractures in burn patients, Arch. Phys. Med. Rehab. **54:**515, 1973.

Salisbury, R.E., and Palm, L.: Dynamic splinting for dorsal burns of the hand, Plast. Reconstr. Surg. **51:**226-228, 1973.

Salisbury, R.E., Reeves, S., and Wright, P.: Acute care and rehabilitation of the burned hand. In Hunter, et al., editors: Rehabilitation of the hand, ed. 2, St. Louis, 1984, The C.V. Mosby Co.

Tanegawa, M.C., Oleta, K.O., and Donnell, B.S.: The burned hand: a physical therapy protocol, J. Am. Phys. Ther. Assoc. **54**(9):953-959, 1974.

Van Straten, O., and Mahler, D.: Hexcelite splints and adaptions for burned and traumatized hands, Burns Incl. Therm. Inj. **8**(3):188-190, 1982.

Von Prince, K.M.P., Curren P.W., and Pruitt, B.H., Jr.: Application of fingernail hooks in splinting of burned hands, Am. J. Occup. Ther. **24:**556-559, 1970.

Von Prince, K.M.P., and Yeakel, M.H.: The splinting of burn patients, Springfield, 1974, Charles C Thomas, Publisher.

Willis, B.: The use of orthoplast isoprene in the treatment of the acutely burned child: preliminary report, Am. J. Occup. Ther. **23:**57, 1969.

Willis, B.: The use of orthoplast isoprene in the treatment of the acutely burned child: follow-up, Am. J. Occup. Ther. **23:**187, 1970.

CONGENITAL DEFORMITY

Butts, D.E., and Goldberg, M.J.: Congenital absence of the radius: the occupational therapist and a new orthosis, Am. J. Occup. Ther. **31:**95-100, 1977.

Curtis, R.M.: Fundamental principles of tendon transfer, Orthop. Clin. North Am. **5:**231-242, 1974.

Flatt, A.E.: The care of congenital hand anomalies, St. Louis, 1977, The C.V. Mosby Co.

Sherik, S.K., Weiss, M.W., and Flatt, A.A.: Functional evaluation of congenital hand anomalies, Am. J. Occup. Ther. **25:**98, 1971.

Weiss, M.W., and Flatt, A.: Functional evaluation of the congenitally anomalous hand. Part II, Am. J. Occup. Ther. **25:**139, 1971.

FRACTURE

Bell, C.H.: Construction of orhoplast splints for humeral shaft fractures, Am. J. Occup. Ther. **33:**114, 1979.

Brown, P.W.: The management of phalangeal and metacarpal fractures, Surg. Clin. North Am. **53:**1393-1437, 1973.

McElfresh, E.C., Dobyns, J.H., and O'Brien, E.T.: Management of fracture-dislocation of the proximal interphalangeal joints by extension-block splinting, J. Bone Joint Surg. [Am.] **54.8:**1705-1711, 1972.

Rockwood, C., and Green, D.: Fractures, vols. 1 and 2, Philadelphia, 1975, J.B. Lippincott Co.

Strickland, J.W., et al.: Factors influencing digital performance following phalangeal fractures. Presented at American Society for Surgery of the Hand, Annual Symposium, 1979, San Francisco.

Watson-Jones, R.: Fractures and joint injuries, vol. 1, ed. 4, Baltimore, 1952, The Williams & Wilkins Co.

Weeks, P.M., et al.: Acute bone and joint injuries of the hand and wrist, St. Louis, 1981, The C.V. Mosby Co.

Wilson, R.L., and Carter, M.S.: Management of hand fractures. In Hunter, et al., editors: Rehabilitation of the hand, ed. 2, St. Louis, 1984, The C.V. Mosby Co.

HAND REHABILITATION; REHABILITATION

Ahuja, M.: Elevation board, Am. J. Occup. Ther. **36**(8):534-536, 1982.

American Occupational Therapy Association, Practice Division: Hand, Rockville, Md., 1984, The Society.

Arras, N., and Van Beek, A.: Characteristics and results in replantation patients (abstract), J. Hand Surg. **6:**299, 1981.

Bear-Lehman, J.: Factors affecting return to work after hand injury, Am. J. Occup. Ther. **37**(3):194-198, 1983.

Becker, C.G.: Adaption of Bunnell block, Am. J. Occup. Ther. **29:**108, 1975.

Berlin, S., and Vermette, J.: An exploratory study of work simulator norms for grip and wrist flexion, Voc. Eval. Work Adjust. Bull. Summer 1985.

Brand, P.W.: Rehabilitation of the hand in leprosy. In Cramer, L.M., and Chase, R.A., editors: Symposium on the hand, vol. 3, St. Louis, 1971, The C.V. Mosby Co.

Brand, P.W.: Rehabilitation of the hand with motor and sensory impairment, Orthop. Clin. North Am. **4:**1135-1139, 1973.

Bright, D., and Wright, S.: Postoperative management in replantations. In American Academy of Orthopaedic Surgeons: *Symposium on Microsurgery,* St. Louis, 1979, The C.V. Mosby Co.

Brown, D.M., and Clark, S.: Elevation crutch in the treatment of the edematous hand, Am. J. Occup. Ther. **32:**320-321, 1978.

Buntine, J.A., and Holthouse, R.L.: Simple physiotherapy for hand injuries, Med. J. Aust. **2:**187-190, 1970.

Cailliet, R.: Hand pain and impairment, Philadelphia, 1975, F.A. Davis Co.

Callahan, A.D.: Occupational therapy and hand rehabilitation, Am. J. Occup. Ther. **37:**166, 1983.

Curtis, R.M., and Engaletcheff, J., Jr.: A work simulator for rehabilitating the upper extremity—preliminary report, J. Hand Surg. **6**(5), 1981.

Curtis, R.M., Clark, G.L., and Snyder, R.A.: The work simulator. In Hunter, et al. editors: Rehabilitation of the hand, ed. 2, St. Louis, 1984, The C.V. Mosby Co.

Fess, E.E.: Rehabilitation of the patient with an upper extremity replantation. In Hunter, et al., editors: Rehabilitation of the hand, ed. 2, St. Louis, 1984, The C.V. Mosby Co.

Hollis, L.I.: Functional restoration—hand rehabilitation. In Hopkins, H.L., and Smith, H.D., editors: Willard and Spackman's occupational therapy, ed. 6, Philadelphia, 1983, J.B. Lippincott Co.

Hunter, J., et al., editors: Rehabilitation of the hand, St. Louis, 1978, The C.V. Mosby Co.

Hunter, J., et al., editors: Rehabilitation of the hand, ed. 2, St. Louis, 1984, The C.V. Mosby Co.

Ketchum, L.D., Hibbard, A., and Hassaneiu, K.M.: Follow-up report on the electrically driven hand splint, J. Hand Surg. **4**(5):474-481, 1979.

Kottke, F., Stillwell, G., and Lehman, J.: Krusen's Handbook of physical medicine and rehabilitation ed. 3, Philadelphia, 1982, W.B. Saunders Co.

Laseter, G.F.: Management of the stiff hand: a practical approach, Orthop. Clin. North Am. **14:**749, 1983.

Laseter, G.F.: Postoperative management of capsulectomies. In Hunter, et al., editors: Rehabilitation of the hand, ed. 2, St. Louis, 1984, The C.V. Mosby Co.

Leont'ev, A.N., and Zaporozhets, A.: Rehabilitation of hand function, New York, 1960, Pergamon Press.

Loma Linda Hand Manual, Loma Linda University Hand Center, Loma Linda, CA, 1981.

Mackin, E.J. editor: Hand rehabilitation, Hand clinics, vol. 2, no. 1, Philadelphia, 1986, W.B. Saunders Co.

Mackin, E.J., Callahan, A.D., and Baxter, P.: Current concepts in hand therapy. In Tubiana, R., editor: The hand, vol. 4, Philadelphia, 1985, W.B. Saunders Co.

Marshall, E., editor: Hand rehabilitation and teaching syllabus, Brookfield, Ill., 1977, Fred Sammons, Inc.

McEntee, P.M.: Therapist's management of the stiff hand. In Hunter, et al., editors: Rehabilitation of the hand, ed. 2, St. Louis, 1984, The C.V. Mosby Co.

Rusk, H.A.: Rehabilitation medicine, ed. 4, St. Louis, 1977, The C.V. Mosby Co.

Schoenhals, L.H.: Rehabilitation following hand injury, J. Okla. State Med. Assoc. **74:**8-11, 1981.

Weber, E.R., and Davis, J.: Rehabilitation following hand surgery, Orthop. Clin. North Am. **9**(2):529-542, 1978.

Weckesser, E.: Treatment of hand injuries—preservation and restoration of function, Chicago, 1974, Yearbook Medical Publishers, Inc. (The Press of Case Western Reverse University, Ltd.).

Wilson, R.L., and Carter, M.: Joint injuries in the hand: preservation of proximal interphalangeal joint function. In Hunter, et al., editors: Rehabilitation of the hand, ed. 2, St. Louis, 1984, The C.V. Mosby Co.

Wood, H.L.: Prevention of deformity in the insensitive hand: the role of the therapist, Am. J. Occup. Ther. **23:**487-560, 1969.

Wynn Parry, C.B.: Management of the stiff joint, Hand **3:**169-171, 1971.

Wynn Parry, C.B.: Restoration of hand function rehabilitation of the injured hand, Trans. Med. Soc. Lond. **90:**101-104, 1974.

Wynn Parry, C.B.: Rehabilitation of the hand, ed. 4, London, 1981, Butterworths.

PERIPHERAL NERVE

Barr, N.: Peripheral nerve lesions of the upper limb and lively splints, Physiotherapy **57:**533-538, 1971.

Blakeney, A.B., Bergtholdt, H.T., and Ramsammy, H.W.: Static splinting and temperature assessment of the injured insensitive hand. In Hunter, et al., editors: Rehabilitation of the hand, ed. 2, St. Louis, 1984, The C.V. Mosby Co.

Callahan, A.D.: Rehabilitation and sensory re-education. In Lamb, editor: The paralyzed hand, New York, 1985, Churchill Livingstone.

Colditz, J.C.: Radial palsy splinting (abstract), J. Hand Surg. **9A:**609, 1984.

Dellon, A.L.: Evaluation of sensibility and reeducation of sensation in the hand, Baltimore, 1981, The Williams & Wilkins Co.

Fess, E.E.: Rehabilitation of the patient with peripheral nerve injury, Hand Clinics, **2**(1):207, 1986.

Kopell, H.P., and Thompson, W.A.L.: Peripheral entrapment neuropathies, Baltimore, 1963, The Williams & Wilkins Co.

Matsen, F., III: Compartmental syndromes, New York, 1980, Grune & Stratton.

Michon, J., and Moberg, E., editors: Traumatic nerve lesions of the upper limb, Group d'Etude de la Main Monographs 2, Edinburgh, 1975, Churchill Livingstone.

Moberg, E., and Michon, J.: Traumatic nerve lesions of the upper limb, New York, 1975, Churchill Livingstone.

Namasivayam, P.R.: A spiral splint for claw fingers, Lepr. India **48:**258-260, 1976.

Omer, G.E.: Acute management of peripheral nerve injuries, Hand Clinics **2**(1);193, 1986.

Omer, G.E., and Spinner, M.: Management of peripheral nerve problems, Philadelphia, 1980, W.B. Saunders Co.

Pearson, S.O.: Splinting the nerve injured hand. In Hunter, et al., editors: Rehabilitation of the hand, ed. 2, St. Louis, 1984, The C.V. Mosby Co.

Penner, D.: Dorsal splint for radial palsy, Am. J. Occup. Ther. **26:**46, 1972.

Rayan, G.M., and O'Donoghue, D.H.: Ulnar digital compression neuropathy of the thumb caused by splinting, Clin. Orthop. **175:**170-172, 1983.

Seddon, H.: Surgical disorders of the peripheral nerves, Baltimore, 1972, The Williams & Wilkins Co.

Spinner, M.: Injuries to the major branches of the peripheral nerves of the forearm, Philadelphia, 1972, W.B. Saunders Co.

Sunderland, S.: Nerves and nerve injuries, ed. 2, New York, 1978, Churchill Livingstone.

Von Prince, K.: Occupational therapy's interest in sensory function following peripheral nerve injury, M. Bull. U.S. Army (Europe) **23**(4), 1966.

Wynn Parry, C.B., Harper, D., Fletcher, I., Dean, P.E., Knight, P.N., and Robinson, P.R.: New types of lively splints for peripheral nerve lesions affecting the hand, Hand **2:**31-38, 1970.

PHYSIOLOGY

Brand, P.W.: Clinical mechanics of the hand, St. Louis, 1985, The C.V. Mosby Co.

Brand, P.W.: The forces of dynamic splinting: ten questions before applying a dynamic splint to the hand. In Hunter, J.M., Schneider, L.C., Mackin, E.J., and Callahan, A.D., editors: Rehabilitation of the hand, ed. 2, St. Louis, 1984, The C.V. Mosby Co.

Brand, P.W.: Hand rehabilitation: management by objectives. In Hunter, J.M., Schneider, L.C., Mackin, E.J., and Callahan, A.D., editors: Rehabilitation of the hand, ed. 2, St. Louis, 1984, The C.V. Mosby Co.

Bryant, W.M.: Wound healing. CIBA Clinical Symposia, vol. 29, no. 3, Summit, N.J., 1977, CIBA Pharmaceutical Co.

Colditz, J.C.: Dynamic splinting of the stiff hand. In Hunter, J.M., Schneider, L.C., Mackin, E.J., and Callahan, A.D., editors: Rehabilitation of the hand, ed. 2, St. Louis, 1984, The C.V. Mosby Co.

Curtis, R.M.: Management of the stiff hand. In Hunter, J.M., Schneider, L.C., Mackin, E.J., and Callahan, A.D., editors: Rehabilitation of the hand, ed. 2, St. Louis, 1984, The C.V. Mosby Co.

Hirsch, G.: Tensile properties during tendon healing, Copenhagen, 1974, Einar Munksgaard.

Kapandji, I.A.: The physiology of the joints, vol. I: Upper limb, Edinburgh, 1970, Churchill Livingstone.

Madden, J.W.: Wound healing: the biological basis of hand surgery, Clin. Plast. Surg. **3**(1):3-13, 1976.

Madden, J., and Arem, A.: Wound healing: biologic and clinical features. In Sabiston, J.: Davis-Christopher textbook of surgery, ed. 12, Philadelphia, 1981, W.B. Saunders Co.

Mason, M.L., and Allen, H.S.: The rate of healing of tendons: an experimental study of tensile strength, Ann. Surg. **113:**424-459, 1941.

Peacock, E.E.: Wound repair, ed. 3, Philadelphia, 1984, W.B. Saunders Co.

Schultz, K.S.: The effect of active exercise on edema, Proceedings American Society of Hand Therapists, J. Hand Surg. **8:**625, 1983.

Watson, H.K.: Stiff joints. In Green, D.P., editor: Operative hand surgery, New York, 1982, Churchill Livingstone.

Weeks, P.M., and Wray, R.C.: The management of acute hand injuries: a biological approach. St. Louis, 1973, The C.V. Mosby Co.

Wright, V., and Johns, R.J.: Physical factors concerned with the stiffness of normal and diseased joints, Bull. Johns Hopkins Hosp. **106:**215-231, 1960.

Wynn Parry, C.B.: Rehabilitation of the hand, ed. 4, London, 1981, Butterworths.

QUADRIPLEGIA, TETRAPLEGIA

Abrahams, D., et al.: A functional splint for the C5 tetraplegic arm, Paraplegia **17**(2);198-203, 1979.

Allen, V.R.: Follow-up study of wrist driven flexor hinge splint use, Am. J. Occup. Ther. **25:**420, 1971.

Allen, V.R.: Role of occupational therapy in rehabilitation of the spinal cord injured patient. In Cull, J.G., and Hardy, R.E., editors: Physical medicine and rehabilitation approaches in spinal cord injury, Springfield, Ill., 1977, Charles C. Thomas, Publisher.

Cravier, P.N.: Typing splints for the quadriplegic patient, Am. J. Occup. Ther. **29**:551, 1975.

Engel, W.H., Kmiotek, M.S., Hoht, J.P., French, J., Barnerias, M.J., and Siebens, A.A.: A functional splint for grasp driven by wrist extension, Arch. Phys. Med. Rehabil. **48**:43-52, 1967.

Engel, W., Peyrot, A., and Knox, C.: Prosthetics, orthotics and devices: an assistive device for forearm lift, Arch. Phys. Med. Rehab. **52**:567, 1971.

Goodman, C.R., Delaney, H.F., and Patterson, P.T.: The use of the Prenyl RIC splint in the early rehabilitation of the upper extremity, Am. J. Occup. Ther. **24**:119-121, 1970.

Grahn, E.C.: A power unit for functional hand splints, Bull. Prosthet. Res. **10**:52-56, 1970.

Jones, R.F., and James, R.: A simple functional hand splint for C5-6 quadriplegia, Med. J. Aust. **1**:988-1000, 1970.

Kay, H.W.: Clinical evaluation of the Engen plastic hand orthosis, Artif. Limbs **13**:13-26, 1969.

Lamb, C.R., Booth, A.J., and Godfrey, M.E.: Flexor hinge splint: modification to allow radial deviation, Arch. Phys. Med. Rehab. **55**:322, 1974.

McCluer, S., and Conry, J.E.: Modifications of the wrist-driven flexor hinge splint, Arch. Phys. Med. Rehabil. **52**:233-235, 1971.

Malick, M.: Manual on management of the quadraplegic upper extremity, Pittsburgh, 1978, Harmarville Rehabilitation Center.

Meyer, C., et al.: A method of rehabilitating the C6 tetraplegic hand, Paraplegia **17**(2):170-175, 1979.

Moberg, E.: Surgical treatment for absent single-hand grip and elbow extension in quadriplegia. J. Bone Joint Surg. [Am.] **57**:196, 1975.

Moberg, E.: Reconstructive hand surgery in tetraplegia, stroke, and cerebral palsy: some basic concepts in physiology and neurology, J. Hand Surg. **1**:129-134, 1976.

Nichols, P.J., et al.: The value of flexor hinge hand splints, Prosthet. Orthot. Int. **2**(2):86-94, 1978.

Patterson, R.P., Halpern, D., and Kubicek, W.G.: A proportionally controlled externally powered hand splint, Arch. Phys. Med. Rehabil. **52**:434-438, 1971.

Ruch, C., and Dommisse, G.F.: A myo-electric hand splint for quadriplegia, S. Afr. J. Surg. **5**:97-103, 1967.

Silverstein, F., French, J., and Siebens, A.: A myoelectric hand splint, Am. J. Occup. Ther. **28**:99-101, 1974.

Smith, A.G.: Early complications of key grip hand surgery for tetraplegia, Paraplegia **19**(2):123-126, 1981.

Treehafer, A.A.: Tendon transfers to improve grasp in patients with cervical spinal cord injury, Paraplegia **13**(1):15-24, 1975.

Truong, X.T., White, C.F., and Canterbury, R.A.: Modification of flexor tenodesis splint, Arch. Phys. Med. Rehabil. **50**:97-99, 1969.

Zrubecky, G., and Stoger, M.: The orthosis for restoration of prehensile function in tetraplegics, Paraplegia **11**:228-237, 1973.

SERIAL CASTING

Bell, J.A.: Plaster cylinder casting of the interphalangeal joints of the fingers. In Hunter, et al., editors: Rehabilitation of the hand, St. Louis, 1984, The C.V. Mosby Co.

Bowers, W.H.: Management of small joint injuries in the hand, Orthop. Clin. North Am. **14**:793, 1983.

Brand, P.W.: Reconstruction of the hand in leprosy, Ann. R. Coll. Surg. Engl. **11**:350, 1952.

Brand, P.W.: Clinical mechanics of the hand, St. Louis, 1985, The C.V. Mosby Co.

Brand, P.W.: External stress on joint motion. In May, J., and Littler, W.J., editors: Converse textbook of plastic surgery: the hand and upper extremity, vols. 7 and 8, Philadelphia, 1985, W.B. Saunders Co.

Goldspink, G.: The adaptation of muscle to a new functional length. In Anderson, D.J., and Matthews, B., editors: Mastication, Bristol, England, 1977, Wright.

Kolumban, S.L.: The use of dynamic and static splints in straightening contracted proximal interphalangeal joints in leprosy patients: a comparative study, Paper presented at the 47th Annual Conference of the APT Association, Washington, D.C., 1960.

Kolumban, S.L.: The role of static and dynamic splints, physiotherapy techniques and time in straightening contractures of the interphalangeal joints, Lepr. India, Oct. 1969, pp. 323-328.

Puddicombe, B.E., Mathewson, K.R., and Hubbard, L.F.: Flexion contracture of the PIP joint—treatment by serial casting, Paper presented at the annual conference of the ASHT, Las Vegas, 1985.

Yamada, H.: Strength of biological materials, Baltimore, 1970, The Williams & Wilkins Co.

SPASTICITY, HEMIPLEGIA, UPPER MOTOR NEURON. CP

Berberian, A.: Splinting for the wrist and hand (letter), Phys. Ther. **58**(7):901, 1978.

Blashy, M.R. and Fuchs, R.: Orthokinetics: a new receptor facilitation method, Am. J. Occup. Ther. **13**:226, 1959.

Bloch, R., and Evans, M.G.: An inflatable splint for the spastic hand, Arch. Phys. Med. Rehab. **58**(4):179-180, 1977.

Bobath, B.: Adult hemiplegia: evaluation and treatment, ed. 2, Longon, 1978, William Heinemann Medical Books, Ltd.

Brennan, J.: Response to stretch of hypertonic muscle groups in hemiplegia, Br. Med. J. **1:**1504-1507, 1959.

Brunnstrom, S.: Associated reactions of the upper extremity in adult patients with hemiplegia—an approach to training, Phys. Ther. Rev. **36:**225-236, 1956.

Caldwell, C.B., Wilson, D.J., and Braun, R.M.: Orthopedic management of stroke. In Nickel, V.L., editor: Clinical Orthopedics and Related Research, **63:**80, 1969.

Charait, S.E.: A comparison of volar and dorsal splinting of the hemiplegic hand, Am. J. Occup. Ther. **22:**319-321, 1968.

Courte, S.: Modified resting pan splint, Am. J. Occup. Ther. **17:**153, 1963.

Doubilet, L., and Polkow, L.S.: Theory and design of a finger abduction splint for the spastic hand, Am. J. Occup. Ther. **31**(5):320-322, 1977.

Exner, C.E., and Bonder, B.R.: Comparative effects of three hand splints on bilateral hand use, grasp, and arm hand posture in hemiplegic children, Occupational Therapy Journal of Research, **3**(2):75-92, 1983.

Farber, S., and Huss, A.J.: Sensorimotor evaluation and treatment procedure for allied health, Indiana University: Purdue University Press, 1974.

Farber, S.E., and Huss, J.A.: Sensorimotor evaluation and treatment procedures for allied health personnel, Indianapolis, Indiana University, Purdue University—Indianapolis Medical Center, 1974.

Fuchs, E.M., and Fuchs, R.L.: Corrective bracing, Am. J. Occup. Ther. **8:**88, 1954.

Gillette, H.E.: The treatment of cerebral palsy, Phys. Ther. Rev. **32:**56-59, 1952.

House, J.H., Cowathmey, F.W, and Fidler, M.O.: A dynamic approach to the thumb-in-palm deformity in cerebral palsy, J. Bone Joint Surg. **63A**(2):216-225, 1981.

Jamison, S.L., et al.: A hard hand-positioning device to decrease wrist and finger hypertonicity: a sensorimotor approach for the patient with nonprogressive brain damage, Nurs. Res. **29**(5):285-289, 1980.

Kaplan, N.: Effect of splinting on reflex inhibition and sensorimotor stimulation in treatment of spasticity, Arch. Phys. Med. Rehabil. **43:**565-569, 1962.

King, T.: Plaster splinting as a means of reducing elbow flexor spasticity: a case study, Am. J. Occup. Ther. **36:**671-674, 1982.

Largent, P., and Waylett, J.: Follow-up study on upper extremity bracing of children with severe athetosis, Am. J. Occup. Ther. **29:**341, 1975.

Leavitt, L.A., and Beasley, W.C.: Clinical application of quantitative methods in the study of spasticity, Clin. Pharmacol. Ther. **5:**918-941, 1964.

Long, C., Thomas, D., and Crochetiere, W.J.: Objective measurement of muscle tone in the hand, Clin. Pharmacol. Ther. **5:**909-917, 1964.

Mathiowetz, V., Bolding, D., and Trombly, C.: Immediate effects of positioning devices on the normal and spastic hand measured by electromyography, Am. J. Occup. Ther. **37:**247-254, 1983.

Mayer, P.: Orthopedic treatment of hemiplegia, current medical literature, J. Am. Med. Assoc. **65:**366, 1915.

McPherson, J.J.: Objective evaluation of a splint to reduce hypertonicity, Am. J. Occup. Ther. **35:**189-194, 1981.

McPherson, J.J., et al.: A comparison of dorsal and volar resting hand splints in the reduction of hypertonus, Am. J. Occup. Ther. **36**(10):664-670, 1982.

Merletti, R., Cvilak, G.: Electrophysiological orthosis for the upper extremity in hemiplegia: feasibility study, Arch. Phys. Med. Rehabil. **56:**507-513, 1975.

Neuhaus, B.E., et al.: A survey of rationales for and against hand splinting in hemiplegia, Am. J. Occup. Ther. **35**(2):83-90, 1981.

Ogden, R.: Systematic therapeutic exercise in the management of the paralysis in hemiplegia, J. Am. Med. Assoc. **70:**828-833, 1918.

Rood, M.: Neurophysiological reactions as a basis for physical therapy, Phys. Ther. Rev. **34:**444-449, 1954.

Rood, M.S.: Neurophysiological mechanisms utilized in the treatment of neuromuscular dysfunction, Am. J. Occup. Ther. **10:**220-224, 1956.

Rosenada, J.P., and Ellwood, P.M.: Review of physiology, measurement and management of spasticity, Arch. Phys. Med. **42:**167-174, 1961.

Snook, J.H.: Spasticity reduction splint, Am. J. Occup. Ther. **33**(10):648-651, 1979.

Stolov, W.C.: The concept of normal muscle tone: hypotonia and hypertonia, Arch. Phys. Med. Rehabil. **47:**156-168, 1966.

Twitchell, T.: The restoration of motor function following hemiplegia in man. In Payton, Hirt, and Newton, editors: Scientific bases for neurophysiological approaches to therapeutic exercises—an anthology, Philadelphia, 1977, F.A. Davis Co.

Varian, J.P.: The ridged plaster volar slab, Hand **7:**78-80, 1975.

Waylett, J., and Barber, L.: Upper extremity bracing of the severely athetoid mental retardate, Am. J. Occup. Ther. **25:**402-407, 1971.

Wilson, D.J., and Caldwell, C.: Central control insufficiency. III. Disturbed motor control and sensation: a treatment approach emphasizing upper extremity orthoses, Phys. Ther. **58:**313-320, 1978.

Wolcott, L.E.: Orthotic management of the spastic hand, South. Med. J. **59:**971-974, 1966.

Zislis, J.M.: Splinting of the hand in spastic hemiplegia patient, Arch. Phys. Med. Rehabil. **45**:41, 1964.

SURGERY

Agee, J.M.: Unstable fracture dislocations of the proximal interphalangeal joint of the fingers: a preliminary report of a new treatment technique, J. Hand Surg. **3**(4):386-389, 1978.

American Academy of Orthopaedic Surgeons: Instructional Lecture Course Series, vol. 27, St. Louis, 1978, The C.V. Mosby Co.

Bank, B.K., Wakefield, A.R., and Hueston, J.T.: Surgery of repair as applied to hand injuries, ed. 3, Baltimore, 1968, The Williams & Wilkins Co.

Beasley, R.W.: Hand injuries, Philadelphia, 1981, W.B. Saunders Co.

Bilos, Z.J., and Eskestrand, T.: External fixator use in comminuted gunshot fractures of the proximal phalanx, J. Hand Surg. **4**(4):357-359, 1979.

Bora, W.F., editor: The pediatric upper extremity, Philadelphia, 1986, W.B. Saunders Co.

Boyes, J.H., editor: Bunnell's surgery of the hand, ed. 4, Philadelphia, 1964, J.B. Lippincott Co.

Boyes, J.H., editor: Bunnell's surgery of the hand, ed. 5, Philadelphia, 1970, J.B. Lippincott Co.

Brand, P.W.: The reconstruction of the hand in leprosy, Ann. R. Coll. Surg. Engl. **11**:350, 1952.

Brand, P.W.: Biomechanics of tendon transfer, Orthop. Clin. North Am. **5**:205-230, 1974.

Brand, P.W.: Clinical mechanics of the hand, St. Louis, 1985, The C.V. Mosby Co.

Bunnell, S.: Surgery of the hand, Philadelphia, 1944, J.B. Lippincott Co.

Bunnell, S.: Splinting the hand. In American Academy of Orthopaedic Surgeons: Instructional course lectures, vol. IX, Ann Arbor, 1952, J.W. Edwards.

Bunnell, S., and Howard, L.: Additional elastic hand splints, J. Bone Joint Surg. [Am.] **32**:226-228, 1950.

Cramer, L.M., and Chase, R.A.: Symposium on the hand, vol. 3, St. Louis, 1971, The C.V. Mosby Co.

Daniel, R., and Terzis, J.: Reconstructive microsurgery, Boston, 1977, Little, Brown & Co.

Eaton, R.G.: Joint injuries of the hand, Springfield, Ill., 1971, Charles C Thomas, Publisher.

Eaton, R.G., and Littler, J.W.: Joint injuries and their sequelae, Clin. Plast. Surg. **3**:87-98, 1976.

Flatt, A.: Care of the arthritic hand, ed. 4, St. Louis, 1983, The C.V. Mosby Co.

Flatt, A.E.: The care of minor hand injuries, ed. 4, St. Louis, 1979, The C.V. Mosby Co.

Flynn, J.E.: Hand surgery, Baltimore, 1966, The Williams & Wilkins Co.

Gingrass, R.P., Fehring, B., and Matloub, H.: Intraosseous wiring of complex hand fractures, Plast. Reconstr. Surg. **66**(3):383-394, 1980.

Gould, J.S., and Nicholson, B.G.: Capsulectomy of the metacarpophalangeal and proximal interphalangeal joint, J. Hand Surg. **4**:482, 1979.

Green, D., editor: Operative hand surgery, New York, 1982, Churchill Livingstone.

Lindsay, W.K.: Hand injuries in children, Clin. Plast. Surg. **3**:65-75, 1976.

Littler, J.W., and Cramer, L.M., and Smith, J.W., editors: Symposium on Reconstructive Hand Surgery, St. Louis, 1974, The C.V. Mosby Co.

Manktelow, R.T., and McKee, N.H.: Digital replantation: a functional assessment, Can. J. Surg. **22**(1):47-53, 1979.

May, J.W. Jr., Toth, B.A., and Gardner, M.: Digital replantation distal to the proximal interphalangeal joint, J. Hand Surg. **7**(2):161-166, 1982.

Milford, L.: The hand, ed. 2, St. Louis, 1982, The C.V. Mosby Co.

Seddon, H.: Surgical disorders of the peripheral nerves, Baltimore, 1972, The Williams & Wilkins Co.

Skoog, T.: Plastic surgery: new methods and refinements, Stockholm, 1974, Almqvist & Wilksell.

Smith, R.: Intrinsic muscles of the fingers: function, dysfunction, and surgical reconstruction, Am. Acad. Orthop. Surg. Instructional Course Lectures, **24**, St. Louis, 1975, The C.V. Mosby Co., 1974, p 200.

Staden, D.V.: An approach to the extensively injured hand, S. Afr. Med. J. **47**:380-381, 1973.

Sunderland, S.: Nerves and nerve injuries, Baltimore, 1968, The Williams & Wilkins Co.

Swanson, A.B.: Flexible implant resection arthroplasty in the hand and extremities, St. Louis, 1973, The C.V. Mosby Co.

Taleisnik, J.: The wrist, New York, 1985, Churchill Livingstone.

Thompson, L., Gosling, C., and Hayes, E.: A facial moulage technique for the plastic surgeon. Presented at the Annual Meeting of the American Society of Plastic and Reconstructive Surgeons, October 5, 1971, Montreal.

Tubiana, R., editor: The hand, vol. 1, Philadelphia, 1981, W.B. Saunders Co.

Tubiana, R., editor: The hand, vol. 2, Philadelphia, 1985, W.B. Saunders Co.

Tupper, J.W.: A compression arthrodesis device for small joints of the hands, Hand **4**:62-64, 1972.

Wadsworth, T.G.: The traction hand splint, Hand **5**:268-269, 1973.

Weeks, P.M., and Wray, R.G.: Management of acute hand injuries: biological approach, ed. 2, St. Louis, 1973, The C.V. Mosby Co.

Wilson, C.S., et al. : Replantation of the upper extremity, Clin. Plast. Surg. **10**:85-101, 1983.

Zancolli, E.: Structural and dynamic bases of hand surgery, Philadelphia, 1968, J.B. Lippincott Co.

TENDON, LIGAMENT

Abouna, J.M.: Splint for mallet finger, Nurs. Mirror PVII, 1966.

American Academy of Orthopaedic Surgeons: Symposium on Tendon Surgery in the Hand, St. Louis, 1975, The C.V. Mosby Co.

Auchincloss, J.M.: Mallet-finger injuries: a prospective controlled trial of internal and external splintage, Hand **14**:168-173, 1982.

Blue, A.I., Spira, M., and Hardy, S.B.: Repair of extensor tendon injuries of the hand, Am. J. Surg. **132**:128-132, 1976.

Cannon, N.M., and Strickland, J.W.: Hand therapy for flexor tendon problems, Hand Clin. North Am. **1**:147-165, 1985.

Doyle, J.R., and Blythe, W.: The finger flexor tendon sheath and pulleys: anatomy and reconstruction. In American Academy of Orthopaedic Surgeons: Symposium on Tendon Surgery in the Hand, St. Louis, 1975, The C.V. Mosby Co.

Doyle, J., and Blythe, W.: Anatomy of the flexor tendon sheath and pulleys of the thumb, J. Hand Surg. **2**(2):149, 1977.

Duran, R.J., Houser, R.G., and Stover, M.G.: Management of flexor tendon lacerations in zone 2 using controlled passive motion post-operatively. In Hunter, J.M., et al., editors: Rehabilitation of the hand, St. Louis, 1978, The C.V. Mosby Co.

Elliott, R.A., Jr.: Splints for mallet and boutonniere deformities, Plast. Reconstr. Surg. **52**:282-285, 1973.

Fess, E.E.: Splinting for tendon transfers: In Hunter, et al., editors: Another decade of tendons. St. Louis, 1986, The C.V. Mosby Co.

Fisher, T.R.: The mallet finger and its treatment, Nurs. Mirror IV-VI, 1966.

Fritschi, E.P.: A new operation hand splint for intrinsic replacement tendon transfers, Lepr. Rev. **50**(1):21-24, 1979.

Gibbs, B.L.: Functional splint after flexor pollicis longus repair, Am. J. Occup. Ther. **23**:344-345, 1969.

Hirsch, G.: Tensile properties during tendon healing, Copenhagen, 1974, Einar Munksgaard.

Idler, R.S.: Anatomy and biomechanics of the digital flexors, Hand Clinics **1**(1):3-13, 1985.

Kleinert, H., Kutz, J., and Cohen, M.: Primary repair of zone 2 flexor tendon lacerations. In American Academy of Orthopaedic Surgeons: Symposium on tendon surgery in the hand, St. Louis, 1975, The C.V. Mosby Co.

Kofkin, J., Tobino, M., and Dellon, A.L.: Dynamic elbow splint following tendon transfer to restore triceps function, Am. J. Occup. Ther. **34**:680, 1980.

Lister, G.D., et al.: Primary flexor tendon repair followed by immediate controlled mobilization, J. Hand Surg. **2**(6):441-451, 1977.

Lopez, M.S., and Hanley, K.F.: Splint modification for flexor tendon repairs, Am. J. Occup. Ther. **38**:398, 1984.

Mackin, E.J., and Maiorano, L.M.: Postoperative therapy following staged flexor tendon reconstruction. In Hunter, et al., editors: Rehabilitation of the hand, St. Louis, 1978, The C.V. Mosby Co.

Mason, M.L., and Allen, H.S.: The rate of healing of tendons: an experimental study of tensile strength, Ann. Surg. **113**:424-459, 1941.

Mayfield, J.K.: Patterns of injury to carpal ligaments: a spectrum, Clin. Orthop. **187**:36-42, 1984.

McFarlane, R.M., and Hampole, M.K.: Treatment of extensor tendon injuries of the hand, Can. J. Surg. **16**:366-375, 1973.

Mikic, Z., and Helal, B.: The treatment of the mallet finger by the Oakley splint, Hand **6**:76-81, 1974.

Milford, L.: Retaining ligaments of the digits of the hand, Philadelphia, 1968, W.B. Saunders Co.

Reis, N.D.: Dynamic profundus splint for flexor profundus repair, Hand **9**(3):265-267, 1977.

Schneider, L.H.: Flexor tendon injuries, Boston, 1985, Little, Brown & Co.

Shrewsbury, M., and Johnson, R.: Ligaments of the DIP joint and the mallet position, J. Hand Surg. **5**(3):214, 1980.

Snow, R.S.: Constructing an improved splint for mallet finger deformity, Plast. Reconstr. Surg. **52**:586-588, 1973.

Splint modification for flexor tendon repairs, Am. J. Occup. Ther. **38**(6):398-403, 1984.

Strickland, J.W., editor: Flexor tendon surgery, Hand Clinics, vol. 1, Philadelphia, 1985, W.B. Saunders Co.

Strickland, J.W., and Glogovac, S.V.: Digital function following flexor tendon repair in zone II: a comparison of immobilization and controlled passive motion techniques, J. Hand Surg. **5**(6):537-543, 1980.

Tsuyuguchi, Y., Tada, K., and Kavaii, H.: Splint therapy for trigger finger in children, Arch. Phys. Med. Rehabil. **64**(2):75-76, 1983.

Verdan, C.: Tendon surgery of the hand, New York, 1979, Churchill Livingstone.

Wilson, R.L., et al.: Flexor profundus injuries treated with delayed two-staged tendon grafting, J. Hand Surg. **5**:74, 1980.

MISCELLANEOUS

Hueston, J.T., and Tubiana, R.: Dupuytren's disease, New York, 1974, Grune & Stratton, Inc.

Kobe, C.T.: Shunt splint for adult renal patients, Am. J. Occup. Ther. **35:**195, 1981.

Perry, J., Hsu, J., Barber, L., and Holler, M.M.: Orthosis in patients with brachial plexus injuries, Arch. Phys. Med. Rehabil. **55:**134-137, 1974.

Saferin, E.H., and Posch, I.L.: Secretan's disease: post-traumatic hard edema of the dorsum of the hand, Plast. Reconstr. Surg. **58:**703-707, 1976.

Splint index

Index